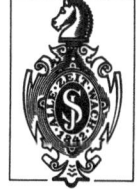

 Current Concepts in Critical Care

Already published in the Series:

Shock and the Adult Respiratory Distress Syndrome
Edited by Wolfgang Kox and David Bihari

Forthcoming:

Acute Renal Failure in the Intensive Therapy Unit
Edited by David Bihari and Guy Nield

W. Kox, J. Boultbee and R. Donaldson (Eds)

Imaging and Labelling Techniques in the Critically Ill

With 167 Figures

Springer-Verlag
London Berlin Heidelberg New York
Paris Tokyo

W. Kox, MD
Senior Lecturer/Head of Department, Department of Anaesthesia, Charing Cross and Westminster Medical School; and Honorary Consultant Anaesthetist (Director Intensive Care Unit), Charing Cross Hospital, Fulham Palace Road, London W6 8RF

J. Boultbee, FRCP
Department of Radiology, Charing Cross Hospital, Fulham Palace Road, London W6 8RF

R. Donaldson, MD, MRCP
Consultant Cardiologist, National Heart Hospital, Westmoreland Street, London W1M 8BA

Cover illustrations are taken from figures within this book

British Library Cataloguing in Publication Data
Kox, Wolfgang, *1946–*
    Imaging and labelling techniques in the critically ill.
    1. Medicine. Diagnosis. Imaging I. Title   II. Boultbee, J. (Joseph), *1939–*   III. Donaldson, R. (Robert), *1946–*
    616.07'54

Library of Congress Cataloging-in-Publication Data
Imaging and labelling techniques in the critically ill/W. Kox, J. Boultbee and R. Donaldson (eds.).
    p.   cm.
    Includes bibliographies and index.
    ISBN-13: 978-1-4471-1442-0   e-ISBN-13: 978-1-4471-1440-6
    DOI:10.1007/ 978-1-4471-1440-6

    1. Diagnostic imaging.   2. Critical care medicine.   I. Kox, W. (Wolfgang), 1946– .   II. Boultbee, J. (Joseph), 1939– . III. Donaldson, R. (Robert) [DNLM: 1. Critical Care.   2. Diagnostic Imaging.   WN 200 I31]
    RC78.7.D53143 1988 616.07'57—dc19 DNLM/DLC
    for Library of Congress
                                                                                            88–12165 CIP

© Springer-Verlag Berlin Heidelberg 1988
Softcover reprint of the hardcover 1st edition 1988

2128/3916–543210 (Printed on acid-free paper)

Foreword

It gives me great pleasure to have this opportunity to write a Foreword for this new book.

In the past two decades we have witnessed very significant advances in the management of the very ill patient. The great success in this field of medical endeavour is largely due to the establishment of intensive care units, but a great deal of progress can also be attributed to the major developments in technology, which affect patient management and care as well as the many sophisticated techniques of diagnosis and patient monitoring. *Imaging and Labelling Techniques in the Critically Ill* covers this new important and difficult field of diagnosis and visual monitoring.

By establishing the criteria and algorhythms for the choice of the different methods available for this purpose, defining the diagnostic signs on images and resolving some of the misconceptions and pitfalls, this book will go a long way to help the reader, particularly those involved in the care of patients in the intensive care units. This book brings together many different methods of investigation and discusses the advantages and limitations of these techniques in different clinical circumstances. Some of the techniques are well established and their usefulness in the intensive care unit is in no doubt. Some of the newer techniques such as PET scanning or NMR imaging have not yet found a defined position of usage in the critically ill patient. There is, however, little doubt that in due course this situation will change.

After observing, over many years, the development of the various imaging techniques which can be used in diagnosis of the very ill patient, one will appreciate the advantages of having all this diagnostic information put together in one volume. I have no doubt about the success of this book's future.

London
September 1988

R. E. Steiner
Emeritus Professor of Diagnostic Radiology

Foreword

Techniques of patient imaging are evolving rapidly. A number have become established in the practice of intensive care medicine, others remain to be evaluated. The contributions of X-rays, ultrasound, nuclear imaging and CAT scanning to the diagnosis and management of the many varied problems that beset the very sick patient are well recognised. Critical illness is now dominated by the ravages of trauma and infection, affecting an even older population, and it is the acquisition of detailed structural and functional information, in a noninvasive fashion, that makes imaging such an important and elegant process in the intensive therapy unit.

This book, *Imaging and Labelling Techniques in the Critically Ill*, the second published in the "Current Concepts in Critical Care" series, describes the use of the various imaging methods in an appropriately systematic fashion, highlighting neural, respiratory, cardiovascular and abdominal pathology. A final section is concerned with special techniques and recent advances.

Each chapter has been prepared by an expert or experts in the particular field and the whole edited by an intensivist, a cardiologist and a radiologist. The complete work represents a most important addition to the literature of intensive care medicine. It portrays the important integration of different disciplines, a theme so fundamental to the efficient and successful care of the critically ill patient.

London
September 1988

Jack Tinker
Regional Postgraduate Dean,
North East Thames R.H.A.,
British Postgraduate Medical Federation;
previously Director, Intensive Therapy Unit,
The Middlesex Hospital, London

Preface

The care of the critically ill patient not only comprises sophisticated monitoring and life-supporting equipment, but also depends on meaningful diagnostic techniques in order to instigate swift intervention when necessary. This can only be achieved when the choice and use of these diagnostic techniques can be rationalised and those involved in the decision for their application are fully aware of the possibilities and limitations of any such technique. It was the intention of the editors to relate diagnostic imaging and labelling techniques to specific organ systems – the brain and the nervous system, the lungs, the cardiovascular system as well as the abdomen – and to clarify their role in aiding the diagnostic process. In addition, techniques which are at present used as research tools are introduced as possible methods for clinical routine in the near future. Obviously, over the last decade, the imaging developments of the sixties and seventies have become standard investigative procedures in the general hospital environment. Some of these technologies take a large portion of the hospital budget, and they need to be used selectively after careful clinical assessment, particularly when related to patients with poor prognosis.

Ten years ago a CT (body) scanner was considered beyond the means of most general hospitals, whereas today most large hospitals have installed, or have reasonable access to, this type of technology. The same might be said for the other imaging technologies such as MR scanning in years to come. We realise that some of the techniques described in this book are not always available to the intensivist; we make no apology for including them in this book as we feel we should all be aware of and ready to use them when they become more freely available.

Some of the imaging modalities, such as ultrasound and gamma cameras, can be mobile and easily applicable to the severely ill patient in the intensive care ward. However, there are restrictions in the use of other modalities which cannot be brought to the patient's bedside. Sometimes, the benefit achieved by yet another diagnostic procedure may be offset by the deterioration in the patient, due to the move to another department. The ideal – bringing the mountain to Mohammed – has been achieved in the use of portable radiography and mobile ultrasonography. Thus, they are now first-line procedures and should always be freely utilised before embarking on the more complicated and hence expensive techniques.

We hope this review will be of value to those involved in the management of critically ill patients.

London
February 1988

Wolfgang Kox
Joe Boultbee
Robert Donaldson

Contents

SECTION IV: The Abdomen

SECTION V: Special Techniques and Recent Advances

Contributors

S. Baglioni
Institute of Anaesthesia, University of Milan, Via Francesco Sforza 35, 20122 Milan, Italy

J. Boultbee
Department of Radiology, Charing Cross Hospital, Fulham Palace Road, London W6 8RF, UK

A. K. Dixon
Department of Radiology, University of Cambridge, Addenbrooke's Hospital, Cambridge CB2 2QQ, UK

R. Donaldson
Department of Cardiology, The National Heart Hospital, Westmoreland Street, London W1M 8BA, UK

R. S. J. Frackowiak
MRC Cyclotron Unit, Hammersmith Hospital, Ducane Road, London W12 0HS, UK

D. Firmin
Magnetic Resonance Unit, The National Heart and Chest Hospitals, 30 Britten Street, London SW3 6NN, UK

R. Fumagalli
Institute of Anaesthesia, University of Milan, Via Francesco Sforza 35, 20122 Milan, Italy

L. Gattinoni
Institute of Anaesthesia, University of Milan, Via Francesco Sforza 35, 20122 Milan, Italy

R. Garlick
Department of Neurosurgery, The Royal Free Hospital, Pond Street, Hampstead, London NW3 2QG, UK

K. Hillman
Department of Anaesthetics, Intensive Care and Coronary Care, The Liverpool Hospital, Liverpool 2170, Sidney, NSW, Australia

G. Iapichino
Institute of Anaesthesia, University of Milan, Via Francesco Sforza 35, 20122 Milan, Italy

R. F. Jewkes
Department of Nuclear Medicine, Charing Cross, Fulham Palace Road, London W6 8RF, UK

W. Kox
Department of Anaesthesia, Charing Cross and Westminster Medical School and Intensive Care Unit, Charing Cross Hospital, Fulham Palace Road, London W6 8RF, UK

M. Langer
Institute of Anaesthesia, University of Milan, Via Francesco Sforza 35, 20122 Milan, Italy

J. P. Lavender
Department of Nuclear Medicine, Hammersmith Hospital, Ducane Road, London W12 0HS, UK

L. Loh
Department of Anaesthesia, John Radcliffe Hospital, Oxford OX3 9DU, UK

R. Marcolin
Institute of Anaesthesia, University of Milan, Via Francesco Sforza 35, 20122 Milan, Italy

D. Mascheroni
Institute of Anaesthesia, University of Milan, Via Francesco Sforza 35, 20122 Milan, Italy

C. N. McCollum
Department of Surgery, Charing Cross and Westminster Medical School, Charing Cross Hospital, Fulham Palace Road, London W6 8RF, UK

J. McIvor
Department of Radiology, Charing Cross Hospital, Fulham Palace Road, London W6 8RF, UK

I. Moseley
Lysholm Department of Radiology, National Hospital for Nervous Diseases, Queen Square, London WC1, UK

A. Pesenti
Institute of Anaesthesia, University of Milan, Via Francesco Sforza 35, 20122 Milan, Italy

S. Rees, Magnetic Resonance Unit, The National Heart and Chest Hospitals, 30 Britten Street, London SW3 6NN, UK

F. Rossi
Institute of Anaesthesia, University of Milan, Via Francesco Sforza 35, 20122 Milan, Italy

G. P. Rossi
Institute of Anaesthesia. University of Milan, Via Francesco Sforza 35, 20122 Milan, Italy

J. E. Tooke
Department of Physiology, Charing Cross Hospital, Fulham Palace Road, London W6 8RF, UK

A. Torresin
Institute of Anaesthesia, University of Milan, Via Francesco Sforza 35, 20122 Milan, Italy

P. S. Treweeke
Department of Radiology, Charing Cross Hospital, Fulham Palace Road, London W6 8RF, UK

R. Underwood
Department of Nuclear Medicine, The National Heart Hospital, Westmoreland Street, London W1M 8BA, UK

A. R. Valentine
Royal Free Hospital, Pond Street, London NW3 2QG, UK

S. Vesconi
Institute of Anaesthesia. University of Milan, Via Francesco Sforza 35, 20122 Milan, Italy

J. R. Weinberg
Department of Medicine, Charing Cross Hospital, Fulham Palace Road, London W6 8RF, UK

Section I

The Brain and Nervous System

Chapter 1

Radiography, Angiography and Computed Tomography of the Central Nervous System

A. R. Valentine

Patients who require cranial imaging while undergoing intensive care fall into two broad categories: patients with a primary intracranial lesion, and patients with intracranial manifestations or complications of a primary extracranial disease. Those patients in the first category suspected of harbouring lesions which may be amenable to neurosurgical treatment will almost certainly be investigated by computed tomography (CT) after referral to a neurosurgical unit. Those patients in the second category may frequently be treated in a hospital without a CT service, although access to a local hospital with CT scanning is very likely to exist. When CT scanning is available, the roles of skull radiography and angiography are limited.

Skull Radiography

Plain radiography of the skull remains the preliminary radiological investigation of neurological disease in many centres, and is readily available in many parts of the world. However, there has been considerable reduction in its use since the introduction of CT, and many clinicians have largely dispensed with it in favour of CT.

Plain radiography is the production and recording of an X-ray picture in the form of a radiographic film, exposed to an X-ray beam which has traversed the subject. The X-ray beam consists of photons which may be considered as small packets of electromagnetic energy, derived from the kinetic energy of electrons suddenly decelerated by the anode or target of an X-ray tube after extreme acceleration

under high voltage from the cathode. The X-ray tube is housed in a metal jacket, with only a small window allowing egress of photons in the form of a collimated (focussed) beam. Considerable heat is generated within this jacket and a system for cooling is required. The X-ray beam emerging from the patient differs from the incident beam because of interaction of the photons with the patient's tissues at atomic level, the photons interacting with the orbiting electrons. This phenomenon results in an effective removal of photons from the X-ray beam, a process described as attenuation. The pattern of photons emerging from the subject and incident on the radiographic film is a two-dimensional representation of the patient in terms of electron density. The radiographic film records the incident beam as a pattern of blackening so that those areas of the body which attenuate the beam less effectively are shown as dark areas on the film and those areas of more active attenuation are represented as lighter areas. A radiographic film bears a coating (emulsion) which is sensitive to, and therefore blackened by, exposure to X-rays. The emulsion is, however, more sensitive to light than to X-rays and therefore to increase the "speed" of the film, intensifying screens are included in the X-ray cassette. These are sheets of a sensitive phosphor which emits small flashes of light when X-ray photons are incident, and the recording radiographic film registers the pattern of flashes. Following an exposure, the radiographic film must be developed and fixed. Such radiographic exposure requires only a very short period of X-ray production, such as 0.01 to 0.3 s for different parts of the body. Serial X-ray film changers are available for the rapid sequential exposure of film required in angiography. If the

radiographic cassette is replaced by a fluorescent
screen linked to an image intensifier and television
monitor, a method of continuous imaging is available, described as fluoroscopy or screening.

Radiographic Projections

There are four standard projections in routine skull
radiography. These are the lateral, the postero-
anterior, the inclined antero-posterior (Townes)
and the submento-vertical (basal) projections.
Some authorities advocate the use of two lateral
projections, the X-ray beam exposed from one side
of the head, then the other, to demonstrate and
lateralise fractures, the edge of the fracture being
sharper when closer to the recording film.

The Use of Plain Skull Radiography in the Context of the Critically Ill Patient

The role of skull radiography in the critically ill
patient is limited by its inherent failure to visualise
normal brain substance. Similarly, plain radiography is a very insensitive detector of intracranial
pathological tissue, requiring the presence of calcification or ossification. The presence of an intracranial mass may otherwise only be inferred from
side to side, or occasionally rostrocaudal displacement of a calcified pineal gland. Other physiological calcifications are unhelpful. Choroid plexus
calcification may be very asymmetrical and dural
membranes, such as falx and tentorium, which may
calcify are only very occasionally displaced. There
are no radiographic manifestations of an acute rise
in intracranial pressure, although very specific evidence of raised intracranial pressure may be evident
in the sella turcica within a few weeks. Radiographs
are, however, effective in the demonstration of fractures and relatively efficient in the demonstration
of any depressed fragments. They may demonstrate
radio-opaque intracranial foreign bodies, and intracranial air–fluid interfaces within the cranial cavity
or in the paranasal sinuses. It should be noted that
with the exception of undisplaced fractures, CT is
more effective than radiography in demonstration
of these abnormalities. CT is, however, very susceptible to artefact from dense opacities, for
example intracranial metallic fragments, and skull
radiographs may have some advantage over CT in
this situation for purposes of localisation (Fig. 1.1).

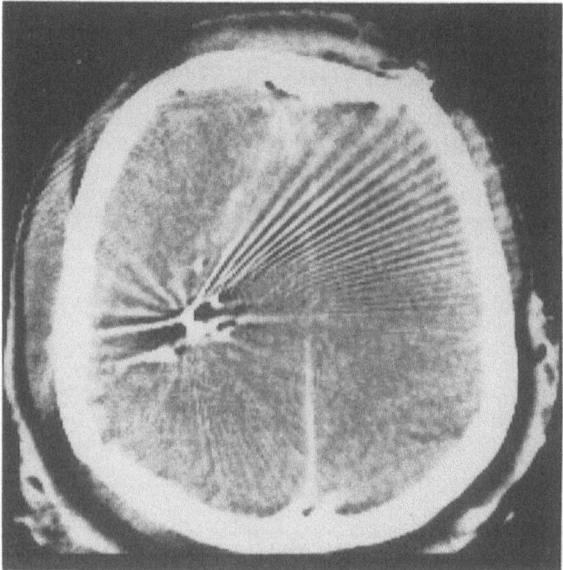

Fig. 1.1. CT scan following gunshot injury. Bullet fragments
causing considerable artefact which hinders precise localisation,
and obscures adjacent anatomy.

Such CT artefact is very much increased by patient
movement, and here the very short radiographic
exposure compared to CT scanning times is advantageous. The "plan" view produced by a radiographic examination also confers some advantage,
particularly in the region of the craniovertebral
junction, which is included on a routine skull radiograph but not usually in a routine brain scan. The
general availability of radiographic examination
compared to CT is, of course, well known.

Computed Tomography

This method of cross-sectional imaging is the
product of applying computer technology to X-ray
examination. The X-ray beam traverses the patient,
but the beam is very accurately collimated so that
only a narrow slice of very precise thickness is
irradiated, the emerging pattern being registered
by a sophisticated detector system rather than on
radiographic film. The electrical output of the detector system is processed by computer and the resulting data reconstructed into an image representing
the cross-sectional anatomical display.

Types of CT Scanner

The first five commercial CT scanners were
produced by EMI Limited and were installed in

British and North American hospitals in 1972/3. Since then there has been dramatic improvement in the image quality, scanner versatility, and speed of image acquisition. Major changes in scanning technology with respect to X-ray production and detection have led to descriptions of new "generations" of scanner. This is a rather misleading concept as a new generation may not necessarily confer a significant improvement in image quality. Scanner types are best described in terms of the coupling of the X-ray tube and detector across the patient aperture, and their relative movements.

1. *Translate-rotate.* In this system, the X-ray source and detectors face each other across the gantry aperture. Tube and detector pass across the periphery of the aperture, tangentional to its circumference (translation) before rotating through a small angle and repeating the translation. A series of translations and rotations result in the accumulation of considerable data. The first generation of scanners utilised a simple pencil beam of X-rays coupled to a detector. The so-called second generation scanners used a diverging fan beam coupled to a small arc of detectors, allowing a larger angle of rotation between each translation as well as larger number of readings per translation. This led to a faster accumulation of data.

2. *Rotate-rotate system.* This refers to rotation of the X-ray tube during exposure, and linked arc array of detectors during exposure. This type of system is often referred to as third generation.

3. *Rotate-stationary system* (*Rotating X-ray source, stationary detectors*). In this the detectors are arranged in a complete circle around the aperture, the X–ray tube rotating within the detector array. This is often described as fourth generation. A sophisticated modification of this array system involves rotation of the X-ray source outside the detector array, those detectors closest to the tube moving aside while the beam irradiates the contralateral detectors.

4. *Stationary system* (*neither X-ray source nor detector system rotates*). These are not in general use. They employ multiple X-ray sources around the aperture, or the use of a scanning electron beam. They are very fast scanners and seem most appropriate to dynamic studies such as cardiac CT, but are inappropriate to neurological application because of poor spatial resolution.

Virtually all modern scanners are capable of producing a scanned projection radiograph (a "digital radiograph"). In this the subject is propelled through the scanner aperture by the motor-driven tabletop while pulsed X-ray exposures are made. The resulting image looks very similar to a conventional radiograph. Its main use is in prospective planning of scanning planes and, following a CT study, such an image may be recorded showing the actual planes of examination. This is particularly helpful in spinal examinations but is also useful in cranial imaging.

Modern scanners frequently have large patient apertures within the gantry, some of 70 cm. It is also possible to tilt the gantry, and therefore the plane of X-ray exposure, by 20° or 30°. A combination of gantry tilt and appropriate positioning of the patient's head allows versatility in the plane of scanning. Direct coronal scanning, for example, is relatively easily obtained in cooperative patients; even sagittal scanning is possible with some machines. The alternative, however, is to reconstruct the data derived from transverse axial plane scanning into the various coronal, sagittal or oblique planes by further computer processing. This requires preliminary acquisition of data in narrow and contiguous transverse axial sections.

CT Scanning in the Context of the Critically Ill Patient

Although the patient must be transferred to the scanning unit, other disturbance to the patient is relatively slight. Routine scanning is performed with the patient supine. Anaesthetic apparatus may be employed in close proximity to the scanner without any interference in the image (cf. magnetic resonance imaging (MRI)), and the intensive care specialist may remain in close contact with the patient; the exposure to stray radiation within the room during scanning is infinitesimal. It is, however, customary for the attendant to wear a lead apron. Modern scanners acquire data for image reconstruction in a few seconds, typically 4–10 s. It is not necessary for respiration or ventilation to be suspended. Simple head restraint such as a "Velcro" band is helpful. The tabletop is propelled by a motor, and in almost all systems may be raised or lowered relatively quickly. The patient in need of urgent attention may be withdrawn from the scanner in a very short period of time. No scanner tables are capable of tilting. Most modern scanners have a facility for "fast" scans from which sufficient detail may be achieved in the restless, uncooperative patient. In these images, detail is less than in standard scans, but significant lesions such as major infarction, haemorrhage or tumour, extra-cerebral collections or hydrocephalus may be adequately demonstrated or excluded.

Basic Principles of Image Interpretation

The CT image is in the form of a reconstruction derived from the application of a grey scale, reflecting X-ray attenuation numbers, to the many picture elements (pixels) comprising the image. Each pixel reflects the calculated attenuation number of each small component of the subject, referred to as a volume element (voxel). The precise number of voxels in any given scan slice depends on the matrix incorporated in the scanner design. A typical modern scanner matrix would be 512×512 voxels, each represented by a pixel. Increasing X-ray attenuation value is represented by increasingly lighter shades of grey to an end point of white. Conversely, less attenuating tissues are represented by darker shades of grey. The full attenuation range encompassed with the grey scale is designed to include all those tissues which will be encountered in diagnostic scanning. Water is arbitrarily allocated the value of zero. Dense bone and metal may achieve an attenuation value of $+1000$. Air and gases show an attenuation value of -1000 or so. Tissues which are predominantly fatty show an attenuation value in the negative range between -20 and -100. Pathological tissues tend to have a very broad range of density but sometimes this is relatively specific, for example, a blood clot will measure $+50$ to $+95$ Hounsfield units. Knowledge of the spectra of attenuation numbers is essential to interpretation of scans. Calcification may appear of similar "whiteness" on the scan to haemorrhage but may measure in excess of $+95$ Hounsfield units on specific measurement. If this is the case, then one must exclude simple intracerebral haemorrhage as an explanation for the scan appearance, and consider calcified lesions in the differential diagnosis.

When describing CT scan appearances, it is customary to refer to tissue as hyperdense when the described tissue is of higher attenuation than adjacent normal brain substance. It is generally accepted that a mean value between the attenuation of grey and white matter be utilised in this context. Isodensity refers to tissue of the same attenuation as adjacent brain tissue and isodense pathology may only be evident from areas of differing density associated with them, such as oedema, or by virtue of associated mass effect. Tissue of lower attenuation than adjacent normal brain substance is referred to as hypodense. As X-rays interact with body tissues at atomic level, the photons being attenuated by interaction with orbiting electrons, the ultimate physical property of the tissue affecting X-ray attenuation is that of electron density, or in other words, effective atomic numer (Z) × number of atoms per unit volume of traversed tissue. It is variation in electron density which allows the scanner to differentiate, for example, grey from white matter. Although high attenuation (very light grey or white pixels) suggest the possibility of haemorrhage or calcification in the lesion, this is not necessarily the case. A typically hyperdense lesion is the colloid cyst, arising from the roof of the third ventricle and at excision these lesions are indeed found to be cystic, containing neither blood nor calcium. Conversely, very well-circumscribed low-density lesions may suggest and, indeed, reflect a cystic nature, but some lesions of this appearance are solid at neurosurgical exploration. However, one of the great advantage of CT scanning is its specificity, in addition to its sensitivity as a detector of intracranial disease. For example, in the clinical setting of a patient deteriorating after subarachnoid haemorrhage, possible explanations include recurrent bleeding, the onset of ischaemia due to vasospasm or the advent of hydrocephalus. CT examination can distinguish between these possibilities in a rapidly achieved, non-invasive test. Such precision was unattainable even from invasive tests prior to the advent of CT scanning.

CT Manifestations of Life-Threatening Intracranial Disease

Haemorrhage

Intracranial haemorrhage may occur in an extracerebral space, in the form of extradural, subdural or subarachnoid haemorrhage. Within the neuraxis, the haematoma may involve the cerebrum, cerebellum or brainstem. In addition, haemorrhage may be predominantly intraventricular, representing intravasation following an adjacent intracerebral haemorrhage, or secondary to rupture of an adjacent aneurysm or angiomatous malformation through ventricular walls. Blood may also enter the ventricular system by reflux against the flow of CSF by way of the 4th ventricle.

Extradural Haematoma (Fig. 1.2a). This is typically of a well-demarcated lentiform configuration, lying against the inner table of the vault, with a convex medial aspect impressing the brain. Usually following tear of a middle meningeal artery in the process of skull fracture, the extracerebral haematoma rapidly clots, resulting in a high-density mass on CT scanning. If trauma is severe, areas of contusion or intracerebral haemorrhage may be evident. There is often considerable swelling of the hemisphere adding to the displacement of intracranial tissues. Considerable sub-falcial herniation may be evident; obliteration of the suprasellar cistern may indicate uncal herniation. In coning, some patients show ischaemic low density in posterior cerebral artery territory due to compression of the posterior cerebral artery as it crosses the tentorial edge.

Subdural Haematoma (Fig. 1.2b). In an acute presentation, the extracerebral mass is of high density. The subdural collection dissects relatively freely through the potential space existing between dura and arachnoid, and subdural collections tend to be more diffuse than extradural. The collection tends to form a layer whose inner surface parallels the

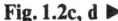

Fig. 1.2c, d ▶

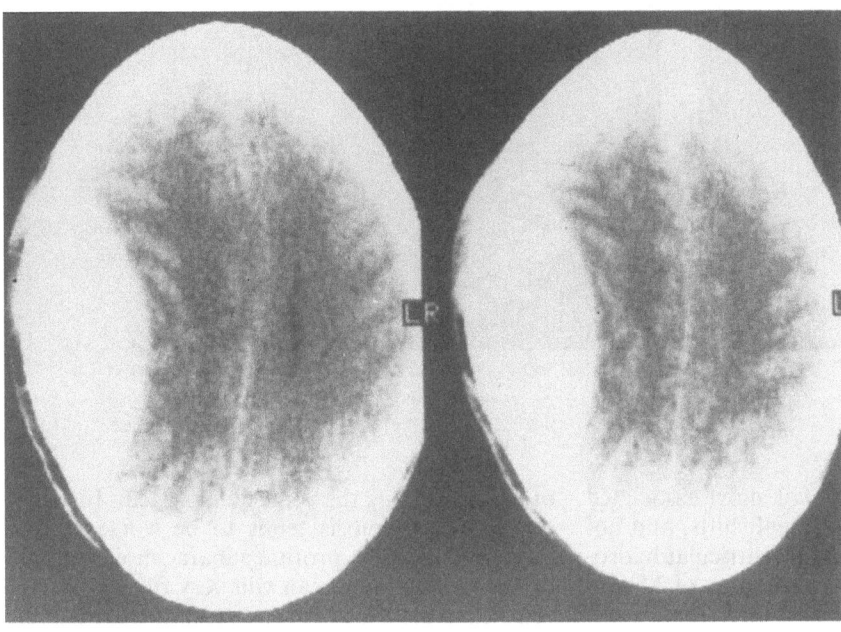

a

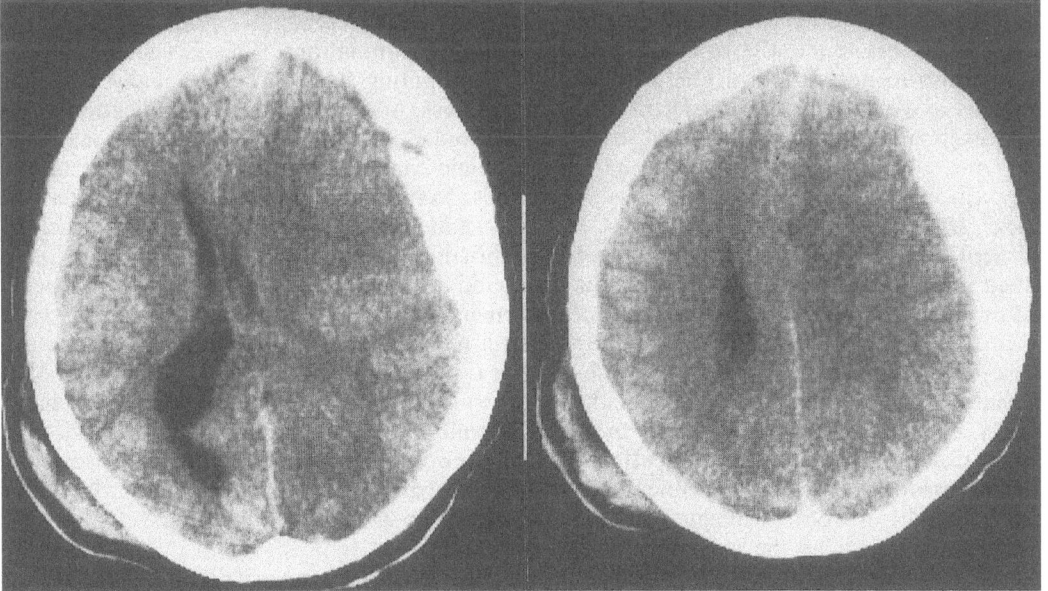

b

Fig. 1.2.a Extradural haematoma of typical lentiform configuration. **b** CT scans showing acute subdural haematoma as a peripheral high density (white) mass. Note the considerable displacement of the ventricular system, and the swelling of the ipsilateral hemisphere. **c** CT scan showing diffuse subarachnoid blood. There is also blood within the 3rd ventricle and the trigones of the lateral ventricles. **d** CT scan showing haematoma in left sylvian region due to ruptured middle cerebral artery aneurysm. Note blood in occipital horns.

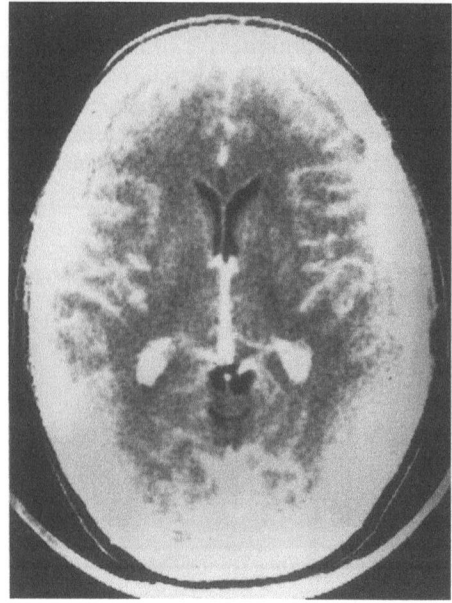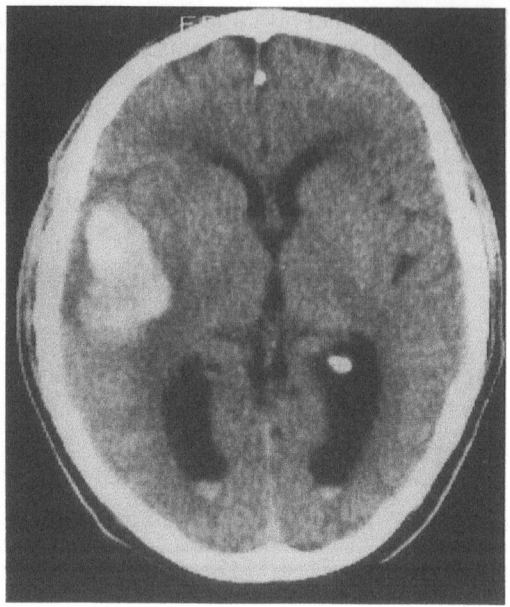

c   d

Fig. 1.2 (*continued*)

inner table. Again, the scan will show associated effects such as marked intracranial shifts, and not infrequently contralateral lateral ventricular hydrocephalus, when kinking of the foramen of Monro leads to ventricular obstruction. Occasionally the shift may seem disproportionate to the size of the collection, and it is useful to remember that the CT scanner tends to underestimate the volume of the collection, but also to note that a degree of contusion may exist in the underlying hemisphere and, on occasion, swelling secondary to venous obstruction.

Subarachnoid Haemorrhage (Fig. 1.2c). The CT scan is efficient in the detection of subarachnoid haemorrhage in the first few days following the event, but the blood subsequently resorbs, and a negative scan after five days or so does not exclude a recent haemorrhage. The cardinal sign of subarachnoid haemorrhage is the replacement of the water density of the subarachnoid spaces, most noticeably the cisterns and fissures, by high attenuation tissue representing blood clot. Forcible haemorrhage may result in focal widening of the subarachnoid space, such as the sylvian fissure, leading to the appearance of an intra-sylvian haematoma. Jetting of blood from the aneurysmal rupture may lead to an intracerebral haematoma in association with subarachnoid blood. Certain aneurysms arise in very close proximity to the ventricular walls. and rupture can then result in a jet

of blood entering the ventricular system. In general terms, the prognosis tends to be worse in those patients with most profuse subarachnoid blood on the early scan. The scan will very frequently demonstrate a state of communicating hydrocephalus following subarachnoid haemorrhage, due to obstruction to cerebrospinal fluid resorption at the arachnoid granulations. This is usually a benign and self-limiting state, but occasionally can persist or progress. A very significant complication of subarachnoid haemorrhage is vasospasm, leading to ischaemic change in the territories of the affected vessels. Many patients who appear to deteriorate fairly suddenly in the days following a subarachnoid haemorrhage have been assumed in the past to have suffered further subarachnoid bleeding. The CT scanner is very useful in this situation, as it can detect recurrent bleeding. In many cases, however, there is no evidence from CT scans of further bleeding, which suggests that the deterioration has an ischaemic rather than haemorrhagic basis. It is worth noting that over half of the patients who suffer subarachnoid haemorrhages die before admission to hospital is possible.

Intracerebral Haematoma (Fig. 1.2d). A mass of clotted blood within brain substance may be spontaneous, usually in vascular hypertensivě patients, post-traumatic or secondary to an underlying lesion such as aneurysm, angioma or occasionally vascular tumour such as glioma, metastasis or meningioma. Haematoma lying in close proximity to a frequent site of aneurysm such as the suprasellar or sylvian region may well prompt angiography.

Cerebral Infarction

The ability of the CT scanner to distinguish reliably those patients who have suffered a stroke due to intracerebral bleeding from those suffering an ischaemic event had a major impact on neurological practice as soon as CT scanners became available. The CT diagnosis of cerebral infarction is sometimes straight forward, when the lesion is represented by an area of hypodensity with a varying degree of swelling and the abnormality corresponds with a recognisable arterial distribution. Frequently, however, only part of a vascular territory is involved, and the lesion may be of relatively non-specific appearance. In this situation other differential diagnoses such as tumour or infection have to be considered. Those patients rendered critically ill by an ischaemic stroke frequently suffer very considerable cerebral swelling complicating the infarct, as well as the extensive ischaemic insult (Fig. 1.3). In this context, CT is extremely valuable in excluding intracerebral haemorrhage and, where possible, distinguishing infarction from other acute life-threatening diseases, which may be difficult to differentiate clinically, such as encephalitis.

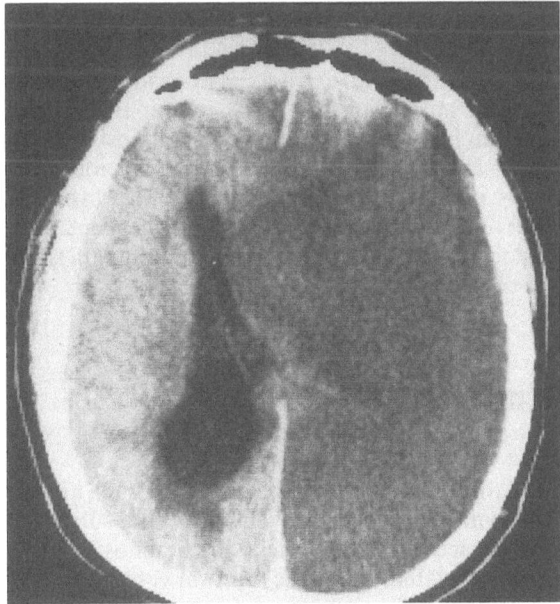

Fig. 1.3. CT scan showing extensive hypodense swelling of the major part of the right cerebral hemisphere. The changes correspond with middle and posterior cerebral territory, with some sparing of the anterior cerebral territory, noted to the right of the falx. Note the massive subfalcial herniation of brain to the left.

Infection

Intracerebral abscess remains a neurosurgical emergency with high mortality. In those patients with a documented history of an inflammatory focus, such as in chest, middle-ear or paranasal sinuses, the index of suspicion is high, but it should be noted that most patients with cerebral abscess presenting to a neurosurgical unit have no identifiable source of infection. The inflammatory cerebral focus progresses rapidly from cerebritis to abscess. One of the greatest practical benefits of CT is in the management of patients harbouring an abscess when demonstration of the state of the ventricles prior to lumbar puncture may avert disaster.

Neurosurgical units frequently admit such patients showing signs of coning following lumbar puncture. In the absence of CT it remains a dilemma in management whether to proceed to lumbar puncture or to risk the delay before definite diagnosis by arranging transfer to a specialised centre with CT. As well as demonstrating complications of intracranial abscess, such as obstruction of the ventricular system, CT is a sensitive and specific detector of an abscess, the capsule of which almost invariably demonstrates a uniform and marked enhancement after intravenous contrast injection. As well as establishing its precise localisation, CT may demonstrate that the abscess is multi-locular, indicating to the neurosurgeon the need to drain more than one area of the mass (Fig. 1.4a).

Prior to CT, the multi-locular nature of an abscess was rarely demonstrable. At angiography the capsule was only occasionally demonstrated, and frequently uncertainty existed about the relative contribution to the mass of abscess and associated oedema. There is no doubt that the use of CT in intracranial sepsis has significantly improved the prognosis of the condition. CT can also demonstrate intraventricular and extracerebral sepsis (eg subdural empyema) (Fig. 1.4b).

Tumour

There is a very wide spectrum of clinical presentation of intracranial tumour. Tumours may present as a stroke, for example, when complicated by haemorrhage. A patient may harbour an indolent glioma for many years, which suddenly exhibits behaviour of a very aggressive malignant tumour; sometimes rapidly generating considerable oedema. CT is extremely precise in the localisation of tumour and frequently allows differentiation of tumour mass from associated oedema (Fig. 1.5). This is, however, not possible when the tumour is substantially of low density, similar to the oedematous

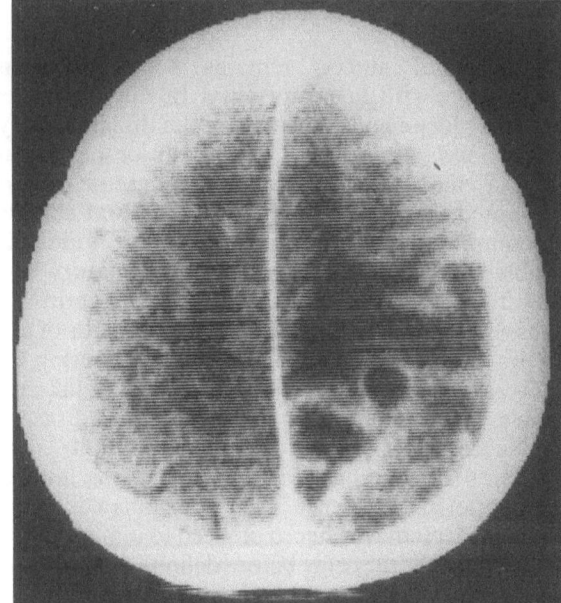

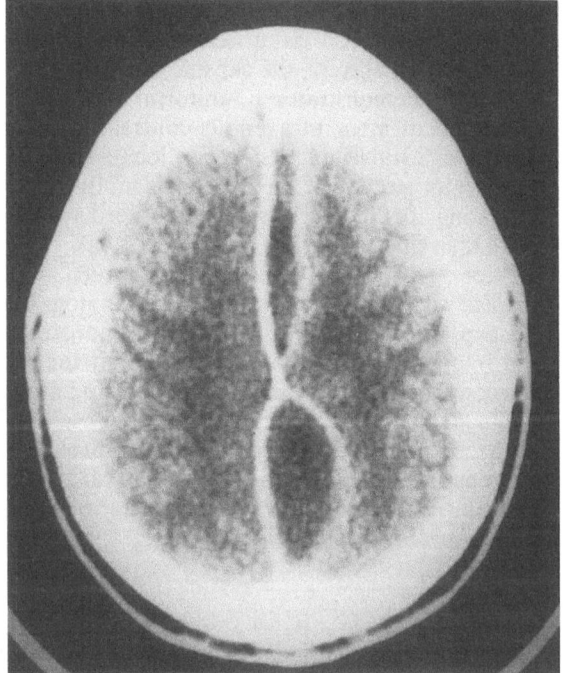

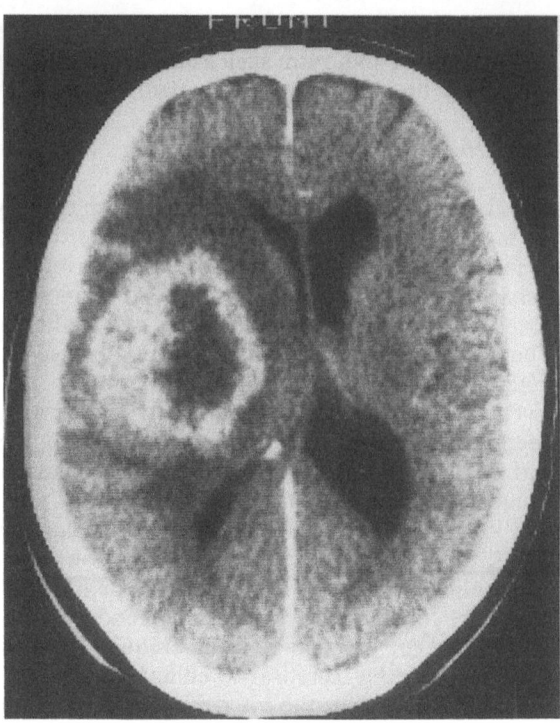

Fig. 1.5. CT scan showing precise localisation of a malignant glioma. It would be reasonable to infer that the solid element of the tumour is represented by the hyperdense (enhanced) tissue, and the zone of low density around is predominantly oedema. Note the co-existing mild hydrocephalus of the right lateral ventricle.

lesion, although an extra-axial mass may show such marked burrowing into the neuraxis that it simulates an intra-axial tumour. The diagnosis of metastatic intracranial tumour is usually made on the basis of multiplicity of lesions. In this event, the differential diagnosis of other multifocal enhancing lesions, such as lymphoma and granulomata should be considered.

Angiography

Fig. 1.4.a Pyogenic abscess with "rim" enhancement outlining three loculi. **b** Enhancing membranes enclosing loculated interhemispheric subdural empyema.

tissue. The administration of intravenous contrast, resulting in enhancement of the tumour mass, sometimes allows this distinction. CT demonstration of the advent of hydrocephalus may explain sudden deterioration in a patient. CT is relatively efficient in distinguishing intra-axial from extra-axial mass

The role of angiography in cranial imaging has been much modified by the advent of CT and subsequent experience of its specificity in diagnosis. Angiographic evaluation of the cerebral vessels is usually undertaken by a process of selective injection of vessels following percutaneous catheterisation of the femoral artery at the groin, and the passage of a catheter to the aortic arch and subsequently into the brachiocephalic vessels, under fluoroscopic control.

Angiographic apparatus is now highly sophisticated. Catheters are available in many sizes and configurations. The main shaft of a modern catheter is of small outer diameter, but the wall so thin that high flow rates are possible. There is, of course, the theoretical argument that smaller, more delicate catheters should lead to less endovascular trauma. If angiography is performed for possible intrinsic vascular disease, the radiologist should not allow guide-wire or catheter to traverse the common carotid bifurcation, at least until it has been angiographically demonstrated to be free of stenosis or significant atheromatous plaque. It is generally safer to perform such investigations by injections into the common carotid artery segments. This leads to only slight reduction in quality of images of the intracranial vessels; the simultaneous opacification of the external carotid branches does not usually prove problematic.

Frequently, when one does not suspect atheromatous disease, selective internal carotid artery injections are made. These may be supplemented by external carotid injections if a dural component to the abnormality is suspected as, for example, in extra-axial tumours such as meningioma and superficially placed angiomatous malformations.

All contrast media are neurotoxic to some extent. As many intracranial lesions are associated with disruption of the blood–brain barrier, the use of less toxic media is theoretically safer. The most modern contrast agents are low osmolar, often non-ionic media and although significantly more expensive than the traditional compounds, they cause the patient much less discomfort. Many patients may therefore be subjected to cerebral angiography with only local anaesthesia and modest sedation. General anaesthesia, frequently employed in the past, conferred an advantage due to the control of pCO_2 which has a major influence on the quality of the images and also, of course, in perfect patient immobility, ventilation being suspended during the series of angiographic exposures. Modern angiography frequently involves use of magnification techniques, as well as subtraction techniques and immobility is essential to both.

A fairly recent development in angiography is the application of digital subtraction techniques. In this, the emergent X-ray beam from the patient, instead of being recorded on radiographic film, is incident on an intensifying screen linked to a high-quality TV chain. The electrical signal generated in this system is subjected to analogue-digital conversion. In digital form, the data are amenable to computer manipulation. A short series of images is obtained before contrast injection, and a series after the injection of contrast medium when peak concentration is anticipated in the region of interest. By a process of electronic subtraction, the plain or "mask" image is subtracted from the frame containing peak contrast in the vessels. The data common to both frames are thereby removed, and the difference "isolated", resulting in an image due to the contrast medium. In practice, some small differences in the patient's position are inevitable and some background data persist. In digital form, the data attributable to the contrast medium may be enhanced logarithmically, so that arterial images of good quality are available after venous injection of contrast medium.

Because of the sensitivity of the system, lower concentrations of contrast medium may be used and therefore, in theory at least, smaller catheter sizes. Both factors should lead to a safer examination. Furthermore, the study should be less time-consuming, another improved safety factor.

The risk of endovascular trauma and embolism remains when the apparatus is used for arteriography, but the greatly increased sensitivity of the system over conventional angiography confers the ability to perform arterial imaging after intravenous contrast injection. Following an intravenous bolus injection (peripheral vein, vena cava or right atrium) the contrast medium returns to the right heart, and passes through the pulmonary circulation. By this time, considerable dilution of medium is inevitable. Image detail after venous injection is, of course, much poorer than in selectively injected arteriographic images, but in the extracranial vessels, for example, stenoses and occlusions may be reliably demonstrated. Because the arterial system is not invaded by the radiologist no risk of arterial damage exists. Perhaps the most significant risk is that of severe reaction to intravascular contrast medium. Contrast-induced death has been quantified from intravenous urography (IVU) studies at about 1 in 40 000, but probably less with modern media.

Angiography in the Context of the Critically Ill Patient

Cerebral angiography will usually follow cranial CT study. The most frequent indication in this clinical context is that of a large intracerebral haematoma, which may require neurosurgical evacuation. In this situation, information about underlying aneurysm, angiomatous malformation, or even tumour is sought by the surgeon. Frequently, the scan will dictate and limit the extent of the study. Angiography may be utilised to obtain further specific information when the nature of the scan abnor-

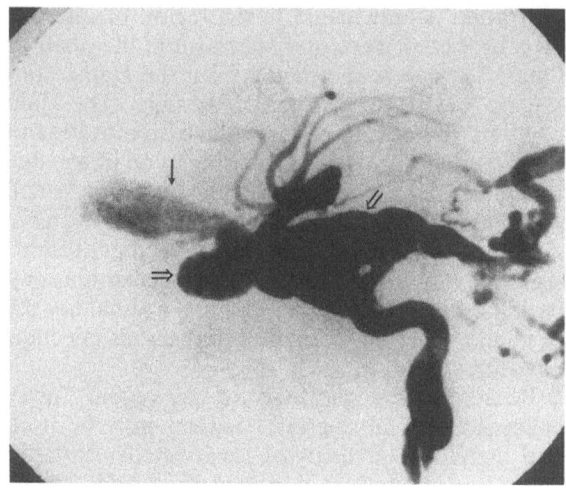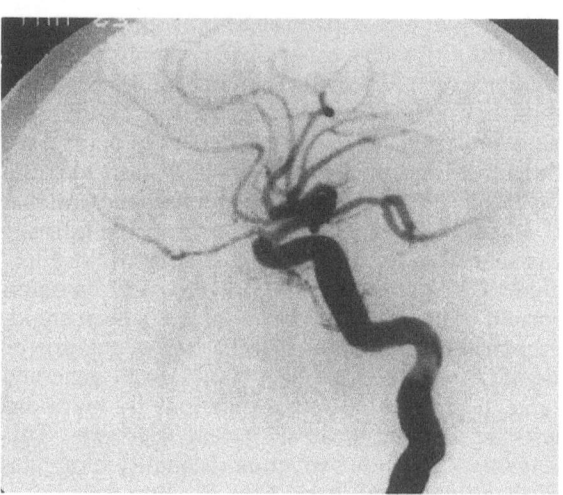

a   b

Fig. 1.6.a Internal carotid angiogram showing extensive arterio-venous shunt of traumatic carotico-cavernous fistula. Single arrow, dilated superior ophthalmic vein; Double arrow, shunt to cavernous sinus and intracranial veins. **b** Internal carotid injection after manipulation of a balloon to close the carotid cavernous fistula.

mality is equivocal. When, for example, a marked state of cerebral swelling is shown at CT and could be explained by cerebral infarction, or encephalitis, angiography may demonstrate a carotid occlusion or middle cerebral embolism in the former condition, and normal vessels in the latter. Occasionally patients are encountered whose most effective therapy is by endovascular therapy in the hands of a radiologist, for example, the infant pre-

senting in cardiac failure with inoperable Vein of Galen aneurysm, or the traumatised patient with carotico-cavernous fistula (Fig. 1.6). At other times endovascular therapy may be undertaken when clinical judgement is that the patient would not withstand major neurosurgical intervention, or to facilitate neurosurgery as in the preoperative embolisation of highly vascular lesions such as some meningiomas, glomus jugulare tumours, etc.

Chapter 2

Nuclear Magnetic Imaging of the Nervous System

I. Moseley and L. Loh

Magnetic Resonance Imaging (MRI)

Nuclear magnetic resonance (NMR) is a property exhibited by paramagnetic nuclei, i.e., those with an odd number of nucleons, in a strong magnetic field. It is induced by the application of bursts of radiofrequency waves, the frequency necessary for excitation depending on the nuclei in question (usually hydrogen in clinical imaging) and the strength of the magnetic field. Use of this property for imaging purposes (MRI) entails detection and spatial coding of the NMR signal, which is itself of radiofrequency. Encoding is achieved by introducing transient gradients across the magnetic field, via passage of electrical currents through coils adjacent to the patient (Pykett et al. 1982).

NMR has certain characteristics which make it an almost ideal imaging technique, but in practice it presents considerable difficulties. Its major advantages are that it does not use ionising radiations (like X- or gamma-rays), with their well-documented biotoxicity; that it permits images to be formed in a number of different planes, either orthogonal or oblique, without physical manipulation of the patient; and that it is uniquely sensitive to biophysical differences between the various normal tissues of the body and between normal and pathological tissues.

Technical Problems

Apart from the enormous capital expense of the imager and its high running and maintenance costs, the major disadvantages of MRI centre on the necessity for a large, very strong magnet, to ensure a uniform high field – imagers currently in use have field strengths from 0.15–2.0 Tesla (the earth's magnetic field is 0.00005 Tesla) – and the duration of the examination, which is rarely less than 15 min and can exceed 1 h.

Constraints Imposed by Static and Changing Magnetic Fields and by Radiofrequency Waves

The potential interaction of the strong magnetic field and ferromagnetic components within or without the body has a number of practical consequences. Metallic clips or inserts within the body, or on its surface, may cause marked distortion and artefactual degradation of the images, to the extent that they become nondiagnostic or highly misleading (Fig. 2.1) (New et al. 1983). Even when metallic components are not within the imaging plane, they may move under the effects of the magnetic field. While this is not problematic where metallic dental fillings are concerned, and does not seem to present difficulties with hip prostheses, intramedullary orthopaedic nails or shunt systems used in the treatment of hydrocephalus (Pusey et al. 1985), arterial clips such as those used in intracranial aneurysm surgery may give rise to concern. Some makes of clip have been shown to be markedly deflected by the magnetic field, and it is possible that they could become dislodged, with disastrous results: the torque acting on certain clips can produce pressures at their tips equivalent to five times arterial blood pressure (New et al. 1983). The previous medical history of obtunded or confused

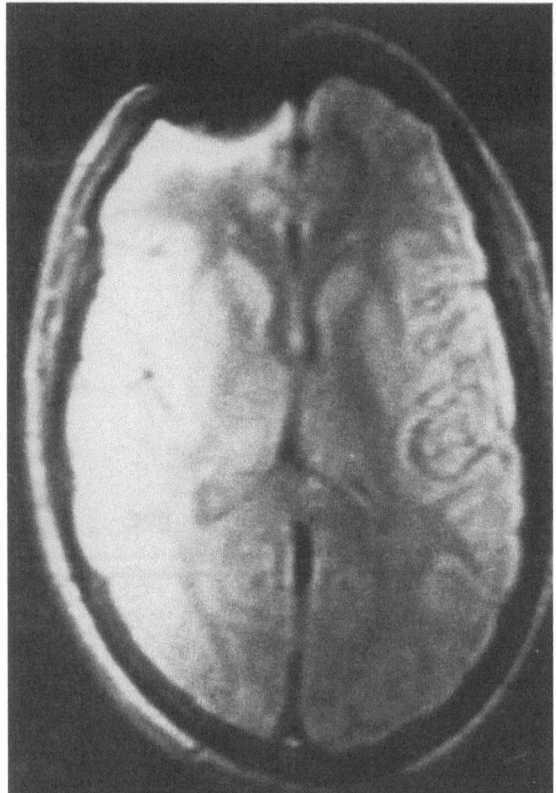

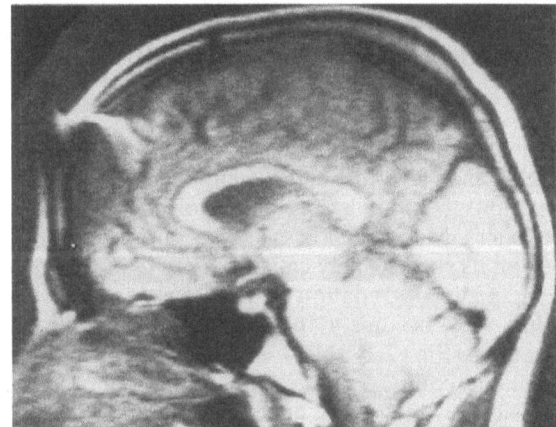

Fig. 2.1. a,b. Artefact caused by ferromagnetic materials in the imaging plane **a** Axial section showing apparent depressed fracture of right frontal bone, with increased signal (brighter) throughout underlying cerebral hemisphere (in this and subsequent axial images the patient's right side is on the observer's left); both the "fracture" and the altered signal are artefacts. **b** Pilot (low resolution) sagittal image reveals the cause: a fragment of shrapnel in the skin of the forehead.

patients admitted directly to an intensive care unit may not be available, and some workers have advocated X-ray fluoroscopic screening for aneurysm clips and prosthetic heart valves before MRI in

cases where there is doubt (Bradley et al. 1984); a metal detector similar to those used in airport security checks is impractical in a busy department (Weinreb et al. 1984).

For similar reasons, catheter mounts, endotracheal tubes, etc., containing ferromagnetic metals are unsuitable for use in patients undergoing MRI; rubber, plastic or nonferrous metals must be used. Plastic can be substituted for metal in tracheal and other tubing connections, and elastomeric cannulae can be employed in place of intravenous needles (Nixon et al. 1987). It has been suggested, rather optimistically, that manufacturers of arterial clips will adopt nickel and titanium alloys to avoid complications with magnets; over ten years ago it was anticipated that titanium or aluminium would be used for such clips, as these metals did not cause severe artefacts on computed tomography (CT), but there do not appear to have been any major changes in industrial practices.

Large metallic objects, such as gas cylinders, anaesthetic machines, or ventilators with substantial metallic components, cannot be used in the immediate vicinity of the magnet; they may be drawn towards it, or deflected. Items containing batteries, such as laryngoscopes, are strongly attracted by the magnet, and can be deflected through more than 45°, while surgical scissors can be turned through almost 90°, or fly through the air towards the magnet (Nixon et al. 1987). Intensity of the magnetic field at a given distance from the magnet approximates to the formula $B = 1 - \cos\theta$, where B is the strength of the field and θ is the angle from the radius of the coil forming the magnet to the point. With the imagers in use at the National Hospital, London, the decay of the magnetic field is most rapid perpendicular to the long axis of the imager so that, when necessary, an anaesthetic machine is placed in this position, but at least 3 m from the magnet. Standard hospital trolleys do not appear to represent a hazard, but they do interefere with imaging, and are therefore removed from the suite during data collection (Nixon et al. 1987). All-plastic trolleys are available (Bradley et al. 1984). The folding-frame aluminium stretchers which ambulance services use are not ferromagnetic, but neither are they very sturdy; Weinreb et al. (1984) suggested that trolleys and/or stretchers can be made rather cheaply from heavy-gauge polyvinyl chloride piping. They also recommended that when emergency resuscitation of previously healthy patients, or of those already requiring intensive care, becomes necessary during an MRI study the patient be removed rapidly to an adjacent room, and the staff be trained to do this as quickly and as efficiently as possible. A standard resuscitation trolley, with the full range of familiar equipment, may then be left in that room, outside the effective field of the magnet (Weinreb et al. 1984).

The radiofrequency signals can cause heating of the tissues. This is not generally sufficient to cause anxiety, but large metallic prostheses, such as hip replacements, can show a detectable increase in temperature (Davis et al. 1981); the magnitude of even this heating effect does not, however, appear to be significant in vitro or in vivo (Bradley et al. 1984). The National Radiological Protection Board (NRPB) does not prohibit examination of patients with clips or prostheses, but recommends that in the latter case the examination should be terminated if the patient experiences discomfort at the site of the implant (NRPB, 1983). The magnitude of the radiofrequency pulses and the gradient currents is related to the static field strength, and the NRPB has set a maximum of 2.5 Tesla for human imaging, while in the US the Food and Drugs Administration has set its upper limit at 2.0 Tesla.

Although no clinical sequelae have been described to date, changes in the T-wave of the electrocardiogram are observed with static fields in excess of 0.3 Tesla (Gaffey et al. 1980). Most cardiac pacemakers of demand type are switched from synchronous (demand) to asynchronous (fixed rate) operation in the static field of the magnet, due to closure of their reed switch; the field strength necessary to close the switch is only 0.0017–0.07 Tesla, depending on the type of pacemaker and its precise orientation relative to the magnet. Should the switch not close, the time-varying magnetic fields, or the electromagnetic interference may be of the order of magnitude required to induce changes in output; this can also occur with the older, fixed-rate pacemakers if they are not encased in metal. Torque forces on an implanted unit can be sufficient to displace it within the chest wall, if there is not considerable surrounding fibrosis (Pavlicek et al. 1983). It is recommended by the NRPB that no individuals bearing pacemakers be allowed within the MRI suite, as patients, staff or visitors.

Mechanical Constraints

Another very inconvenient feature of most current magnetic resonance imagers, particularly troublesome in the acutely ill, is the relative inaccessibility of the patient: this is both direct, as the patient is hidden from view, and indirect, as there are significant obstacles to monitoring. The imager is usually in cylindrical form, about 2 m long, and 2 m in external diameter, with a central aperture about 60 cm in diameter, in which the patient is placed, with the part to be imaged at its centre. The ends of the aperture may be extended by cagework radiofrequency shielding, or closed (Figure 2.2). Direct observation of the patient is therefore extremely limited, particularly when the head and neck are being imaged, and in the case of small children. Some workers have tried to use solid-state closed-circuit television monitoring, but have found that an adequate image was not achieved, because of internal reflections within the 2.5-m-long central bore (Bradley et al. 1984). Verbal communication is not generally possible, particularly because the regular switching of currents through the gradient coils causes a loud drumming noise. Simple alarm systems can be arranged: the conscious patient can, for example, hold a rubber bulb in his hand, which works a small whistle outside the imager; solid-state intercom apparatus is also available (Bradley et al. 1984).

Babies and young children, and adults who are mentally retarded, demented or simply claustrophobic may be unable to lie sufficiently still to permit satisfactory images. Because of the limited observation and access, heavy sedation may be hazardous without adequate airway protection. If an examination by MRI is strongly indicated in such individuals, general anaesthesia, with tracheal intubation, may be justified; it can be maintained in a conventional manner, with volatile anaesthetic agents and spontaneous breathing. When the patient requires assisted ventilation, total anaesthesia with intravenous agents, combined with simple pneumatic ventilation with oxygen-enriched air, represents a useful practical alternative, simplifying the equipment and avoiding atmospheric pollution with anaesthetic vapours.

Commonly used intravenous infusion pumps can be used alongside MRI apparatus (Dunn et al. 1985). However, infusion and other tubing which does not normally reach outside the imager must be disconnected for the duration of the examination or, should this not be feasible, extended (Figure 2.2), possibly increasing the dead space for injections of small volumes of intravenous drugs, for example, which can be particularly inconvenient in small children with severe fluid-balance restrictions. Monitoring devices must also be modified appropriately. Respiratory rate can be monitored using a rubber bellows linked by a pressure line to a pressure transducer, such as a piezoelectric crystal, by an apnoea alarm mattress, or by remote capnography (Nixon et al. 1987), while oscillometry (with nylon connectors) or a direct intra-arterial cannula can be used for blood pressure. Automated noninvasive blood-pressure and heart-rate monitoring devices such as the Datascope Accutorr and

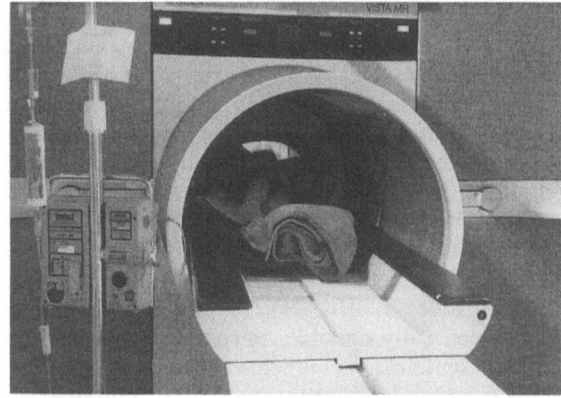

a

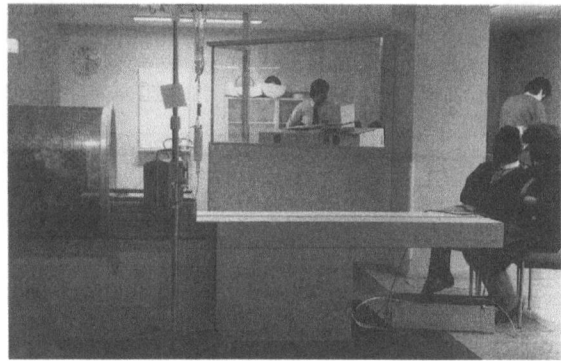

b

Fig. 2.2. a The upper thorax of a child is being examined, using the "body coil" (Fig. 2.3): the inaccessibility of the head and neck is clearly demonstrated. A metallic infusion pump, with extended tubing, is positioned close to the imager. The mesh-work radiofrequency shielding is seen more clearly in **b**, which also shows a relative and a nurse sitting unshielded within a few feet of the magnet.

Critikon Dynamap have been used successfully with a 0.5 Tesla NMR imager (Dunn et al. 1985). Loops of wire, even when nonferrous, can interfere with radiofrequency pulses and the resulting NMR signals, and electrical connections may also introduce radiofrequency noise. Fibreoptic systems can be employed for transmitting the electrocardiogram (ECG) signal, but at increased cost; transducers are required. Radiofrequency pulses and gradient currents can interfere with transmitted signals. The former can be removed by filtering, and gradient interference can be effectively "blanked out", at the cost of flat segments in the ECG record. If the respiratory rate signal is subjected to amplitude modulation, both ECG and respiration-rate data can be carried on a single fibreoptic channel, and some manufacturers will provide monitoring ports on the MRI operator's console (Blakeley and Gangarossa 1985). The static magnetic field can nevertheless grossly distort CRT displays, even at a

distance. It is feasible to continue recording intra-cranial pressure while the patient is in the imager (Dunn et al, 1985), but further difficulties may arise (see below).

When patients must be ventilated during the examination, a low-mass ventilator, without ferrous components, whose performance is not adversely affected by the static magnetic field can be placed near the imager; a Monaghan 225 SIMV fluidic volume ventilator has been used alongside a 0.5-Tesla magnet (Dunn et al. 1985). The alternative is remote placement of a standard ventilator, possibly incorporated in an anaesthetic machine, with long (5–6 m) connecting tubes. Unfortunately, expira-tory resistance increases with tube length: standard 22-mm tubing was found to have a resistance of $7\,Pa^{-1}/m^{-1}$ at $30\,l^{-1}/min^{-1}$, more than doubled at $60\,l^{-1}/min^{-1}$ [6]. Coaxial systems, although more convenient for handling, generally have a high expiratory resistance (Humphrey 1982).

Against these inconveniences can be weighed the fact that an attendant can stay near the patient throughout the examination, free from any known risk, and without the need for the radiation pro-tection required when X-rays are involved (Fig. 2.2). In some cases, parents or medical staff have actually lain in the patient aperture together with a child. However, a further drawback when the head is being examined is that for high-quality images the coils which emit the radiofrequency pulses and receive the NMR signals should be as close to the part of interest as possible, to maximise the signal-to-noise ratio. As commercially available head coils are often cylindrical, with an internal diameter of 30 cm or less (Fig. 2.3), patients with large head-dressings, intracranial pressure monitors, or even standard endotracheal tube fittings, may not fit

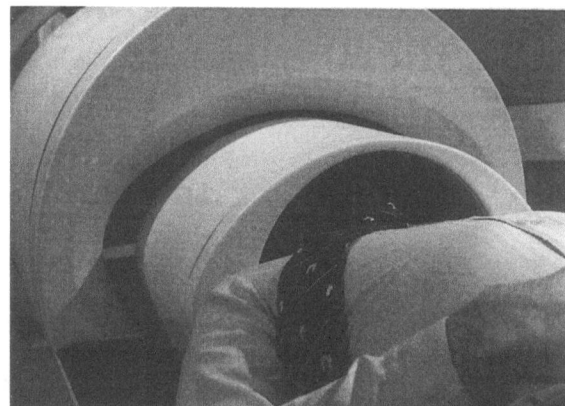

Fig. 2.3. The head has been positioned in the "coil" containing the radiofrequency transmitter and receiver. The small diameter of the coil, which fits concentrically within the larger "body coil", is evident, as is the masking of the facial area.

within the coil. If MRI is essential under these conditions, it may be necessary to remove inessential artefacts temporarily and to use a soft, flexible endotracheal tube; Nixon et al. (1987) recommended a Rae pattern oral tube with a 15 mm connector. The current trend is towards coils fashioned in a helmet form which, while leaving the face relatively free, may prove even more troublesome over the cranium.

Constraints Imposed by the Duration of the Examination

In MRI, data are collected continuously during an extended period, in which respect the procedure resembles early CT, where data collection took 5 min or more per pair of images. On the imager currently in use at the National Hospital, London, a typical spin echo sequence covering the entire head would take 18.2 min of uninterrupted scanning time, during which the patient must remain immobile; data are collected simultaneously for up to 16 images, but the overall times required for eight or four comparable images are 9.4 and 5.1 min respectively. Similar inversion recovery sequences take 26, 20.5 or 17.9 min, while a single "planning" scan, equivalent to the "scout" of a CT scanner, takes more than 1 min. It is not feasible therefore to obtain a whole series of single images while suspending the ventilation, for example, or to aspirate secretions regularly between data collections, as one might during a CT study. When the thoracic or lumbar spine is being examined, cardiac and respiratory movement both cause major artefacts. "Gating", i.e., using only data obtained during certain segments of the cardiac and/or respiratory cycles is currently employed but, understandably, effectively doubles the total duration of the examination.

Clinical Use of MRI

When considering the practical advantages of MRI, it is most appropriate to compare it with CT, since of available methods it is the most similar in the diagnostic information it provides. Of the two, MRI is much more sensitive to tissue composition, and to differences between abnormal and healthy tissues, and in certain regions, where the quality of CT images is reduced by artefacts or poor inherent radiographic contrast, such as the posterior cranial fossa and the thoracic spine (Fig. 2.4), it also gives superior morphological information.

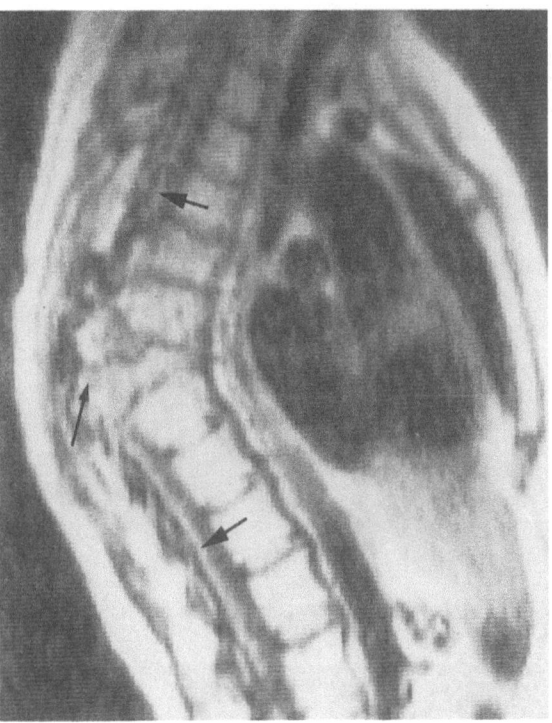

Fig. 2.4. Spinal trauma. Sagittal NMR image, showing a compression fracture of the eighth thoracic vertebra, which protrudes backwards into the spinal canal; there appears to be a loose fragment posteriorly (*vertical arrow*). The spinal cord, visible above and below (*arrows*), could not be identified at this level in any of a series of sagittal sections.

The magnetic fields and radio waves to which the patient and staff are exposed in MRI are without known deleterious effects, other than those described above, which do not concern the majority of individuals. It is therefore permissible to carry out MRI during pregnancy, and even specifically to examine the foetus, although on a totally empirical basis, the NRPB has indicated that it should not be performed during the first trimester (NRPB 1983).

Accurate positioning of the acutely ill patient is somewhat less critical with MRI than with CT, and minor movements during the examination tend to produce merely a generally inferior image (Fig. 2.5), rather than the grossly degraded scan which may well be the end result of CT in such patients. Because selection of both the level and the orientation of the image plane in MRI is electronic rather than mechanical as in CT, the most suitable plane can be adopted *ab initio* if the probable nature of the clinical problem is known, and images in further planes can be obtained to supplement the data it provides. Once the patient is placed in the imager, further manipulation is usually unnecessary (Fig. 2.5).

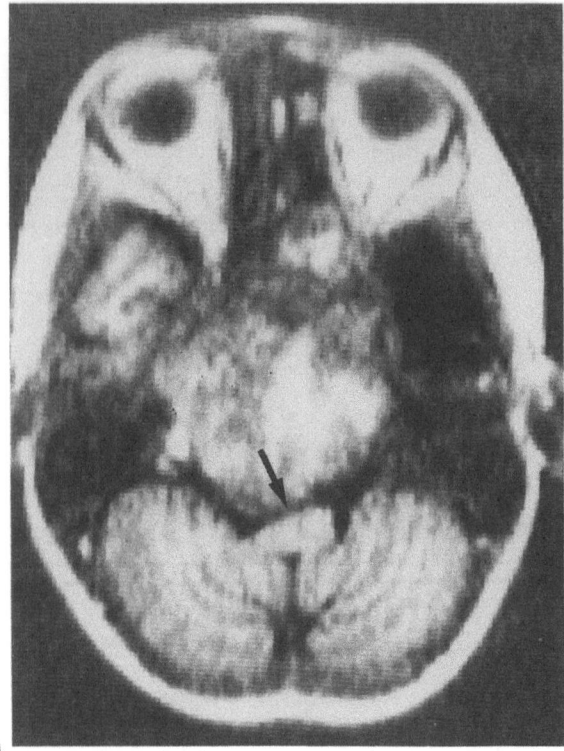

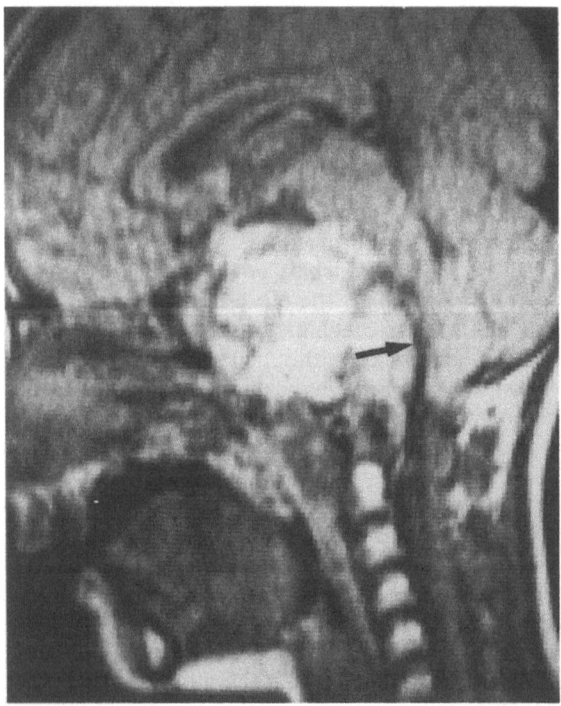

Fig. 2.5. a,b. Malignant tumour of the skull base, causing gross extrinsic compression of the brainstem (*arrows*). **a** Axial and **b** sagittal NMR images, obtained without change in position of the patient: **b** is of diagnostic quality, despite multiple linear artefacts due to movement.

Most examinations with MRI do not involve intravenous or intrathecal contrast media such as are used in CT; the latter preparations, which usually contain iodine, are contraindicated in patients with impaired renal and/or hepatic function, and are associated with well-documented morbidity – nausea and vomiting, or ECG disturbances in 7%–8%, urticaria, hypotension or bronchospasm in 1%, and less frequently angioneurotic oedema or cardiorespiratory arrest – even in normal individuals. Prospective studies have revealed a mortality rate of 1 in 40 000 (Ansell et al. 1980). Avoidance of these potentially noxious substances is an even greater advantage in the patient whose condition is already precarious. Contrast media which are being developed for use in MRI are devoid of similar biotoxicity (Runge et al. 1983), but they are unnecessary for the majority of studies, and even information on flow in major vessels is available without them (Fig. 2.6).

Indications

Given the practical problems discussed above, it may be asked why one should persist with this very expensive imaging technique in patients whose conditions already gives cause for concern. The urgency of imaging of the brain and spinal cord is inversely related to the threat posed to life or the quality of recovery by conditions requiring intensive care; in the case of CT, it was spelt out by the Consensus Development Conference held at the National Institutes of Health in 1981 that the examination is rarely so strongly indicated that it should be allowed to prejudice the intensive care process, and its presumptive benefits must be weighed against the risks of removing the patient from a dedicated unit (Consensus Development Conference 1982). Whenever possible, the imaging procedure is delayed until the patient's condition is less acutely critical. This is particularly true in the case of young children, although Thalaysingham et al. (1985) have described a specially adapted incubator, in which a baby may be examined without interrupting intensive care.

Indications for examinations of the central nervous system can be divided into those for the brain and those for the spinal cord.

The Brain. In the context of intensive care, MRI may be called into play in the emergency assessment of acute head injuries, in suspected intracranial infections, vascular accidents, demyelination and following cranial surgery. Sensitivity to most of the abnormalities mentioned above is as great or

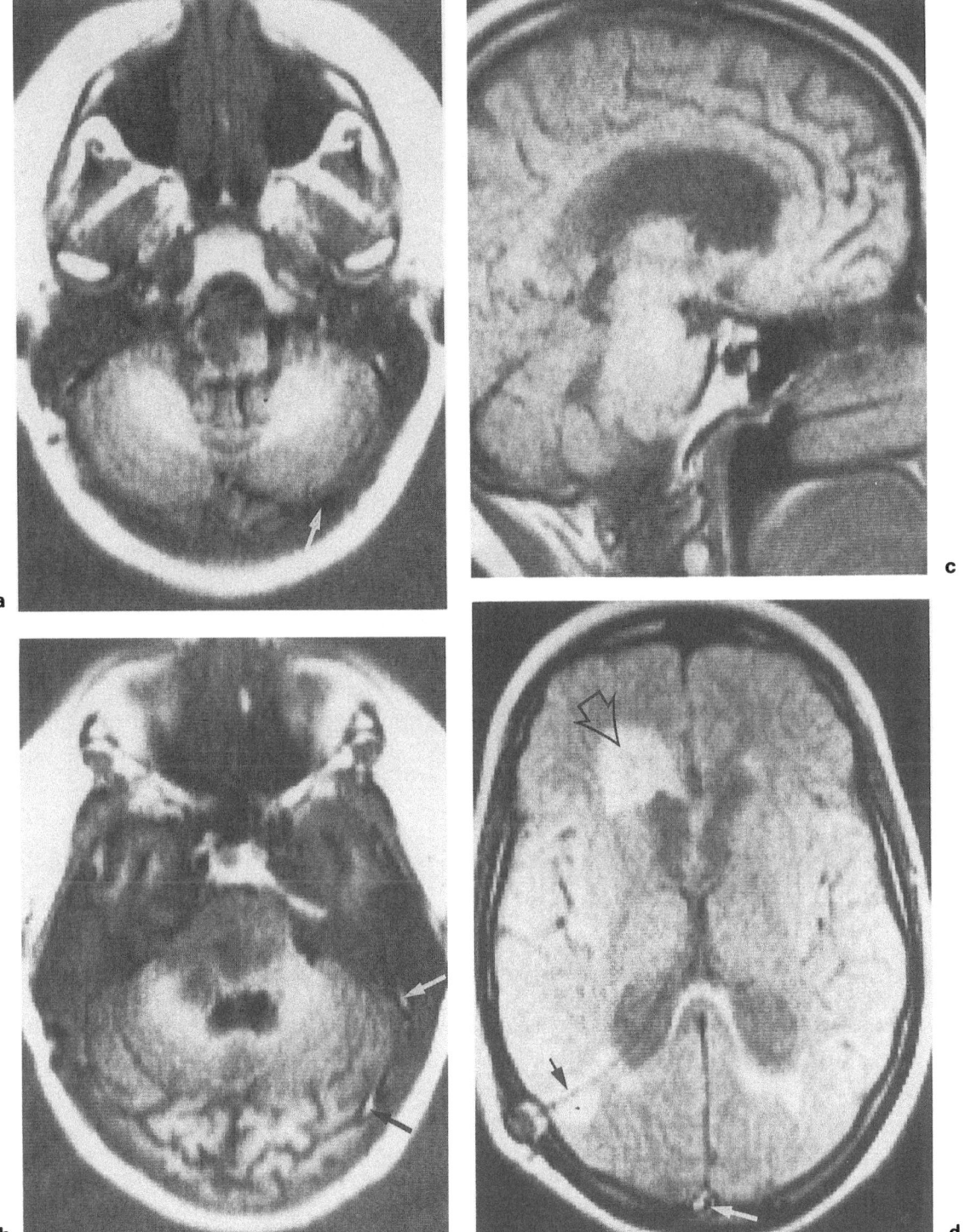

Fig. 2.6. a–d. Intrinsic tumour of the brainstem (presumed glioma). **a,b** Axial inversion recovery and **c** sagittal spin echo images indicate clearly the intra-axial nature and thereby the inoperability of this tumour (cf Fig. 2.5). **d** A spin echo section through the lateral ventricles shows increased signal (bright) around the ventricles and the path of the ventricular catheter (*small arrow*), but also reveals the presence of a mass, probably metastatic, compressing the right frontal horn (*open arrow*). Note the absence of artefact from the shunt system, and the areas of very bright and/or dark signal caused by laminar blood flow in the dural venous sinuses in **a, b** and **c** (*arrows*).

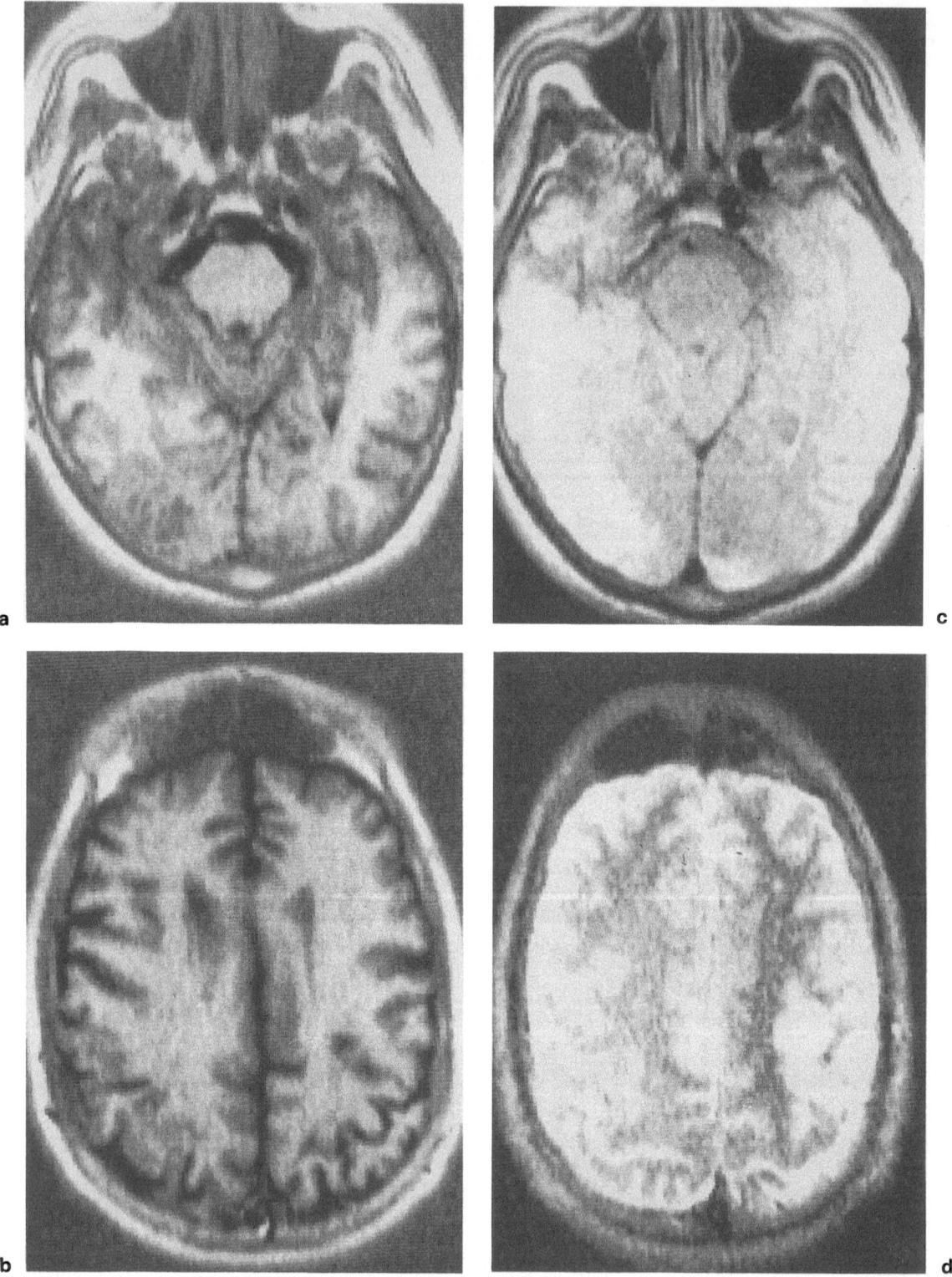

Fig. 2.7 a–d. Acute cerebral infarction. **a,b** Inversion recovery. **c,d** Spin echo images. Areas of altered signal (darker grey than the adjacent white matter on inversion recovery and white on spin echo) are visible in the right temporo-occipital and left parietal lobes.

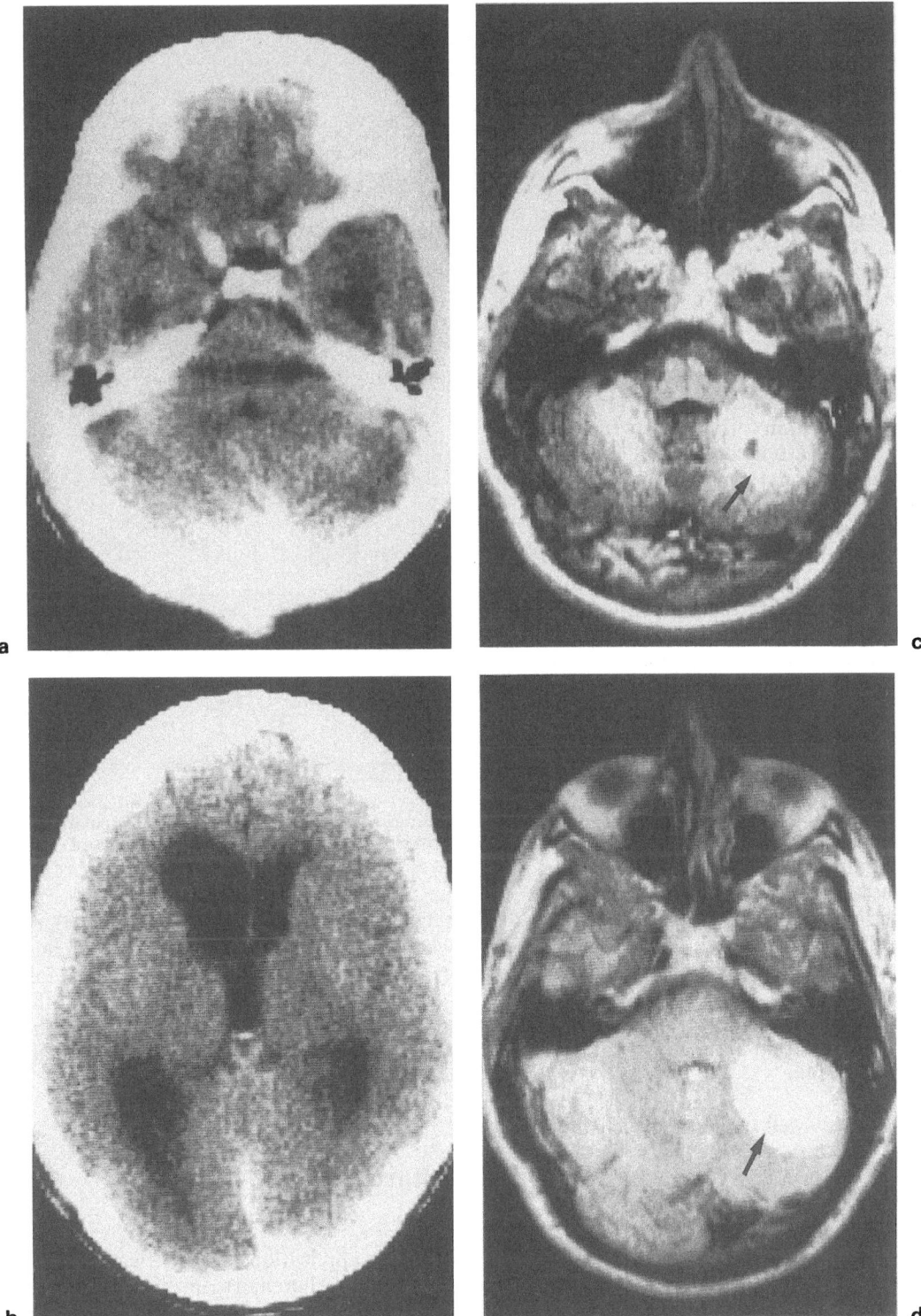

Fig. 2.8. a–d. MRI and CT in a patient with persistent cerebellar and brainstem disturbance after a head injury. **a** CT of the posterior fossa, originally interpreted as normal, shows poorly defined low density in the left cerebellar hemisphere and minimal distortion of the fourth ventricle. There is nevertheless mild dilatation of the lateral and third ventricles. **b.** MRI performed one day later. **c** Inversion recovery and **d** spin echo images: a rounded area of increased signal (*arrows*), representing a resolving haematoma, occupies much of the left cerebellar hemisphere, encroaching on the middle cerebellar peduncle.

greater than that of CT, with one very significant exception: the NMR characteristics of freshly extravasated blood may be so similar to those of normal cerebral tissues that the nature of a haematoma is not evident. The technique is particularly advantageous for assessment of patients with acute brainstem and/or cerebellar syndromes, with bulbar palsy (Fig. 2.6) or respiratory depression, since CT images of this region are commonly degraded by artefact (Bydder et al. 1983). Acute central pontine myelinolysis, for example, a life-threatening but self-limiting complication of hyponatraemia, often superimposed on a history of alcoholism, tends to be very elusive on CT, but has been shown very clearly with MRI (De Witt et al. 1984).

Cerebral, cerebellar or brainstem infarction (Fig. 2.7) may be visualised within 6 h of onset, even more reliably than by CT and at a time when radionuclide studies are uniformly normal (Sipponen et al. 1983). MRI has been found superior to CT for detection of small traumatic extracerebral collections, and for determination of the extent of larger lesions (Fig. 2.8). The ability to obtain coronal images without additional manipulation of the patient, although it prolongs the examination, is particularly valuable in vertical, peritentorial or subtemporal haematomas. Areas of contusion are clearly visible on MRI when they are seen poorly if at all on CT, although their bland or haemorrhagic nature may not be readily apparent (Han et al. 1984).

In most countries, as in Britain, brain death is a clinical diagnosis, but there are still some countries in which imaging techniques are recommended as a means of establishing the likely cause of irreversible coma, or of decreasing the length of a statutory observation period (Guidelines for the determination of death 1981); MRI may contribute in both these ways. It has already been mentioned that movement of blood causes variations in the NMR signal, which can be related to flow (Fig. 2.6); demonstration that flow is absent in the major cerebral vessels is certainly feasible.

The Spine. MRI is very well suited to investigation of spinal cord compression, as the cord, the subarachnoid space and the adjacent bones and paraspinal tissues can be seen on a single image (Modic et al. 1983). The multiplanar capacity of MRI is particularly important in spinal imaging. Excessive manipulation can be avoided in patients suspected of having critical cervical or thoracic cord compression, but the maintenance of adequate traction during the examination, as can be achieved during spinal CT, is difficult, and may necessitate the design of new traction apparatus using nonmetallic components.

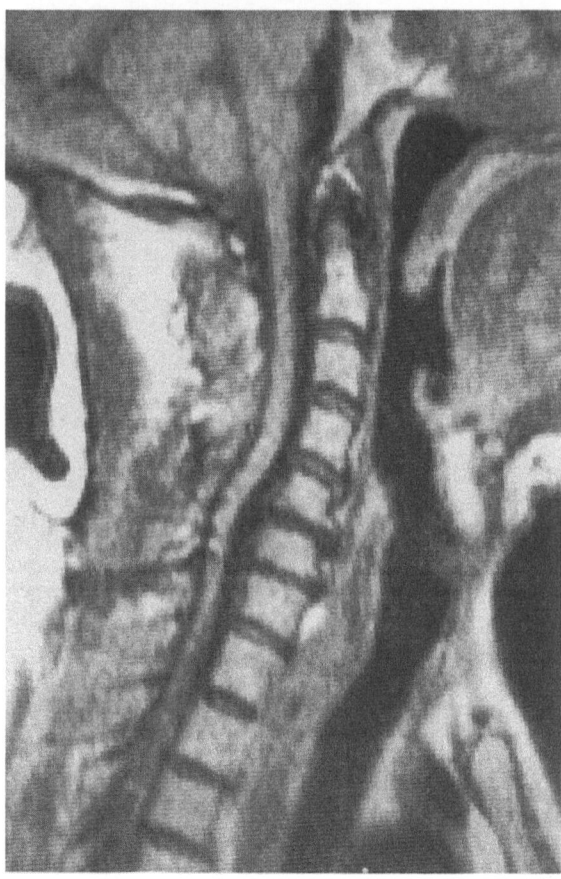

Fig. 2.9. Patient with persistent quadriparesis and intermittent breathing disturbance after cervical laminectomy. Sagittal image showing posterior displacement and apparent tethering of spinal cord at the operation site.

Thus, in the acutely injured patient (Fig. 2.4), or when where is evidence of persistent cord compression and/or respiratory embarrassment following spinal surgery (Fig. 2.9), MRI is the examination of choice, particularly as myelography is especially difficult, and occasionally technically unsatisfactory, in ventilated patients.

The Future

The first major application of NMR was to spectroscopic analysis rather than to imaging. It appears probable that future apparatus for MRI may also be used for in vivo spectroscopy. Nuclei which can be used for this technique include sodium (Hilal et al. 1985), phosphorus and fluorine.

In vivo phosphorus spectroscopy has been used to investigate metabolism in muscle (including demonstration of the pathological changes in McArdle's syndrome (Ross et al. 1981)) and in brain, where changes in the relative concentrations of phosphorus-containing metabolites as a result of disturbances of blood flow can be detected (Ackerman et al. 1980). The potential applications of these methods to management of critical illness are as yet unclear.

Many drugs contain fluorine: they include anaesthetic agents (halothane, enflurane), haloperidol, blood substitutes (perfluotributylamine) and synthetic steroids (dexamethasone). Since it may be feasible to monitor their distribution, and thereby to assess penetration of these substances within the brain (Wyrwicz et al. 1983), the effectiveness of chemotherapeutic regimes may be amenable to very precise in vivo evaluation.

Conclusions

MRI is an extremely valuable imaging technique for investigation of the nervous system. Although its application in intensive care is fraught with technical hurdles, most of these can be overcome satisfactorily. Spectroscopic monitoring of cerebral metabolism and pharmacology is an exciting potential expansion of its role.

References

Ackerman JJF, Bore PJ, Gadian DG, Grove TH, Radda GK (1980) NMR studies of metabolism in perfused organs. Phil Trans R Soc Lond [Biol] 289: 425–436

Ansell GM, Tweedie MCK, West CR, Price Evans DA, Couch L (1980) The current status of reactions to intravenous contrast media. Invest Radiol (1980) 15: S32–S39

Blakeley DM, Gangarossa RE (1985) Implementation of fibre-optic data link for cardiac and respiratory gating/monitoring. Soc Mag Res in Med Fourth Annual Meeting, Book of Abstracts 2: 1073–1074

Bradley WG, Opel W, Kassabian JP (1984) Magnetic resonance installations: siting and economic considerations. Radiology 151: 719–721

Bydder GM, Steiner RE, Thomas DJ, Marshall J, Gilderdale DJ, Young IR (1983) Nuclear magnetic resonance imaging of the posterior fossa: 50 cases. Clin Radiol 34: 173–188

Consensus development conference (1982) Computed tomographic scanning of the brain. Surg Neurol 18: 72–75

Davis PL, Crooks L, Arakawa M, McKee R, Kaufman L, Margulis AR (1981) Potential hazards in NMR imaging: heating effects of changing magnetic fields and RF field on small metallic implants. AJR 137: 857–869

DeWitt LD, Buonanno FS, Kistler JP, Zweffiro T, DeLaPaz RL, Brady TJ, Rosen BR, Pykett IL (1984) Central pontine myelinolysis: demonstration by nuclear magnetic resonance. Neurology 34: 570–576

Dunn V, Kurschinski DT, Scamman FL, Ehrhardt JC (1985) MRI of seriously ill patients requiring monitoring, mechanical ventilation or general anaesthesia. Soc Mag Res in Med Fourth Annual Meeting, Book of Abstracts 2: 920–921

Gaffey CT, Tenforde TS, Dean EE (1980). Alterations in the electrocardiogram of baboons exposed to DC magnetic fields. Bioelectromagnetics 1: 209

Guidelines for the determination of death (1981) Report of the medical consultants on the diagnosis of death to the President's Commission for the study of ethical problems in medicine and biomedical and behavioural research. JAMA 246: 2184–2186

Han JS, Kaufman B, Alfidi RJ, Yeung HN, Benson JE, Haaga JR, El Yousef SJ, Clampitt ME, Bonstelle CT, Huss R (1984) Head trauma evaluated by magnetic resonance and computed tomography: a comparison. Radiology 150: 71–77

Hilal SK, Maudsley AA, Ra JB (1985) In vivo NMR imaging of sodium-23 in the human head. J Comput Assist Tomogr 9: 1–9

Humphrey D (1982) The Lack, Magill and Bain anaesthetic breathing systems. A direct comparison in spontaneously breathing anaesthetised adults. J R Soc Med 75: 513–524

Modic MT, Weinstein MA, Pavlicek W, Boumphrey F, Starnes D, Duchesneau PM (1983) Magnetic resonance imaging of the cervical spine: technical and clinical observations. AJR 141: 1129–1136

National Radiological Protection Board ad hoc Advisory Group on Nuclear Magnetic Resonance Clinical Imaging (1983) Revised guidance on acceptable limits of exposure during nuclear magnetic resonance clinical imaging. Br J Radiol 56: 974–977

New PFJ, Rosen BR, Brady TJ, Buonanno FS, Kistler JP, Burt CT, Hinshaw WS, Newhouse JH, Pohost GM, Taveras JM (1983) Potential hazards and artifacts of ferromagnetic and nonferromagnetic surgical and dental materials and devices in nuclear magnetic resonance imaging. Radiology 147: 139–148

Nixon C, Hirsch NP, Ormerod IEC, Johnson G (1987) Nuclear magnetic resonance: its implications for the anaesthetist. In press.

Pavlicek W, Geisinger M, Castle L, Borkowski GP, Meaney TF, Bream BL, Gallagher JH (1983) The effect of nuclear magnetic resonance on patients with cardiac pacemakers. Radiology 147: 149–153

Pusey E, Bradley W, Brown RKJ, Shoemaker S, Waluch V, Bassett L (1985) Safety of MR scanning in patients with metallic prostheses. Soc Mag Res in Med Fourth Annual Meeting, Book of Abstracts 2: 923–924

Pyckett IL, Newhouse JH, Buonanno FS, Brady TJ, Goldman MR, Kistler JP, Pohost GM (1982) Principles of nuclear magnetic resonance imaging. Radiology 143: 157–168

Ross BD, Radda GK, Gadian DG (1981) Examination of a case of suspected McArdle's syndrome by ^{31}P nuclear magnetic resonance. N Engl J Med 304: 1338–1342

Runge VM, Clanton JA, Lukehart CM, Partain CL, James AE (1983) Paramagnetic agents for contrast-enhanced NMR imaging. AJR 141: 1209–1215

Sipponen CT, Kaste M, Ketonen L, Sepponen RE, Katevuo K, Sivula A (1983) Serial nuclear magnetic resonance (NMR) imaging in patients with cerebral infarction. J Comput Assist Tomogr 7: 585–589

Thalayasingham S, Chu A, Delpy DT (1985) An infant incubator for use during NMR spectroscopy and imaging. Soc Mag Res in Med Fourth Annual Meeting, Book of Abstracts 2: 927–928

Weinreb JC, Maravilla KR, Peshock R, Payne J (1984) Magnetic resonance imaging: improving patient tolerance and safety. AJR 143: 1285–1287

Wyrwicz AM, Pszenny MH, Schofield JC, Tillman PC, Gordon RE, Martin PA (1983) Noninvasive observation of fluorinated anesthetics in rabbit brain by ^{19}fluorine nuclear magnetic resonance. Science 222: 429–430

Chapter 3

Positron Emission Tomography in the Investigation of Cerebral Disease

R. S. J. Frackowiak

Principles

Positron emission tomography (PET) is often regarded as another imaging technique. In fact, imaging is only a minor by-product of PET which is actually concerned with measurement of tissue function. In principle PET is the application of tracer techniques to the measurement of tissue function in living man by what is essentially a non-invasive technique (Phelps et al. 1986).

The tracers are detected by specialised systems designed to record the distribution of positron-emitting isotopes regionally and quantitatively in the brain. The ability to make such measurements is dependent on the physics of radioisotope decay by positron emission. Standard single photon-emitting isotopes such as technitium can also be detected tomographically. However, true quantitation with such instruments is not possible. Decay by positron emission results in the production of two photons per disintegration which have the property of leaving the point of positron annihilation at 180° to each other. The two gamma rays so formed both have an energy of 511 KeV and so in passing through the tissue they experience the same degree of attenuation by similar density material. The detection of the two gamma rays within a narrow time window constitutes the essential element of the detecting apparatus. Single events which might arise from outside the field of view subtended by the two detectors placed on opposite sides of the body are thus ignored. Likewise, scattered radiation is also largely eliminated. The field of view is very clearly defined by the area of the crystal faces on opposite sides of the body. In effect, this results in a form of electronic collimation. The sensitivity of detection is quite uniform throughout the field of view. This is because only events which are a result of the passage of each photon of the pair to its respective detector are recorded, which is equivalent to saying only those events where a photon has traversed the complete distance between the two detectors are significant. One must contrast this with single photon detection where the sensitivity rapidly decreases with distance from the detector face, events occurring deeper in the tissues being much less likely to reach the correct detector than those arising at the periphery. The combination of well-defined field of view, uniform sensitivity and considerable elimination of noise contribute greatly to the ability to quantitate these isotopes with tomography. Another consideration is the question of correction for attenuation. Whenever photons traverse tissue they may be stopped depending on the depth of tissue traversed and its absorbing properties. In PET this attenuation effect can be precisely measured by recording with a positron-emitting source between the body and detectors. Registration of two simultaneous events in this transmission mode will result in an estimation of the attenuating capacity through the full thickness of the tissue as one photon traverses it, whilst the other simply passes through a small gap of air before reaching its detector. The accumulation of sufficient angular data allows for reconstruction of the attenuation coefficients point-for-point through the tomographic plane. This information can then be used on the tomographic reconstruction obtained in the emission mode, with the positron tracer introduced into the body, to obtain a corrected distribution. It is important to note that this correction for attenuation is measured and unique for each patient and each plane that comes under study, and represents a quantitative operation which is not available to single photon tomography. The combination of these various properties means that the positron camera is capable of measuring exact distributions of positron labelled ligands introduced into the tissue. It then remains to calibrate the pixel response of the camera with an independent measure of radioactivity, to convert the camera-derived measurements into units of $\mu Ci^{-1}ml^{-1}$.

The ability to quantitate radioactivity regionally in the brain in absolute units means that tracer techniques can be applied and measurements of tissue function can be made in a meaningful and comparable manner. It is frequently stated that a major disadvantage of PET resides in the fact that the positron-emitting isotopes need to be produced by a cyclotron or a similar particle accelerating machine. This results in major cost and considerable difficulties in isotope manipulation. In fact this disadvantage is comparatively minor given the fact that the longest-lived gamma-emitting isotopes of nitrogen, oxygen and carbon are all positron emitters. The ability to trace molecules of physiological, biochemical or neurochemical interest with isotopes of oxygen, carbon or nitrogen is a very major advantage. For example, the substitution of a stable carbon atom by carbon-11 in a molecule of interest means that its biological properties will remain conserved. Thus inferences made from measurements of tracer kinetics of the carbon-11-labelled molecule will remain valid for the stable molecule. Another relative disadvantage is the short half-life of these isotopes. Oxygen-15 has a half-life of 2.1 min, carbon-11 of 20 min and fluorine-18 of 110 min. Fluorine-18 is frequently used to substitute for hydrogen in larger molecules and appears to have little effect on the biological properties of the majority of molecules. Its use as a tracer however demands that the biological fate of the fluorinated compound becomes compared to that of the unfluorinated so that inferences made from measurement of the tracer can be translated into real life. The short half-life can frequently also be used to advantage. A particularly good example of this is in the steady-state inhalation technique for measuring cerebral blood flow, oxygen extraction and consumption with oxygen-15-labelled compounds. There are therefore many good reasons for preferring positron-emitting isotopes to label tracers which in principle considerably outweigh the disadvantage which remains a scientifically trivial one, that of cost.

The application of tracer techniques to man opens up a range and versatility of measurements which is unparalleled. It is already clear that 15%–20% of the Pharmacopoeia can potentially be labelled with positron-emitters by existing techniques of radiochemistry. The difficulty lies in identifying appropriate tracers to study the physiological pathway of interest and subsequently developing these tracers and their use in a technique that will result in a measurement of the appropriate function. With PET the only data available following the injection of a tracer into the body is a measurement of radioactivity in the tissue of interest (possibly also as a function of time) and a measurement of radioactivity in blood. Any positron-based method must therefore be capable of expressing the desired physiological, biochemical or pharmacological function with reference to these measurable variables. This is one of the main limiting steps of positron-based tracer techniques.

A number of such techniques have become developed over the last six or seven years since PET has been applied to the measurement of tissue function in man. I will describe some of these in the remainder of this chapter in relation to physiological functions which may be of interest to intensive care medicine. I will also attempt to indicate lines of enquiry which have not as yet been pursued but which could be resolved with the techniques at present established. This chapter concerns itself with the brain, but it is pertinent that tracer measurements can be made in any organ of the body. In relation to intensive care medicine, this is of obvious interest with respect to the lungs and heart and also perhaps the metabolic function of the liver, although I shall not consider these organs further in this article.

Energy Metabolism

In the past, the only tracer methods of making observations of the physiology of the brain with any regional specificity have been related to cerebral blood flow (CBF). Over the last six years considerable effort has been expended on a study of cerebral energy metabolism in the human brain in health and disease by using PET. A number of techniques have been used. The best established and most widely used in clinical research at present is the steady-state inhalation technique (Frackowiak et al. 1980). This method was ideally adapted to the first- and second-generation positron cameras which had considerably lower sensitivity and temporal resolution than the most modern instruments now being developed. This meant that in order to obtain sufficient data to give statistically meaningful measurements, a method had to be devised to freeze the distribution of isotope, as a function of the physiological variable in time.

The steady-state technique depends on the consecutive, continuous inhalation of oxygen-15-labelled carbon dioxide and oxygen, followed by a bolus inhalation of carbon-11-labelled carbon monoxide or continuous inhalation of carbon-15-labelled carbon monoxide. The general principles of the tracer method are conceptually simple (Frackowiak et al. 1980; Lammertsma, and Jones, 1983; Lammertsma et al. 1983, 1981, 1982). The inhalation of trace amounts of $C^{15}O_2$ results in the labelling of circulating water in the pulmonary capillaries. This is a rapid, virtually complete process of high efficiency. The oxygen-15-labelled circulatory water is then distributed throughout the body as a function of blood flow. In the brain the cerebral capillaries are virtually completely permeable to water at normal physiological flow levels. This results in a deposition in the tissue of all the water delivered to a given region. The labelled water in tissue, delivered as a function of flow, then suffers two fates both resulting in disappearance of the label from its site of deposition. In the first instance the very short half-life of the isotope means that a considerable proportion of it decays. Secondly, because of the great permeability of the tissue to water, a further proportion is washed out of the tissue and hence back to the heart. With continuous inhalation of $C^{15}O_2$ within three or four half-lives of the ^{15}oxygen (5–6 min), a steady-state isotope concentration is established in the brain. This steady state is the result of the delivery of labelled water in the arterial blood balanced by its disappearance through radioactive decay and venous washout. Measurements of arterial and tissue ^{15}O-labelled water concentrations by PET allow one to solve simply for CBF.

In the next part of the measurement, the patient continuously breathes molecular oxygen labelled with oxygen-15. In vivo labelling of haemoglobin with oxygen-15 occurs in the pulmonary capillaries. The labelled oxyhaemoglobin is delivered to the cerebral tissues via the capillaries, where a constant proportion is extracted by the brain for the purpose of aerobic glucose metabolism. The extracted oxygen functions as an electron acceptor at the end of the cytochrome chain with the resultant production of water. This metabolically generated water is therefore itself labelled with oxygen-15. In this instance continuous inhalation of the $^{15}O_2$ molecule results in the deposition of metabolically generated oxygen-15-labelled water in the tissue. This also suffers the two fates of radioactive decay and wash-out. Indeed, in this case the washed-out, metabolically generated water constitutes a confusing signal because it then circulates and redistributes as a function of the flow. The previous procedure has already given the distribution of water of circulation as a function of flow and this information can be used to subtract the contaminating signal from the $^{15}O_2$ readings. In the normal brain only about 40% of the delivered oxygen is used for metabolic purposes. This is expressed in classical physiological terms by the arterio–venous difference. The unextracted oxygen resides within the cerebral blood pool and therefore constitutes a further contaminating signal. This also has to be subtracted before a distribution of radioactivity due solely to metabolically generated water can be derived. This is done simply by the third component of the method, which involves inhalation of carbon monoxide. This tracer attaches to haemoglobin irreversibly and therefore will reside in the blood volume exclusively. Measurements of regional activity with labelled carbon monoxide will therefore give measurements of cerebral blood volume (CBV). This can then be used to subtract the unextracted oxygen signal. The distribution of metabolically generated water gives information about the fraction of oxygen extracted for metabolic purposes. The combination of fractional extraction, CBF and a measurement of stable arterial oxygen content results in the derivation of the cerebral oxygen consumption rate ($CMRO_2$). In this way, the sequential use of three tracers results in the measurement of four physiological variables which give a very complete picture of cerebral energy metabolism and haemodynamics (Figs. 3.1, 3.2).

The steady-state inhalation method is a good example of a positron tracer technique. However, there are many other ways of looking at the problem of energy metabolism. One of these uses oxygen-15-labelled water and molecular oxygen to obtain dynamic measurements of the variables discussed. This method was made possible by technological advances in the design and performance of positron cameras and by the development of different strategies of administration and analysis of the resulting signal. Thus, for example, with cameras that are capable of much finer temporal resolution it is possible to conceive of tracer methods which rely on kinetic modelling and depend on rapid sampling of tissue radioactivity with time (Raichle et al. 1983,

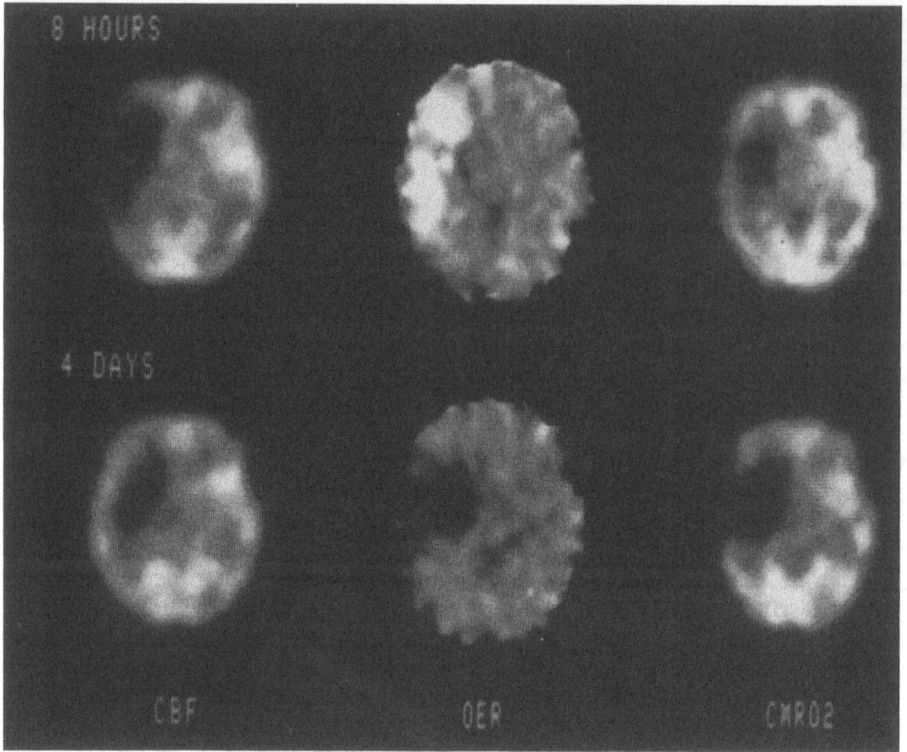

Fig. 3.1. PET scans of a subject 8 h (top) and 4 days (bottom) after a right hemiplegia and aphasia. The oxygen extraction in the early hours after the stroke is greatly elevated indicating ischaemia. It can be seen that the defect in cerebral blood flow (CBF) is proportionally greater than that of cerebral metabolism (CMRO2). With time, however, the oxygen extraction (OER) falls to subnormal levels indicating infarction in the presence of a large defect of metabolism. Despite this, perfusion in the cortex has normalised but this flow is redundant.

Herscovitch et al. 1983; Mintun et al. 1984; Phelps et al. 1986).

A further strategy is that developed by Sokoloff and relates to the use of positron-labelled substrate analogues. The fluorodeoxyglucose technique (^{18}FDG) is an example of this type of method (Sokoloff et al. 1977). In conceptual terms, fluorodeoxyglucose (FDG) is a substrate for facilitated transport across the blood–brain barrier and indeed is a competitive inhibitor of the transport of glucose. Given in trace quantities it will not perturb normal glucose transport but will reflect its kinetics as long as the relationship between FDG and glucose transport kinetics is known. In the tissue, the FDG resides in a tissue pool in the manner analogous to glucose and is a substrate for hexokinase, the first enzyme in the glycolytic chain. Unlike glucose, however, the product of hexokinase-catalysed phosphorylation of FDG can no longer be metabolised down the remainder of that chain. It therefore accumulates in the tissue and reflects hexokinase activity. If the kinetics of hexokinase-catalysed phosphorylation of FDG are known in

relation to that of glucose, then again inferences about glucose uptake can be derived. In its details, the model is considerably more complex than this simple conceptual description. However, the method has been used very successfully, particularly in the description of glucose consumption, especially in normal subjects and some pathologies. If used alone, the FDG method gives limited information. In conjunction with measurements of CBF or indeed oxygen metabolism, information can be obtained about the stoichiometry of glucose and oxygen metabolism which can certainly be deranged in hypoxic states and also in malignant tissue (Wise et al. 1983b).

Cerebral Ischaemia

The application of these two techniques to cerebral ischaemic disease has provided a considerable amount of new information (Frackowiak and Wise 1983; Frackowiak 1985b). It has become clear that the coupling of cerebral blood flow to oxygen util-

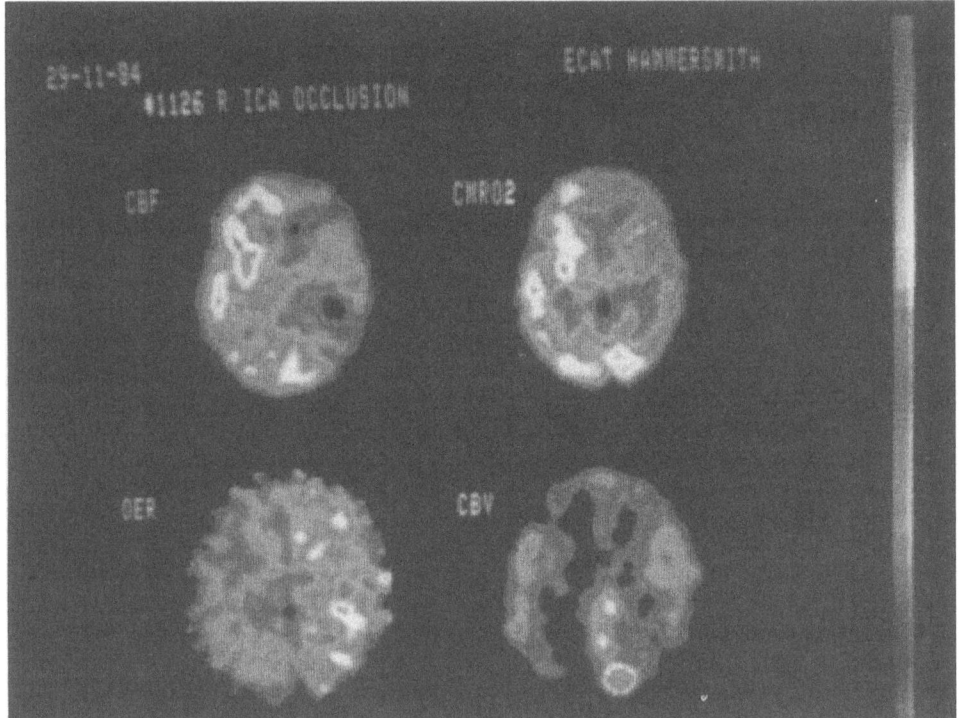

Fig. 3.2. PET scan of a subject who has undergone a right hemisphere infarction following right internal carotid artery occlusion. The patient has a mild left hemiparesis with neglect and visuospacial disturbances. A relative decrease in cerebral metabolic rate (CMRO2) in the territory of the middle cerebral artery in the right hemisphere is noted. The defect in perfusion is, however, much greater. Metabolism is maintained by compensatory vasodilatation seen as a local increase in cerebral blood volume (CBV) and also by a compensating increase in oxygen extraction to submaximal levels. The OER in this instance is 60% in the affected hemisphere and 45% in the normal hemisphere. This represents a state of critical perfusion.

isation is quite uniform throughout the normal brain (Frackowiak 1985b). The effects of acute impairment of blood flow in man are attenuated by homeostatic mechanisms which have been described and which appear to act in series (Frackowiak 1985a). The first of these mechanisms is a vasodilatation and consequent decline in peripheral resistance in response to a sudden fall in perfusion pressure. This vasodilatation can be quantified by PET measurements of CBV. Studies of patients with extracranial vascular occlusions have shown that the relationship between CBF and CBV is an extremely sensitive indicator of local tissue perfusion pressure and haemodynamic reserve. Thus the ratio CBF/CBV in any tissue region in the brain tends to fall as perfusion pressure falls.

The second mechanism relies on the proportion of oxygen delivered to the cerebral capillaries which is not used in oxidative metabolism (about 60%). If the vasodilatation resulting in a fall in peripheral tissue resistance becomes maximal and yet is inadequate to compensate fully for the fall in perfusion

pressure, then CBF will begin to fall. In this case, the supply of oxygen to the tissue is maintained by an increase in the fraction extracted from the arterial blood which will progressively rise depending on the degree of the impairment of blood flow until maximal extraction of 80%–100% occurs. Should the fall in perfusion be such that this is still insufficient to maintain metabolic function, then the oxygen consumption rate will begin to fall linearly as a function of flow. This is the stage of true ischaemia. Dependent on its depth and duration, tissue infarction will occur to a greater or lesser degree. The question remains as to what happens if perfusion is restored during the ischaemic phase. The answers to this question are as yet unclear due to lack of data. There is some evidence that deeper tissues progress from ischaemia to infarction comparatively early and probably within hours of the onset of ischaemia (Wise et al. 1983a). Superficial cortical regions progress to frank infarction somewhat later. The physiological feature of infarction is a low metabolic rate for oxygen combined with low oxygen extraction (Wise et al. 1983a). This indicates that the tissue is unable to use oxygen, presumably because of a decrease in the number of viable residual neurons. These physiological mechanisms are of considerable importance in assessing patients who have suffered from ischaemic events. However they hold out little promise for salvage therapy unless this can be applied with extreme rapidity. The description of these mechanisms means that pre-ischaemic states can be recognised, raising the possibility of prophylactic therapy. Thus certain patients with extensive extracranial vascular disease show chronic states of vasodilatation, or indeed vasodilatation associated with modest but submaximal elevations of oxygen extraction. Such patients may be entirely asymptomatic but in physiological terms appear to constitute a group at considerably increased risk of ischaemia.

There are a number of unanswered questions which remain in the sphere of energy metabolism and ischaemia. I have already referred to the question of reversibility dependent on depth and possibly duration of ischaemia. There is little information on thresholds of irreversible ischaemia at present (Lenzi et al. 1982). In intensive-care terms, certain surgical procedures such as the establishment of cardiopulmonary bypass have been totally unexplored in physiological terms. It would be of great interest to know what happens to the cerebral circulation, oxygen extraction and consumption supervening on general anaesthesia and establishment of bypass.

Haemodynamics

The haemodynamic status of the brain can also be effectively measured regionally with PET. CBF and CBV are each independently measured using the tracers $C^{15}O_2$ and ^{11}CO (or $C^{15}O$). Normally CBF is maintained constant, despite changes in systemic blood pressure over a wide range, from a mean of around 60 mmHg to an upper mean of around 150 mmHg. This maintenance of CBF in the face of falls in systemic and therefore perfusion pressure is accomplished by a progressive decline in peripheral resistance as perfusion pressure falls. This is achieved by cerebral arteriolar vasodilatation, the main resistive component to blood flow residing in this part of the circulation. However it has been demonstrated that changes in venular calibre mirror those of the arterioles and further it is possible that capillary recruitment occurs which also effectively diminishes peripheral resistance. At the upper limit of autoregulation, it appears that the cerebral

vessels are maximally vasoconstricted. As the blood pressure rises further the flow now varies with pressure. Conversely, at the lower limit of autoregulation, the cerebral vessels are maximally vasodilated and minimal peripheral resistance is achieved. As blood pressure falls below this lower limit the blood flow also falls. It is clear that the relationship between blood flow and blood volume appears to decline progressively with declining perfusion pressure across the whole range of autoregulation but also above and below the upper and lower limits. In this way the CBF/CBV relationship can be regarded as an index of local perfusion pressure. Gibbs et al. (1984) have shown that this holds true in terms of extracranial occlusive vascular disease. Thus normal subjects with patent carotid arteries exhibit CBF/CBV ratios over 10 min⁻¹. Patients with unilateral occlusions exhibit ratios below $10 \, \text{min}^{-1}$ but above $6 \, \text{min}^{-1}$. Patients with bilateral occlusions show the lowest CBF/CBV ratios. The relationship between this ratio, which is an index of perfusion pressure, and oxygen extraction indicates that there appears to be a threshold below which oxygen extraction begins to rise. This is firm evidence that the two homeostatic reserves that maintain cerebral metabolism act in series. Initially a haemodynamic reserve quantifiable in terms of the CBF/CBV ratio operates. If it becomes exhausted a call on the oxygen carriage reserve follows. In this way, the haemodynamic status of the tissue can be assessed regionally and at microvascular level.

Chronic disturbances of haemodynamics have been observed in patients with extracranial occlusive disease. Such patients may present with transient ischaemic events and be found to have occlusions on angiography. They have been shown, on occasion, to exhibit a marked asymmetry of CBV and a considerable decrease in CBF/CBV ratio on the side of the occlusion. Some such patients have been restudied following revascularisation surgery when the CBF/CBV ratio has inevitably risen (Gibbs et al. 1985). Blood flow sometimes also rises, but in addition changes have been observed in the CBF/CBV ratio of the contralateral hemisphere.

This latter finding is not as surprising as it initially seems. The two carotid circulations are usually joined by a patent circle of Willis and thus in response to occlusion of one internal carotid artery, blood will flow into the ipsilateral hemisphere via collaterals, some of which will be coming from the contralateral carotid circulation via the circle of Willis. This will in turn result in a fall in perfusion pressure to the contralateral hemisphere and slight compensatory vasodilatation. The improvement of perfusion pressure by operation will now result in a re-establishment of flow on the ipsilateral side and also an amelioration of the compensating mechanisms which have affected the contralateral side. Our work with extracranial–intracranial bypass patients has consistently shown improvement of CBF/CBV ratio on the bypass side but no consistent improvement in blood flow.

In terms of intensive care medicine, a large number of unanswered questions remain. For example, it is unclear at present whether patients with extracranial vascular occlusive disease need prophylactic carotid surgery prior to going on to cardiopulmonary bypass for coronary artery bypass grafting operations. Opinion is divided. One of the factors contributing to this is the fact that no reliable method of measuring regional haemodynamics has been available to date. A second question relates to patients who have a decreased CBF/CBV ratio and the natural history of their haemodynamic insufficiency. Follow-up studies are required to see whether spontaneous changes are observed. Equally patients with elevated extractions of oxygen need to be followed to see what the variation in this factor is in those who have a chronically elevated but subischaemic level.

There are many other problems in intensive care medicine, for example traumatic head injury, which have not been addressed to date with these powerful new techniques. The main reason for this deficiency is the siting of the positron cameras and their attendant cyclotrons. Severely-ill patients can be moved with difficulty to investigative facilities sited at some distance from intensive care wards. The scope for investigation however is very large. It would seem reasonable to suggest that the siting of a positron camera in an intensive care environment would result in considerable elucidation of many of the pressing questions regarding energy metabolism and haemodynamics in the intensive care situation in medicine today. It should be added that other organs such as the lungs and heart are equally susceptible to sudden and major fluctuations of function in patients who are severely ill (Phelps et al. 1986). The function of these organs can be studied according to the general principle outlined above. This also remains a field of study unexplored as yet by PET.

Other Physiological Parameters

The variety of physiological functions amenable to study is constantly increasing. Methods have recently been described for the measurement of regional cerebral pH by using ^{11}C-DMO and ^{11}CO$_2$

(Brooks et al. 1984b; Syrota et al. 1983). Likewise, the breakdown of the blood–brain barrier to various sized molecules has been examined in a number of pathologies. ^{82}Rubidium is a short-lived isotope of rubidium which behaves biologically very much like potassium and has been used as an analogue for this important biological cation (Brooks et al. 1984a). Rubidium, like potassium, normally does not cross the blood–brain barrier. Maximal, steady-state extraction is around 2%. In certain pathological conditions, for example in gliomas, extraction can rise as high as 20%. This indicates a profound breakdown of the blood–brain barrier. Barrier function can also be tested to small protein molecules, by the use of carbon-11 labelled albumen. The breakdown of blood–brain barrier function may be of considerable importance with respect to drug delivery.

Dr K. Leenders at the Hammersmith Laboratory has recently demonstrated competition for the transport of ^{18}F-dopa across the blood–brain barrier by large neutral branched-chain amino acids. These amino acids are usually transported into the brain by a specific carrier which is also utilised by dopa, the precursor of dopamine in the brain. The level of branched-chain neutral amino acids in the blood radically alters the transport of the fluorinated dopa. This is of considerable importance as Parkinsonian patients are frequently asked to take their tablets with food. If the protein content of the food is high then one could well imagine inadequate amounts of dopa crossing the blood–brain barrier, with an attenuation of the clinical effectiveness of the drug.

Neurochemistry

The most recent advances in positron based techniques relate to precursor tracers and neurotransmitter receptor ligands, both labelled with positron emitters. The aim of this work has been to assess pre- and postsynaptic function in neurotransmitter pathways. The dopaminergic system has been the main focus of attention. 18F-DOPA has been used to trace dopamine in vesicles in the presynaptic nerve terminals (Garnett et al. 1983). A highly specific signal is obtained which appears to relate to the storage and uptake capacity of the presynaptic striatal nerve endings and correlates with the severity of Parkinson's disease (Leenders et al. 1986). A number of postsynaptic dopaminergic (D2) receptor ligands have also now been described including ^{11}C-methyl spiperone and ^{11}C-raclopride

(Leenders et al. 1984). Recent studies performed by Farde and his colleagues at the Karolinska Institute in Stockholm have demonstrated that the receptors can be characterised in terms of their density and affinity (Farde et al. 1986). Such measurements in man in vivo are of considerable interest. They provide the perspective of looking at neuro-specific functions in an in vivo context. More recently, opiate receptor ligands namely ^{11}C-carfentanil and ^{11}C-diprenorphine have been used to demonstrate specific uptake into regions of the brain known to contain high concentrations of such receptors (Frost et al. 1985; Jones et al. 1985). This specific uptake can be blocked by pretreatment with opiate receptor antagonists if these are given in saturating doses. These studies suggest that in the future PET may be used to measure receptor occupancy by endogenous neurotransmitters. Likewise, drug potency may be assessable in vivo by displacement or competition experiments with reference positron-labelled ligands. The use of appropriate positron-labelled substrate analogues also raises the perspective of localisation and measurement of the function of enzyme systems intrinsic to the brain. It need only be remembered that FDG is such an analogue measuring the activity of hexokinase. Under certain circumstances positron-labelled substrates of other enzymes could be used in analogous fashion to measure enzymatic activity.

Conclusion

The principal question relevant to this volume must be what relevance does PET have to intensive care medicine? There is at present no definitive answer to this question simply because the siting of positron cameras and facilities thus far have not permitted a systematic investigation of the pathophysiology of patients in intensive care. I hope that in describing the principles, with reference to some examples, of making measurements of tissue physiology, biochemistry or pharmacology with PET, I have made a case for the eventual siting of such a facility in an intensive care environment. There appears to be a large scope for study, not only in the brain but also in organs such as the lung, the heart and the liver. The various changes in regional perfusion, ventilation and metabolism of the human lung under conditions of respiratory failure could thus be addressed. I think it is clear that in the present state of development of tracer techniques, PET is destined to remain a research tool for the foreseeable short-term or even medium-term future.

The reason for this is that the development of a tracer technique is an undertaking of considerable difficulty requiring a number of steps including identification of suitable ligands, the development of methods for the rapid synthesis of positron-labelled species, the description of their distribution and metabolism in the body fluids and organs of interest. Mathematical models must then be described which will allow for the derivation of the function of interest from serial measurement of blood and tissue radioactivity. Finally, validation experiments, possibly in animal models, are also required. These various stages require a multidisciplinary scientific expertise which is not negligible. In addition to this the hardware of a positron camera and cyclotron demands considerable maintenance and expertise in its use. The type of commitment in terms of human and financial resources is not likely to lend itself to the profuse proliferation of such facilities in the near future. The aim of research with positron tomography is the better understanding of the pathophysiology of disease. This should lead to amelioration of therapeutic strategies and an objective way of assessing their effectiveness. Clinical research with PET must be viewed in this wider context at present rather than in the context of obtaining information in individual patients for use in their management. This is not to say that the insights obtained with PET will not be of benefit to clinical medicine. Hopefully, techniques will eventually be developed to obtain information in an easier, perhaps more restricted, manner which will be cross-calibrated against PET measurements. As the technology of cyclotron design and positron camera performance advances, it is not inconceivable that in the longer term considerably cheaper machines may become more widespread in their use.

References

Brooks DJ, Beaney RP, Lammertsma AA, Leenders KL, Horlock PL, Kensett MJ, Marshall J, Thomas DGT, Jones T (1984a) Quantitative measurement of blood brain barrier permeability using rubidium 82 and positron emission tomography. J Cereb Blood Flow Metab 4: 535–545

Brooks DJ, Lammertsma AA, Beaney RP, Leenders KL, Buckingham PD, Marshall J, Jones T (1984b) Measurement of regional cerebral pH in human subjects using continuous inhalation of 11CO2 and positron emission tomography. J Cereb Blood Flow Metab 4: 458–465

Farde L, Hall H, Ehrin E, Sedvall G (1986) Quantitative analysis of D2 dopamine receptor binding in the living human brain by PET. Science 231: 258–261

Frackowiak RSJ (1985a) The pathophysiology of human cerebral ischaemia: a new perspective obtained with positron tomography. Q J Med 57: 713–727

Frackowiak RSJ (1985b) Pathophysiology of human cerebral ischaemia: studies with positron tomography and oxygen-15.

In: Sokoloff L (ed) Brain imaging and brain function. Proc Assocn Res Nerv Ment Dis Raven Press New York 63: 139–162

Frackowiak RSJ, Wise RJS (1983) Positron tomography in ischaemic cerebrovascular disease. Neurol Clinics 1: 183–201

Frackowiak RSJ, Lenzi GL, Jones T, Heather JD (1980) Quantitative measurement of regional cerebral blood flow and oxygen metabolism in man using 15O and positron emission tomography: theory, procedure and normal values. J Comput Assist Tomogr 4: 727–736

Frost JJ, Wagner HN, Dannals RF, Ravert HT, Links JM, Wilson AA, Burns HD, Wong DF, McPherson RW, Rosenbaum AE, Kuhar MJ, Snyder SH (1985) Imaging opiate receptors in the human brain by positron tomography. J. Comput Assist Tomogr 9: 231–236

Garnett ES, Firnau G, Nahmias C (1983) Dopamine visualised in the basal ganglia of living man. Nature 305: 137–138

Gibbs JM, Wise RJS, Mansfield AO, Ross Russell RW, Thomas DJ, Jones T (1985) Cerebral circulatory reserve before and after surgery for occlusive carotid disease. J Cereb Blood Flow Metab 5 suppl, S19–S20

Gibbs JM, Wise RJS, Leenders KL, Jones T (1984) Evaluation of cerebral perfusion reserve in patients with carotid artery occlusion. Lancet I, 310–314

Herscovitch P, Markham J, Raichle ME (1983) Brain blood flow measured with intravenous H2 15O 1. theory and error analysis. J Nucl Med 24: 782–789

Jones AKP, Luthra SK, Pike VW, Herold S, Brady F (1985) New labelled ligand for in vivo studies of opioid physiology. Lancet II 665–666

Lammertsma AA, Jones T (1983) The correction for the presence of intravascular oxygen-15 in the steady state technique for measuring regional oxygen extraction in the brain. 1: description of the method. J Cereb Blood Flow Metab 3: 416–424

Lammertsma AA, Jones T, Frackowiak RSJ, Lenzi GL, Pozzilli C (1981) A theoretical study of the steady state model for measuring regional cerebral blood flow and oxygen utilisation using oxygen-15. J Comput Assist Tomagr 5: 544–550

Lammertsma AA, Heather JD, Jones T, Frackowiak RSJ, Lenzi GL (1982) A statistical study of the steady state model for measuring regional cerebral blood flow and oxygen utilisation using oxygen-15. J Comput Assist Tomogr 6: 566–573

Lammertsma AA, Wise RJS, Heather JD, Gibbs JM, Leenders KL, Frackowiak RSJ, Rhodes CG, Jones T (1983) The correction for the presence of intravascular oxygen-15 in the steady state technique for measuring regional oxygen extraction ratio in the brain. 2: results in normal subjects, brain tumour and stroke patients J Cereb Blood Flow Metab 3: 425–431

Leenders KL, Herold S, Brooks DJ, Palmer AJ, Turton D, Firnau G, Garnett ES, Nahmias C, Veall N (1984) Presynaptic and postsynaptic dopaminergic system in human brain. Lancet: II: 110–111

Leenders KL, Palmer A, Turton D, Quinn N. Firnau G, Garnett S, Nahmias C. Jones T, Marsden CD (1986) DOPA uptake and dopamine receptor binding visualised in the human brain in vivo. In: Fahn S, Marsden CD, Jenner P, Teychenne P (ed.) Recent developments in Parkinsons disease. Raven Press New York, pp 103–113

Lenzi GL, Frackowiak RSJ, Jones T (1982) Cerebral oxygen metabolism and blood flow in human cerebral ischaemic infarction. J Cereb Blood Flow Metab 2: 321–335

Mintun MA, Raichle ME, Martin WRW, Herscovitch P (1984) Brain oxygen utilisation measured with O-15 radiotracers and positron emission tomography. J Nucl Med 25: 177–187

Phelps ME, Mazziotta JC, Schelbert H (1986) Positron Emission Tomography and autoradiography: principles and applications for the brain and heart. Raven Press, New York 690 pp.

Raichle ME, Martin WRW, Herscovitch P, Mintun MA, Markham J (1983) Brain blood flow measured with intravenous H2 15O II: implementation and validation. J Nucl Med 24: 790–798

Sokoloff L, Reivich M, Kennedy C, DesRosiers MH, Patlak CS, Pettigrew KD, Sakurada O, Shinohara M (1977) The (C-14)-deoxyglucose method for the measurement of local glucose utilisation: theory, procedure and normal values in the conscious, anaesthetised albino rat. J Neurochem 28: 897–916

Syrota A, Castaing M, Rougemont D, Berridge M, Baron JC, Bousser MG, Pocidalo JJ (1983) Tissue acid–base balance and oxygen metabolism in human cerebral infarction studied with positron emission tomography. Ann Neurol 14: 419–428

Wise RJS, Bernardi S, Frackowiak RSJ, Legg NJ, Jones T (1983a) Serial observations on the pathophysiology of acute stroke: the transition from ischaemia to infarction as reflected in the regional oxygen extraction. Brain 106: 197–222

Wise RJS, Rhodes CG, Gibbs JM, Hatazawa J, Frackowiak RSJ, Palmer AJ, Jones T (1983b) Disturbance of oxidative metabolism of glucose in recent human cerebral infarcts. Ann Neurol 14: 627–637

Chapter 4

Jugular Venous Bulb Oxygen Saturation and Cerebral Blood Flow Measurement in Intensive Care

R. Garlick

Introduction

The best method of monitoring cerebral deterioration remains clinical assessment (Jennett 1985). There is no physiological or laboratory test that can replace this important clinical skill (McDowall 1976). However, it is not an uncommon situation in intensive care to need to ventilate a patient because of poor pulmonary gas exchange e.g. in some cases of sepsis (Hanson 1978) or as a management option to prevent raised intracranial pressure e.g. severe head injury (Gordon 1971; Becker et al. 1977). Usually, the patient also receives sedative drugs and this makes it difficult to assess patient responsiveness on a coma scale such as the Glasgow Coma Scale. This scale describes the response of the patient to verbal command or painful stimulus in terms of eye opening, verbal and motor response (Teasdale and Jennett 1974). Certainly after severe head injury and, indeed, in any unconscious patient the monitoring that should be undertaken concerns the maintenance of adequate blood pressure. oxygen and blood glucose levels. Values outside the normal range of these physiological measurements can compromise cerebral function (Stoner, and Cremer 1985; Rose et al. 1977; Price and Murray 1972).

Severe cerebral deterioration resulting in brainstem failure causes abnormalities in the pulse rate, blood pressure and pupillary reflexes (Plum and Posner 1972). Irreversible damage is associated with these signs (Overgaard et al. 1973; Bates 1985). Monitoring aims to prevent this happening.

One important pathological mechanism of damage that we hope our monitoring will measure is the presence of ischaemia, which at first may be only on a regional basis. Ischaemic hypoxia is one mechanism of damage in severe head injury (Graham et al. 1978). Other mechanisms include engorgement of the brain with blood, common in children (Bruce et al. 1978) and the formation of oedema by increased permeability of blood vessels (vasogenic oedema) or cell swelling (cytotoxic oedema) (Klatzo and Seitelberger 1967).

Each of these pathological mechanisms can occur in one or more of three anatomical locations: the cerebral cortex, the supratentorial compartment or the brainstem. For example, a post-traumatic haematoma in the supratentorial compartment can enlarge to cause raised intracranial pressure or associated oedema can add to the space occupying effect. Anatomically, these events can be monitored by serial computed tomography (CT) scanning. From the picture obtained inferences can be made about physiological measurements such as raised intracranial pressure and these can indicate the need for further treatment. However, the scan displays no absolute quantitative measurement of the degree of function.

In order to measure the degree of function quantitatively physiological measurements are necessary. Intracranial pressure measurement, introduced over 25 years ago (Lundberg 1960) can be undertaken in most intensive care units. Portable machines have been developed to measure cerebral blood flow (Novocerebrograph, Novo Industries, Copenhagen). Another portable machine can be used to monitor the overall electrical activity of the brain (Cerebral Function Monitor; Maynard et al. 1969). When normal and abnormal values have been established within the setting of the pathophysiology involved, action can be taken to reverse a deteriorating situation. It may also be possible to predict prognosis more accurately. One measurement that has not yet found widespread use is the arteriovenous difference for oxygen across the brain ($AVDO_2$) or the jugular venous bulb oxygen saturation ($JVO_2Sat.$) used in the derivation of the former value.

The information that can be gained from the $AVDO_2$ and $JVO_2Sat.$ will be examined in the context of two groups of sedated and ventilated patients. The first were those who had suffered a severe head injury and the second group contained patients with a septic illness.

A physiological measurement gains much if it can be measured continuously. A fibreoptic catheter (Opticath, Oximetrix, Mountain View CA) has been used to monitor the $JVO_2Sat.$ This value fluctuates rapidly simultaneously with changes in the mean arterial pressure (mABP) and intracranial pressure waves. My conclusions have led me to believe that, in the group of patients studied, knowledge of changes in $JVO_2Sat.$ within an individual patient can provide an indication of global cerebral blood flow (CBF). However, the absolute value of $JVO_2Sat.$ is not only a function of CBF. The metabolic activity of the brain together with arterial oxygen content is also important. Continuous techniques of measuring $JVO_2Sat.$ are shown to be of use in discovering the effects of drugs on cerebral physiology or elucidating pathophysiological mechanisms such as intracranial pressure waves. Examples are described.

Methods

The group of patients for whom results are described were sedated and ventilated as part of the management of severe head injury (most with Glasgow Coma Score < 6 on admission) or severe sepsis (core temperature $> 38.5°C$, white cell count $> 12 \times 10^9 l^{-1}$ and a documented episode of hypotension systolic BP < 90 mmHg) in the 48 h preceding admission to the intensive therapy unit. Sedation was with a phenoperidone infusion (1–4 mg h^{-1}) and pancuronium (2–5 mgh^{-1} was the muscle relaxant used. In individual patients antibiotics and anticonvulsants were prescribed when indicated. The head-injured group were hyperventilated to a mean p_aCO_2 of 31 mmHg. Only patients who had been resuscitated with a mean arterial pressure of 93 mmHg for the group as a whole were studied.

Various measurements were made. The cerebral metabolic rate for oxygen ($CMRO_2$) is an index of cerebral metabolism based on the product of the CBF and the $AVDO_2$. Simultaneous measurements were made of CBF, arterial oxygen content (art.O_2) and jugular venous bulb oxygen content ($JVBO_2$).

CBF was measured with a Novocerebrograph 10a (see Fig. 4.1) and collimators were placed over each somatosensory cortex to detect the clearance of ^{133}Xe injected intravenously. Bicompartmental analysis of the value was carried out (Obrist et al. 1975) using the Risberg version to compute CBF (Risberg et al. 1975).

Samples of blood to measure arterial oxygen content were withdrawn from an indwelling radial artery catheter. Haemoglobin, oxygen saturation (Radiometer OSM 2 oximeter) and pO_2 (Corning 170 blood gas analyser) were estimated. Blood from the jugular venous bulb was sampled by introducing

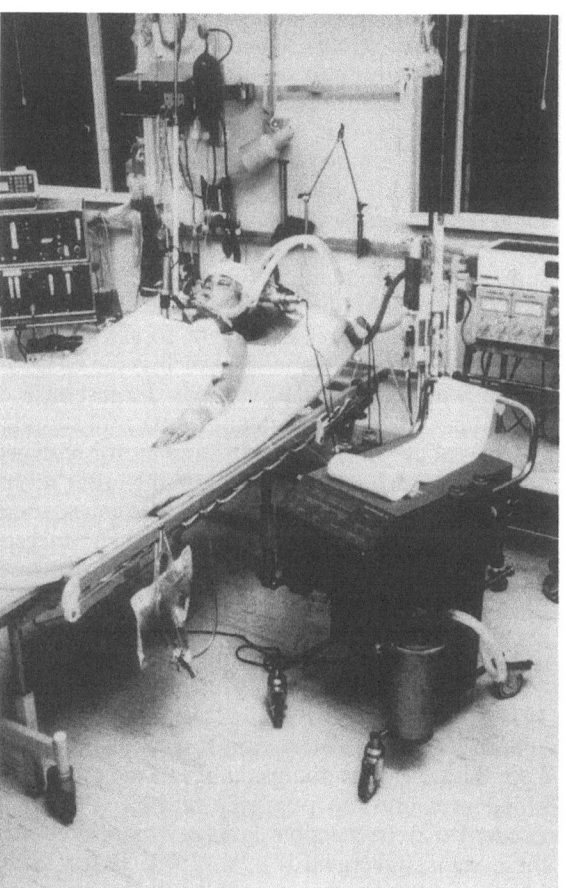

Fig. 4.1. Novocerebrograph 10a by the bed side.

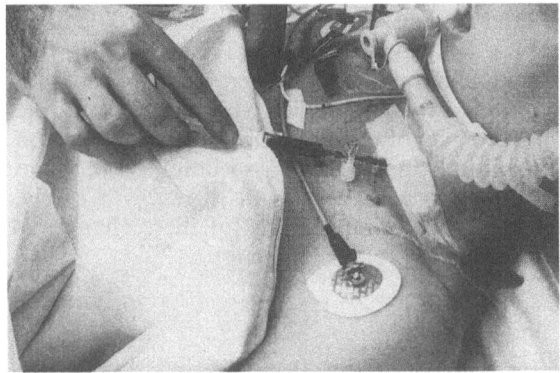

Fig. 4.2. Sampling blood from the jugular venous bulb.

a 16 G catheter retrogradely up the internal jugular vein (Fig. 4.2) after first measuring the length of catheter needed to reach the bulb by placing it up against the skin of the neck.

Continuous measurements were made using a fibreoptic catheter (Fig. 4.3). This catheter is of small size (4 FrG) and is placed in the jugular venous bulb by introducing it through a larger 14 G catheter placed in the internal jugular vein. A sampling channel enables in vivo calibration but the catheter is standardised against its own reference before insertion.

An optical fibre transmits three wavelengths of red and near infrared light to the catheter tip each at 244 pulses s^{-1}. Here the light is reflected, refracted and absorbed by blood flowing past the catheter tip. Some of the light is collected by a second optical fibre where it is transmitted to a photodetector. The colour of the blood and hence the amount of oxygen it contains will alter the intensity of light that returns. After conversion of these transmissions to an electrical signal, the average oxygen saturation for the preceding 5 s is displayed on a digital readout and strip chart recorder. This value is updated every second. Audible and visible alarms indicate when

the intensity of light received is very low and invalid results may appear. This can happen when the catheter tip lies up against the vein wall. Repositioning of the head or correction of a low venous pressure can cure the problem.

In 6 patients intracranial pressure was measured with an intraventricular fluid-filled manometric catheter and transduction of the fluid pulse (Meadox pressure transducers) to an electrical signal. Cardiac output was measured with a flow-directed pulmonary – artery catheter and the thermodilution method. The average of three measurements was taken. Mixed venous blood could be sampled from this catheter. Jugular venous pressure was measured from the jugular venous bulb (Meadox pressure transducers). Mean arterial pressure (mABP) was measured from an indwelling radial artery catheter with electronic derivation of the mean (Hewlett Packard 78353B). All signals were displayed on a Gould 4 channel chart recorder, chart speed 5 mm min^{-1}. The following formulae were used:

Art. O_2 content = Hb × 1.34 × % sat. + $p0_2$ × 0.003

Whole body oxygen extraction ratio (OER) = Whole body $AVDO_2$/Art. O_2 content

Cerebral OER = Cerebral $AVDO_2$/Art. O_2 content

Oxygen uptake index = cardiac index × body $AVDO_2$

Measurements of CBF and $AVDO_2$ were made before and after an increase in a dopamine infusion (mean 8 $\mu g\,kg^{-1}\,min^{-1}$ increase) which caused a mean increase in mABP of 32 mmHg. Results are described as means with standard deviations. Student's t-test was used to test significance.

Results

Arterial oxygen saturation varied within only narrow limits and was high on serial testing. There was a wide variation in JVO_2Sat. however with a significantly lower JVO_2Sat. in the septic group of patients. Similarly, the $AVDO_2$ was wider in the septic group compared with the head injured (Table 4.1). However, there was no significant difference in cerebral blood flow, which was within the normal range for the group of patients of the age group studied (Table 4.2). An increase of 1 °C in the mean temperature of the septic group was reflected in a significantly greater body OER in the septic group

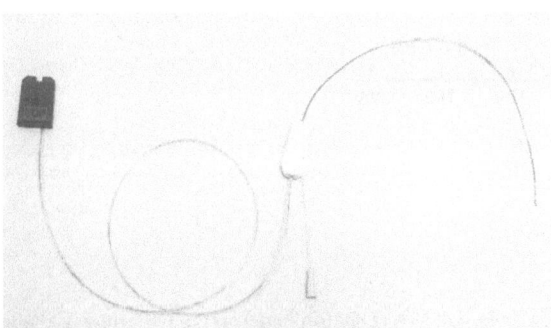

Fig. 4.3. A fibreoptic "Opticath" catheter.

Table 4.1. Art.O_2 saturation and JVO_2Sat.

	Head Injured Cases $n = 10$	Septic Cases $n = 7$
art.O_2Sat. (%)	97.2 ± 2.2 (94–100)	96 ± 4.1 (82–100)
JVO_2Sat. (%)[a]	67.1 ± 10.7 (48–93)	60.9 ± 7.6 (40–70)
$AVDO_2$ (ml dl^{-1})[b]	4.5 (0.94–7.74)	5.4 (2.85–8.52)

[a] $p < 0.02$
[b] $p < 0.05$

Table 4.2. CBF and art.p_aCO_2.

	Head Injured Cases $n = 10$	Septic Cases $n = 7$
CBF (ml 100g^{-1}min^{-1})	73.5 ± 29 (22–133)	71.6 ± 29 (21–147)
art.p_aCO_2 (mmHg)	31 (27–38)	36 (26–56)

Table 4.3. Brain OER and whole body OER.

	Head Injured Cases $n = 5$	Septic Cases $n = 5$
Brain OER (%)[a]	31.2 ± 10.6 (8–50)	40 ± 8.4 (25–58)
Body OER (%)[b]	19.2 ± 4.5 (12–25)	28.4 ± 5.2 (18–41)

[a] $p < 0.001$
[b] $p < 0.001$

compared with the head-injured group (Table 4.3). Increases in the dopamine infusion brought about an increase in cerebral blood flow in some patients and the concomitant changes in $AVDO_2$ are shown in Fig. 4.4.

The traces from continuous measurement of JVO_2Sat., mABP, intracranial pressure (ICP) and jugular venous pressure are shown in a conscious patient who had sustained gunshot pellet wounds to the left temporal lobe (Fig. 4.6). The trace from

the same patient, but on this occasion sedated and ventilated, is shown in Fig. 4.7. The effect of starting dopamine in a patient who had an acute subdural haematoma with no midline shift is shown in Fig. 4.8. The effect of changing this dopamine infusion is shown in Fig. 4.9. The association of waves in the JVO_2Sat. trace with ICP 'B' waves is shown in Fig. 4.7. The implications of these changes is discussed in the following section.

Discussion

Oxygen flux across the brain is a good index of cerebral metabolism as oxygen diffuses rapidly between brain and blood to achieve equilibrium and there are negligible brain stores. If cerebral oxygen uptake and arterial oxygen content remain stable, the amount of oxygen in the jugular venous bulb can be an indicator of cerebral blood flow as indicated by a rearrangement of the Fick equation shown below:

$$JVBO_2 = Art.O_2 - O_2uptake/CBF$$

Loss of CBF autoregulation to changes in mABP can be seen in Fig. 4.4. Changes in $AVDO_2$ correspond to changes in CBF brought about by an increase in a dopamine infusion. Over short periods of time, when cerebral metabolism is assumed to be constant, changes in $AVDO_2$ have been used as a guide to CBF changes in normal subjects (Severinghaus and Lassen 1967), in patients undergoing carotid endarterectomy (Ellis et al. 1986) and for

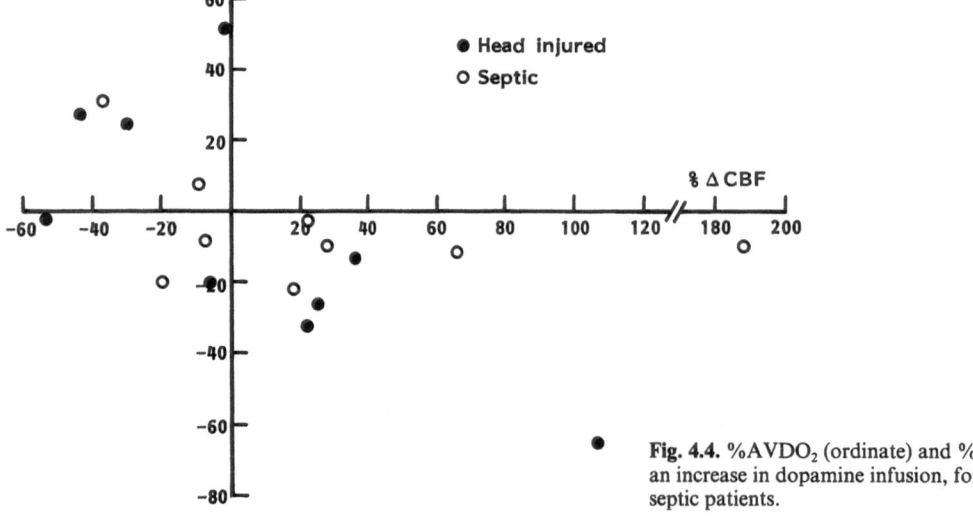

Fig. 4.4. %$AVDO_2$ (ordinate) and % CBF (abscissa) after an increase in dopamine infusion, for head-injured and septic patients.

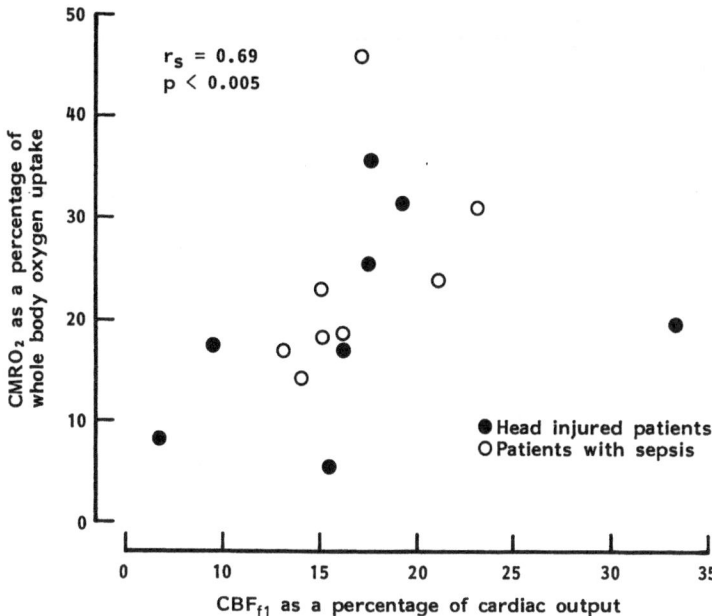

Fig. 4.5. CBF as percentage of cardiac output (abscissa) plotted against CMRO₂ as percentage of oxygen uptake index for head-injured and septic patients.

the serial monitoring of head injuries (Obrist et al. 1983; Cruz and Miner 1986).

However, a wide AVDO₂ need not necessarily be associated with a low CBF. If body OER is high, as in our septic patients, brain OER is similarly high (Table 4.3), yet CBF was within the normal range. A useful way to examine whether the brain is acting in some way "independently" of the body is to look at the CMRO₂ as a percentage of the oxygen uptake index (normally 18%) in relation to the CBF expessed as a percentage of the cardiac

output (normally 15%). Fig. 4.5 shows that there appears to be a close relationship between the two. However, there are two head-injured patients where CBF is in excess of metabolism, a state of hyperaemia described by others (Obrist et al. 1983; Lassen 1966). Normally, regional perfusion of the brain is tightly coupled to the metabolic requirements (Ingvar and Risberg 1967). However, in ischaemic regions the pathological condition of hyperoxygenation can be seen and sometimes red blood will be drawn from the jugular venous bulb.

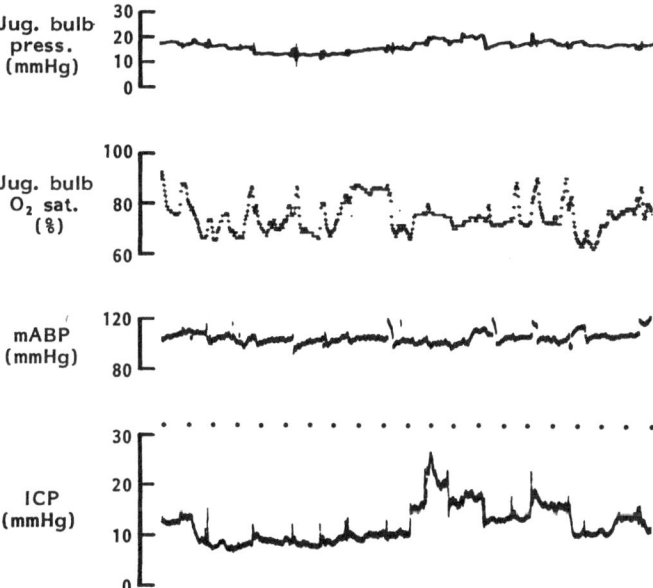

Fig. 4.6. Variations in JVO₂Sat., ICP, mABP and jugular venous pressure in a conscious patient.

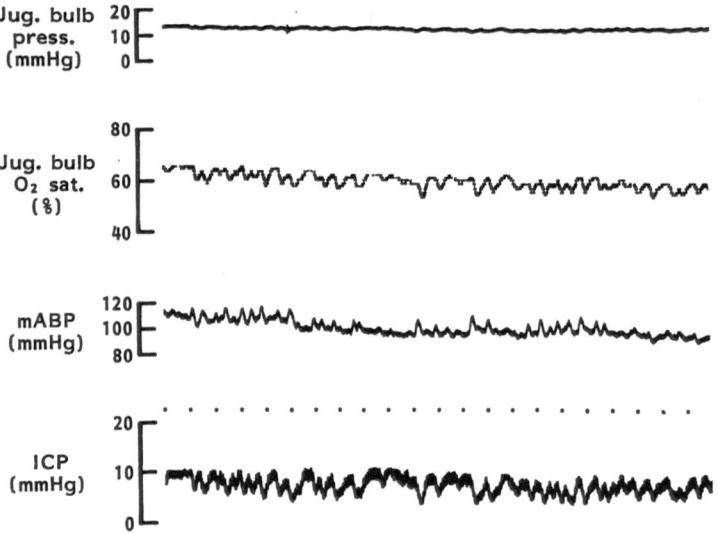

Fig. 4.7. Variations in JVO$_2$Sat., ICP, mABP and jugular venous pressure for the same patient as in Fig. 4.6, sedated and ventilated.

Cerebral ischaemia may exist without a low JVO$_2$Sat. or a wide AVDO$_2$ (Waltz et al, 1972) and JVO$_2$Sat. does not provide a reliable warning of focal ischaemia or inadequate cerebral oxygenation (Larson et al. 1967; Jawad et al. 1976). To be abnormal, the JVO$_2$Sat. has to lie outside the limits of normal cerebral oxygen extraction, which has been shown by positron emission tomography to lie between 30%–40% (Frackowiak et al. 1980). Although some patients are confused or stuporose at a JVO$_2$Sat. of 57%, others exhibit no signs of cerebral ischaemia at a JVO$_2$Sat, of 49% (Meyer et al. 1966).

One reason for this is the regional differences in blood flow in the various areas of brain that contribute to the blood in the jugular venous bulb, where mixing averages out the differences. Poorly perfused areas contribute little and are underrepresented. When there is an increased intercapillary distance, for example in cerebral oedema, oxygen can diffuse from the arterial end of one capillary to the venous end of the adjacent capillary – a diffusion shunt.

Changes in the hydrogen ion concentration of blood in the venous bulb can also cause changes in the observed saturation of the blood by a shift of

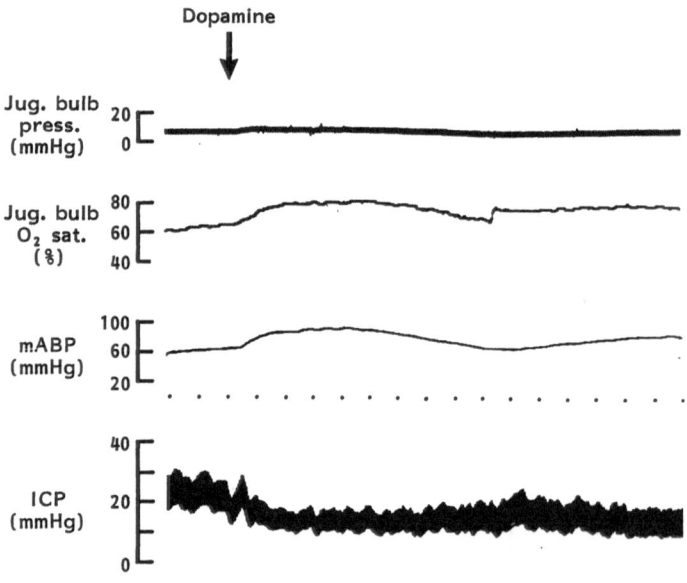

Fig. 4.8. The effect of starting a dopamine infusion.

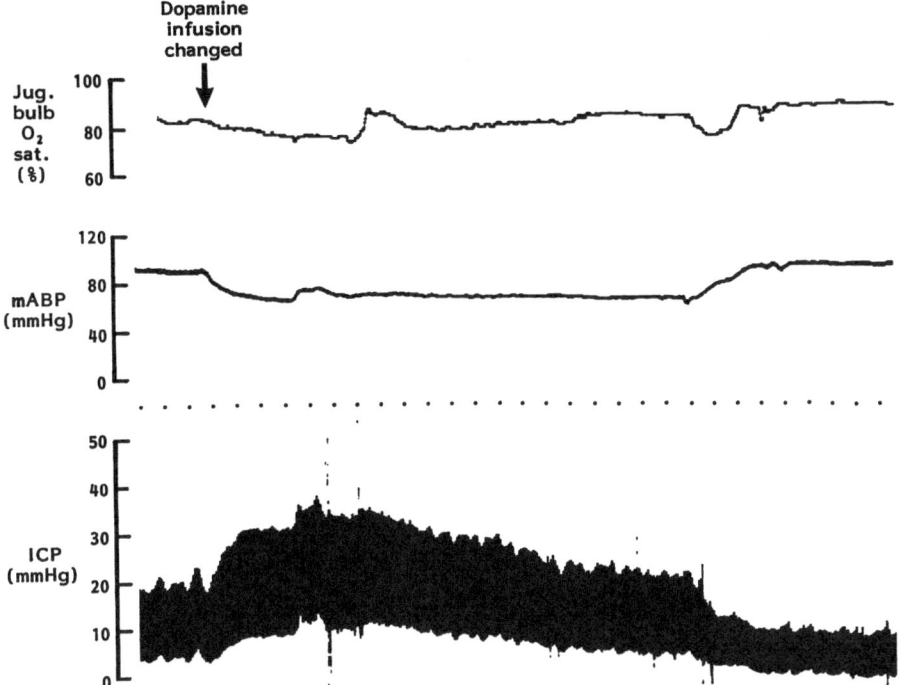

Fig. 4.9. The rapid changes seen when an empty dopamine syringe pump is exchanged for a full one.

the oxyhaemoglobin dissociation curve. However, in our patients, despite jugular venous blood being consistently more acid than arterial blood, there was a mean difference of only 0.05pH units and the mean jugular venous blood pH was 7.41.

Within individual patients the traces of results obtained with continuous monitoring of JVO_2Sat. implicate CBF changes as the cause of the rapid variations in JVO_2Sat. seen on some occasions. Present-day techniques of measuring CBF do not have the response time to appreciate these changes which occur at intervals as short as a second. In the conscious individual, the variations in JVO_2Sat. can be quite marked (Fig. 4.6) and any calculations based on this value can be different depending on when the sample was taken. Studies of patients with severe head injuries have found $CMRO_2$ to correlate poorly with time after injury or outcome (Cold 1978). One reason for this could be the observed large variation in JVO_2Sat. and the effect this would have on derived calculated values. With sedated patients the variations are much less marked (Fig. 4.7). The absolute value of JVO_2Sat. is an unreliable guide to ischaemia but the observation of a reduction in JVO_2Sat. may indicate a falling CBF. It is at this point that a formal CBF measurement using isotope clearance methods could give quantitative and regional data.

The response to therapy is continuously variable and is best measured by continuous means. The mechanism of drug action can also be demonstrated. Fig. 4.8 shows the increase in JVO_2Sat. obtained after the administration of dopamine. The increase in JVO_2Sat. mirrors the increase in mABP. This can be explained on the basis of loss of pressure autoregulation of CBF. The increase in mABP causes an increase in CBF which in turn is seen as an increase in the JVO_2Sat. The JVO_2Sat. and mABP changes are almost perfectly matched. If dopamine were to cause an increase in the metabolic activity of the brain a drop in the JVO_2Sat. value would be expected as oxygen demand was increased. If there were a mixed effect of increasing flow and increasing metabolic activity the increase in JVO_2Sat. would not have the same gradient as the rise in mABP.

Figure 4.7 shows the presence of intracranial pressure "B" waves. They are seen in association with waves in the mABP and JVO_2Sat. traces. No waves are seen in the jugular venous pressure trace where distension of the vein wall dampens the pulse. The waves are all of corresponding frequency, approx. 2 min^{-1}. One explanation of the waves is that variations in mABP with pressor centre instability are the basis of waves seen in the ICP and JVO_2Sat. traces. In a damaged brain which has lost the ability to autoregulate CBF to changes in mABP, changes in mABP will result in an increase or decrease of CBF. This in turn brings about changes in cerebral blood volume which, in a brain less compliant than usual, will register as an ICP wave in this case of frequency 2 min^{-1} – the type known as a "B" wave. We have assumed that when the patient is sedated, the oxygen requirements remain stable.

Summary

The JVO$_2$Sat. is thus a useful measurement in monitoring sedated unconscious patients in the intensive care unit. In a patient with a stable adequate arterial oxygen content it can reflect general body metabolism, together with global CBF.

A falling JVO$_2$Sat. may be secondary to a generalised reduction in CBF or to an increase in whole-body metabolism. This latter change will also be reflected in a reduced mixed venous blood oxyhaemoglobin saturation. If this value has remained constant and JVO$_2$Sat. falls it is useful to measure CBF by a quantitative means such as isotope clearance with multiple detectors to demonstrate regional flow. However, cerebral ischaemia can exist without there being a low JVO$_2$Sat. Indeed, one of the signs after an ischaemic event to the whole brain is red blood in the jugular venous bulb associated with a high JVO$_2$Sat. Continuous measurements can reflect the action of drugs and provide clues to the mechanism of such pathophysiological features as ICP waves.

Acknowledgement. RG was supported by a grant from the Sir Jules Thorn Charitable Trust.

References

Bates D (1985) Predicting recovery from medical coma. Br J Hosp Med 33: 276–280

Becker DP, Miller JD, Ward JD et al. (1977) The outcome from severe head injury with early diagnosis and intensive management. J Neurosurg 47: 491–502

Bruce DA, Schut L, Bruno LA et al. (1978) Outcome following severe head injury in children. J. Neurosurg 48: 679–688

Cold G (1978) Cerebral metabolic rate of oxygen (CMRO$_2$) in the acute phase of head injury. Acta anaeth Scand 22: 249–256

Cruz J, Miner ME (1986) Modulating cerebral oxygen delivery and extraction in head injury patients. Miner ME, Wagner KA (Eds) Neural Trauma Vol. 1. Butterworth, Mass pp 55–73

Ellis R, Muizelaar M, Franks P et al. (1986) The influence of the cerebral metabolic rate on the correlation between jugular venous oxygen saturation and cerebral blood flow during carotid endarterectomy. Anesthesiology 65: 3A

Frackowiak RSJ, Lenzi G-L, Jones T et al. (1980) Quantitative measurement of regional cerebral blood flow in man using ^{15}O and positron emission tomography: theory, procedure and normal values. J Comput Assist Tomogr 4: 727–736

Gordon E (1971) Controlled ventilation in the management of patients with traumatic brain injuries. Acta Anaesthesiol Scand 15: 193–208

Graham DI, Adams JH, Doyle D (1978) Ischaemic brain damage in fatal non-missile head injuries. J Neurol Sci 39: 213–234

Hanson G (1978) Shock and Infection. In: Hanson G, Wright PL (eds) The Medical Management of the Critically Ill. Academic Press, London, pp 367–373

Ingvar DH, Risberg J (1967) Increase of regional cerebral blood flow during mental effort in normals and patients with focal brain disorders. Exp Brain Res 3: 195–211

Jawad K, Miller JD, Fitch W, et al. (1976) Measurement of jugular venous blood gases for prediction of brain ischaemia following carotid ligation. Eur Neurol 14: 43–52

Jennett B (1985) Altered Consciousness and Coma. In: Crockard A, Hayward R, Hoff JT (eds) Neurosurgery. The Scientific Basis of Clinical Practice. Blackwell Scientific Publications, Oxford, UK pp 117–126

Klatzo I, Seitelberger F (1967) Brain Oedema Springer Verlag, New York

Larson CP, Ehrenfield W, Wade J, et al. (1967). Jugular venous oxygen saturation as an.index of the adequacy of cerebral oxygenation. Surgery 62: 31–39

Lassen NA (1966) The luxury perfusion syndrome and its possible relation to acute metabolic acidosis localized within the brain. Lancet ii: 1112–1115

Lundberg N (1960) Continuous recording and control of ventricular fluid pressure in neurosurgical practice Acta Psychiatr Scand [Suppl] 149: 1–193

Maynard DE, Prior PF, Scott DF (1969) Device for continuous monitoring of cerebral activity in resuscitated patients Br Med J 4: 545

McDowall DG (1976) Monitoring the brain. Anesthesiology 45: 117–134

Meyer JS, Gotoh F, Ebihara S (1966) Influence of cerebrovascular disease and state of consciousness on cerebral metabolism. J Am Geriatr Soc 14: 205–220

Obrist WD, Cruz J, Jaggi JL et al (1983) Cerebral blood flow and intracranial pressure in acute head injury. J Cereb Blood Flow Metab 3 [Suppl 1]: 567–68

Obrist WD, Thompson HK Jr, Wang HS et al. (1975) Regional cerebral blood flow estimated by ^{133}Xe inhalation. Stroke 6: 245–256

Overgaard J, Christensen S, Jansen O et al. (1973) Prognosis after head injury based on early clinical examination. Lancet II: 631–635

Plum F, Posner J (1972) The diagnosis of Stupor and Coma 2nd edn. FA Davis, Philadelphia pp 1–59

Price DJE, Murray A (1972) The influence of hypoxia and hypotension on recovery from head injury. Injury 3: 218–224

Risberg J, Ali Z, Wilson EM et al. (1975) Regional cerebral blood flow by ^{133}Xe inhalation. Stroke 6: 142–148

Rose J, Valtonen S, Jennett B (1977) Avoidable factors contributing to death after head injury. Br Med J 2: 615–618

Severinghaus JW, Lassen N (1967) Step hypocapnia to separate arterial from tissue pCO$_2$ in the regulation of cerebral blood flow. Circ Res 20: 272–278

Stoner HB. Cremer JE (1985) Maintenance of metabolic integrity in the brain after trauma. Br Med Bull 41: 246–250

Teasdale G, Jennett B (1974) Assessment of coma and impaired consciousness. A practical scale. Lancet ii: 81–84

Waltz AG, Sundt TB, Michenfelder JD (1971) Cerebral blood flow, jugular venous pO$_2$ and lactate concentrations and arterial venous oxygen content during carotid endarterectomy. Eur Neurol 6: 346–349

Section II

Imaging the Lungs

Chapter 5

The Interpretation of the Portable Chest Film and the Role of Complementary Imaging Techniques

W. Kox, J. Boultbee and K. Hillman

Imaging the chest in critically ill patients is often limited by their clinical state and the environment of the intensive care ward. Simple and repeatable techniques such as plain chest radiography and ultrasonography do not require the patient mobilisation that is necessary in computed tomography (CT) scanning, cardiopulmonary angiography and ventilation perfusion scanning.

The antero-posterior (A–P) chest film made with portable X-ray equipment is one of the most useful tools in critical care medicine. It is a mandatory supplement to the examination of the respiratory system and should be performed daily as a routine on the most seriously ill patients. During examination of the daily chest film the progression of the underlying disease is monitored, the position of lines and endotracheal tubes checked, and iatrogenically induced changes such as barotrauma are looked for. A chest film should also be performed after intrathoracic line placement or intubation, as well as in response to sudden changes in the patient's clinical state, such as fever, hypoxia and increased ventilatory pressures. Many unsuspected abnormalities not detected on clinical examination are seen on chest films and these often lead to major management changes (Strain et al. 1985). However, interpreting A–P chest films taken in less than ideal circumstances on seriously ill patients can be difficult.

Although it is tempting to accept the chest film with the patient supine, it is crucial to gain co-operation of the nursing and radiographic staff and ensure that films are taken in the erect or semi-erect position with a horizontal X-ray beam; failing this a lateral decubitus film with a horizontal beam is always possible, but technically more difficult. Air fluid levels which are only demonstrable with a horizontal X-ray beam may be defined where there is fluid immediately in contact with air such as lung abscess and haemopneumothorax.

Interpretation of the chest film is often limited without previous radiographs or imaging and the relevant pathological and clinical data. In an environment where patients are sedated or even paralysed whilst being ventilated, and therefore potentially uncooperative and immobile, it may be difficult to achieve a diagnosis by chest radiography alone. The main advantage of ultrasonography is the ability to detect and quantify phenomena which otherwise may not be diagnosed: pleural effusions accompanying pulmonary oedema and hypoalbuminaemia, loculated collections or fluid hidden behind the diaphragm (Fig. 5.1), and some cases of basal consolidation or collapse due to mechanical diaphragmatic problems.

Computed tomography (CT) is cross-sectional so that the anatomy is demonstrated without the superimposition of structures that occur on a chest radiograph. It is a sensitive technique based on the density of the patient's tissues to X-rays. Fine structures and small changes in density are easily detectable. These appearances are much better understood by doctors familiar with chest radiography. There may be considerable pressure on CT services, and transporting cardiovascularly or otherwise unstable patients to the scanner suite may be hazardous. An important use of CT scanning in the critically ill is in suspected trauma to the major thoracic vessels and in aortic aneurysm although it has also been used in the diagnosis and management

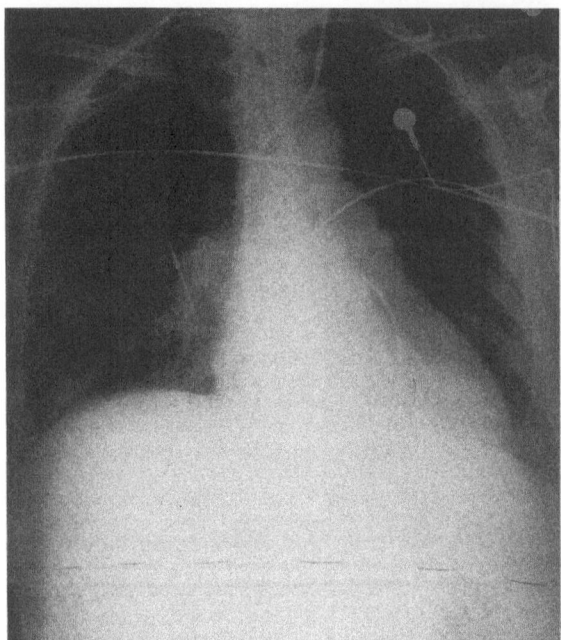

Fig. 5.1. Chest film pre-aspiration of pleural effusions seen on ultrasound, but not demonstrated radiologically. Right side yielded 350 ml aspirate, left side yielded 200 ml aspirate.

of adult respiratory distress syndrome (ARDS) (see Chapter 6) and in the diagnosis of lung abscess and pleural effusions.

Pleural Effusions

Pleural effusions may be difficult to detect on radiographs taken even with the patient sitting upright, because the fluid tends to lie posteriorly in the pleural space. Even in the absence of an effusion the costophrenic angles are often shallow and the diaphragm may appear flattened and elevated (Fig. 5.2). The differentiation of fluid may be diffi-

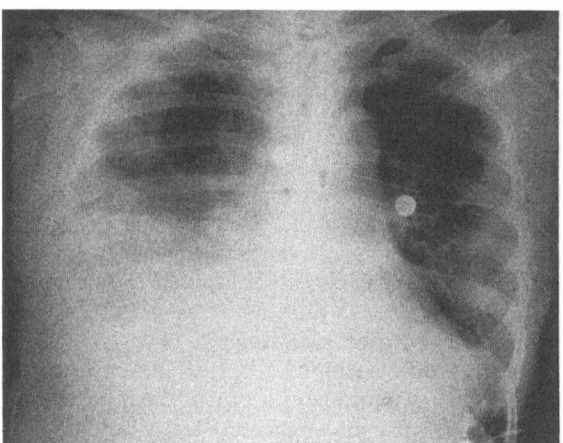

a

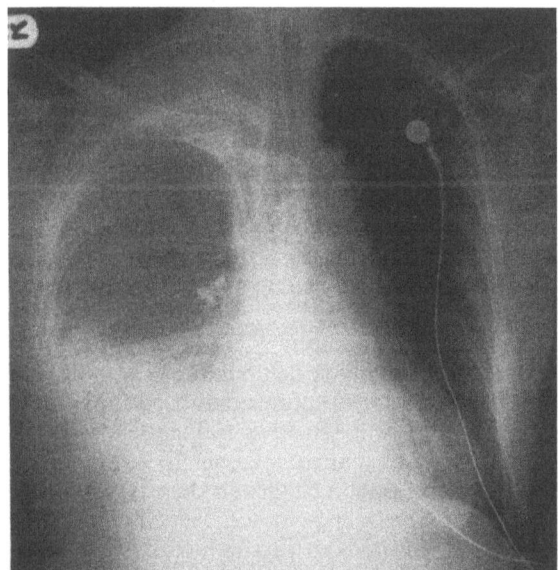

Fig. 5.2. A large pleural effusion from which 800 ml were aspirated. There is increased density throughout the right lung field; the lung markings in the right upper and mid-zones are still present, but there is loss of the right hemidiaphragm with increased shadowing at the right base which is due to some consolidation as well as pleural fluid.

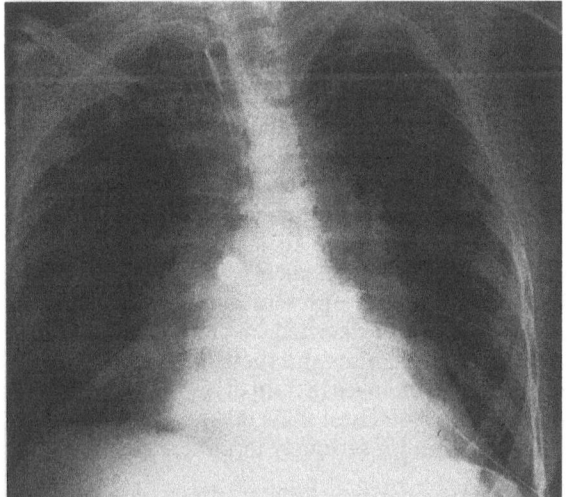

b

Fig. 5.3.a Pleural effusion following chest trauma due to a road traffic accident; fractured ribs 5th and 6th on the right. Significant pleural fluid is present causing shadowing of the right mid and lower zones. **b** After aspiration of a large effusion the right lung field is clear.

cult. Ultrasound can readily detect free effusions and ultrasonically guided thoracocentesis will greatly increase the chances of a successful tap and minimise the risks of inadvertent damage to lung or mediastinal structures (Fig. 5.3a, b). However, attempts to predict the likelihood of a successful tap based on the echogenicity of the focal collection have not been reliable – some echo-free collections will not yield fluid whereas many complex collections do (Laing and Filly 1978) – because some contain micro-gas bubbles which are echogenic, whereas some echolucent areas such as seen in haemothorax do not drain freely when tapped. The ability to tap pleural fluid under ultrasonograph control is of great benefit to the critically ill patient as it provides diagnostic samples for biochemistry and microbiology, and some can have therapeutic benefit when large collections are aspirated. Drainage of large effusions may be associated with an increase in arterial pO$_2$ in acute respiratory failure.

CT will also graphically demonstrate the extent of fluid, its loculations and its relationship to other intrathoracic structures. CT and ultrasound have repeatedly demonstrated that portable radiography grossly misjudges the amount of effusion present (Fig. 5.4a, b, c). Other fluid collections in the chest such as mediastinal or pericardial effusions are also amenable to diagnosis with ultrasound or CT scanning and to drainage under scan control.

A common diagnostic problem in the intensive care unit (ICU) is that occurring when large amounts of pleural fluid are present and are not demonstrated on an A–P film, because they lie posteriorly in the pleural space, behind the hemidiaphragm or an area of collapse or consolidation. Ultrasound may locate loculated collections and increase the chances of a successful tap of the pleural pocket. If doubt remains, CT scanning will give further information.

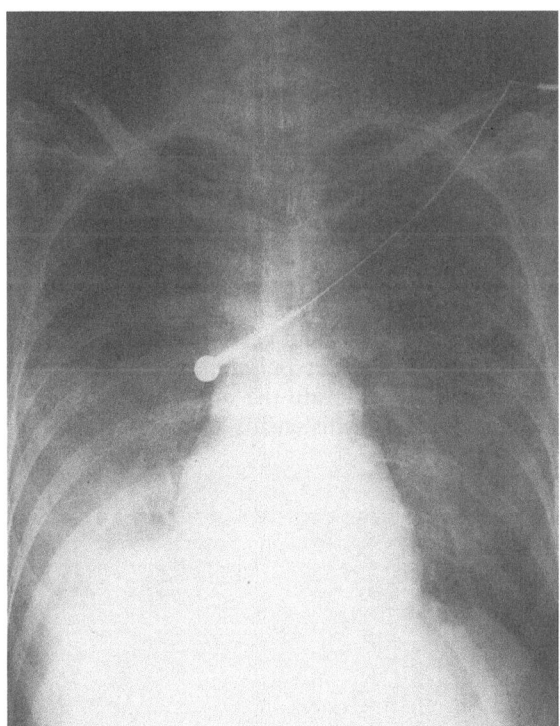

a

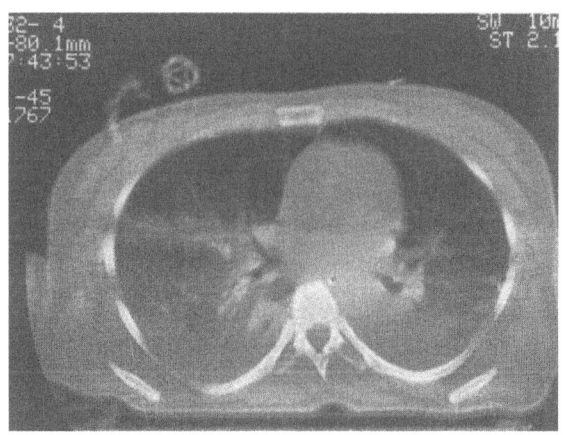

b

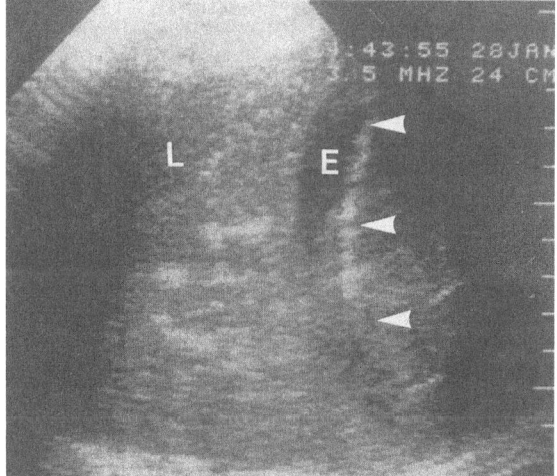

c

Fig. 5.4.a Consolidation with pleural fluid at both bases. There is increased density of the right lower lobe and loss of the outline of the right hemi-diaphragm. The left hemi-diaphragm is present with some increased shadowing at the left base. **b** CT scan below the carina shows shadowing and fluid posteriorly and on the right and left. Note the fluid in the transverse fissure. **c** Longitudinal ultrasound scan through the right base posteriorly. Consolidated lung (*L*) with an effusion (*E*). The white arrow heads represent the right hemidiaphragm.

Pulmonary Oedema and Infiltrates

The balance of fluid distribution between the intra- and extravascular spaces of the lungs is best described by the Starling equation (Starling 1886):

$$QF = Kf\,(Pmv - Ppmv) - \sigma\,(\Pi mv - \Pi pmv)$$

where: QF = net fluid flux, Kf = capillary endothelial permeability coefficient, Pmv = intravascular hydrostatic pressure, Πmv = intravascular oncotic pressure, σ = protein reflection coefficient, Ppmv = interstitial hydrostatic pressure, Πpmv = interstitial oncotic pressure.

There is normally an imbalance favouring fluid efflux from the intravascular space to the pulmonary interstitial spaces; however, because of active lymphatic removal, net fluid accumulation does not occur in health (Staub 1974). Pulmonary oedema will occur with an increase in the Pmv ("cardiac" pulmonary oedema), a decrease in Πmv, or an increase in the permeability of the pulmonary capillaries (σ). Pulmonary oedema fluid usually accumulates initially in the interstitium and later in the alveoli.

It is commonly assumed that the chest radiograph is insensitive in the detection of pulmonary oedema and that significant pulmonary oedema causing tachypnoea and hypoxaemia may exist in the absence of radiographic abnormalities. Indeed Fishman (1976) has suggested that extravascular lung water (EVLW) must be increased by 300%–600% before oedema becomes detectable on chest X-ray (CXR). However, Harrison et al. (1971) stressed the sensitivity of the radiograph in the detection of acute pulmonary oedema after myocardial infarction. They showed that the radiographic appearances of pulmonary oedema may frequently precede clinical signs whereas the radiograph was always abnormal when clinical signs were present. In an attempt to evaluate this problem Snashall et al. (1981) induced acute pulmonary oedema in dogs and measured the ratio of extravascular water to dry lung weight on seven portions of each lung. Baseline and final radiographs were examined by two radiologists and when extravascular water per gram dry lung was increased by more than 35% it was invariably recognised in one or more zones as definite oedema. The chest films of the control dogs were always recognised as normal when compared with the baseline films. The chest radiograph therefore seems to be a reasonably sensitive and early tool in detecting an increase in lung water.

A recurrent problem in the ICU is the patient with acute respiratory insufficiency associated with a radiograph demonstrating a diffuse alveolar or interstitial process. The differential diagnosis may include left ventricular failure, ARDS, severe infection, lung contusion, pulmonary embolism and fat embolism.

Cardiogenic Pulmonary Oedema

It is comforting to know that there is a good correlation between the estimation of EVLW by the thermal dye technique and X-ray (Baudendistel et al. 1982; Laggner et al. 1984; Sibbald et al. 1983). However, as mentioned above, there has to be a 35% increase in EVLW before oedema is seen on the chest film (Snashall et al. 1981). Variations in pulmonary artery wedge pressure (PAWP) correlate well with changes on the chest film (McHugh et al. 1972). The chest film appearances are expected to be normal when the PAWP is less than 12 mmHg. The peripheral vessels dilate, and interstitial oedema occurs when the PAWP is between 18 and 22 mmHg and alveolar filling is seen with PAWP of more than 22 mmHg. However, many of the radiological signs of interstitial oedema are seen best in chronic rather than acute oedema states (Fig. 5.5). Peri-bronchial cuffing remains a good indication of acute pulmonary oedema (Don and Johnson 1977), but many of the classical signs such as perihilar oedema pattern are inconsistent findings.

Unfortunately, the features of an A–P supine film can mimic some of the radiological changes of pulmonary oedema, especially upper lobe diversion of pulmonary vessels and peri-bronchial cuffing. A generalised increase in pulmonary blood volume and flow may obliterate the normal gravitational effect and result in distensio.. of upper and lower

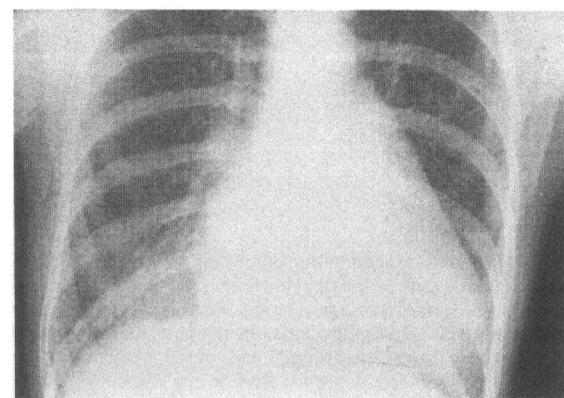

Fig. 5.5. Cardiac failure: Septal lines – horizontal lines seen above the costophrenic angle at the right base.

zone vessels (Milne 1978). The patient's position, abnormalities of parenchyma and the integrity of the pulmonary vascular bed can all affect the distribution of pulmonary oedema. It is common to see atypical pattern of pulmonary oedema in patients with chronic lung disease (Hublitz and Shapiro 1969).

Adult Respiratory Distress Syndrome (ARDS)

In 1967 Ashbaugh et al. first described the clinical syndrome of respiratory distress in twelve adult

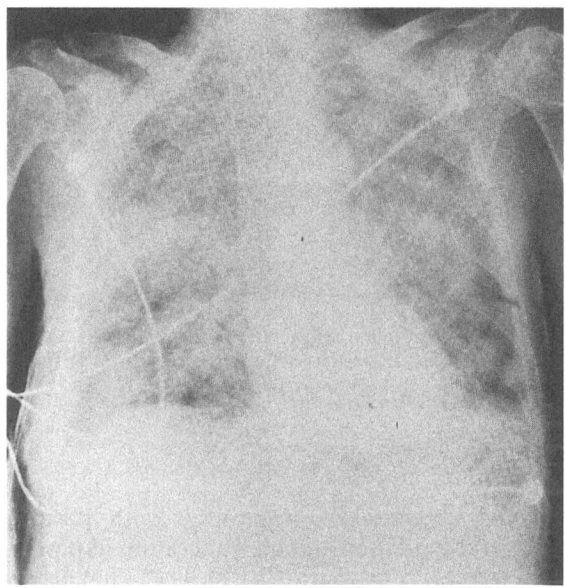

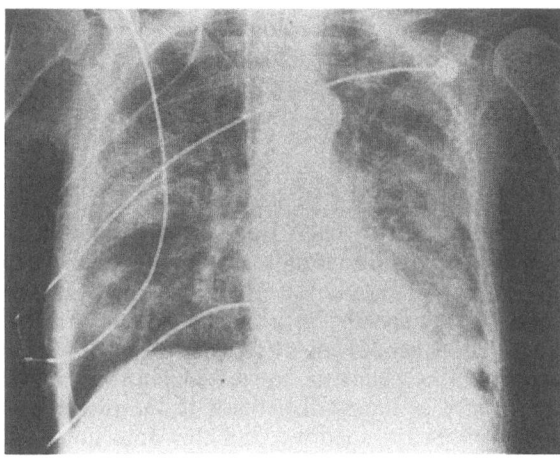

Fig. 5.6a. ARDS. This demonstrates the non-specific nature of the shadowing. Peri-hilar shadows with scattered infiltrates. **b** Clearing of the peri-hilar shadowing and reduction of infiltrate with the appearance of small pneumothoraces.

patients who had dyspnoea, hypoxaemia, reduced lung compliance and diffuse pulmonary infiltrates resembling pulmonary oedema but without evidence of prior lung disease or cardiac failure, which has subsequently become the adult respiratory distress syndrome. The radiographic changes range from a normal chest radiograph in the presence of dyspnoea and tachypnoea through minor radiological changes and diffuse pulmonary infiltrates, to a "white-out" of both lung fields. This is usually associated with refractory hypoxaemia and a metabolic and respiratory acidosis. The picture may be complicated by the fact that in severe ARDS there is often colonisation of the respiratory tract with bacterial and fungal pathogens (Fig. 5.6a, b). Although measurement of the pulmonary capillary wedge pressure can differentiate between cardiogenic and non-cardiogenic pulmonary oedema the distinction between ARDS and severe pneumonia may be very difficult. Esteban et al. (1983) suggested that a decrease in pulmonary longitudinal diameter is suggestive of ARDS and helps differentiate the syndrome from bilateral pneumonia. Bedside balloon occlusion pulmonary angiography through pulmonary artery flotation catheters has shown that pulmonary artery filling defects occur in almost one-half of ARDS patients early in their hospital course (Fig. 5.7).

Other abnormalities seen on the angiogram are reduced background opacification (capillaries not seen), minor-vessel occlusion and tortuosity of peripheral pulmonary vasculature. These vascular occlusions are not restricted to any aetiological type of ARDS and the mortality rate is greatly increased in these patients compared to patients with normal angiograms (Lawler 1986). Gattinoni et al. in Chapter 6 of this book describe the value of CT scanning in patients with ARDS in the detection of lung abscesses or localised tension pneumothoraces in anterior or posterior areas of the lung.

As both cardiogenic pulmonary oedema and ARDS result in an increase in EVLW, it is not surprising that they are indistinguishable on chest X-ray films. Cardiogenic pulmonary oedema usually occurs as a result of a failing heart and raised left atrial pressure, whereas ARDS occurs in the right clinical and aetiological circumstances (eg. sepsis, shock, burns) and in the presence of a normal left atrial pressure. The conditions are clinically differentiated by measuring the PAWP, but the size of the heart on the chest film may also give a clue to the origin of EVLW.

Because both the clinical and radiographic features of ARDS are not specific, it is important to interpret chest films serially. It is this progression of abnormalities that is the hallmark of ARDS

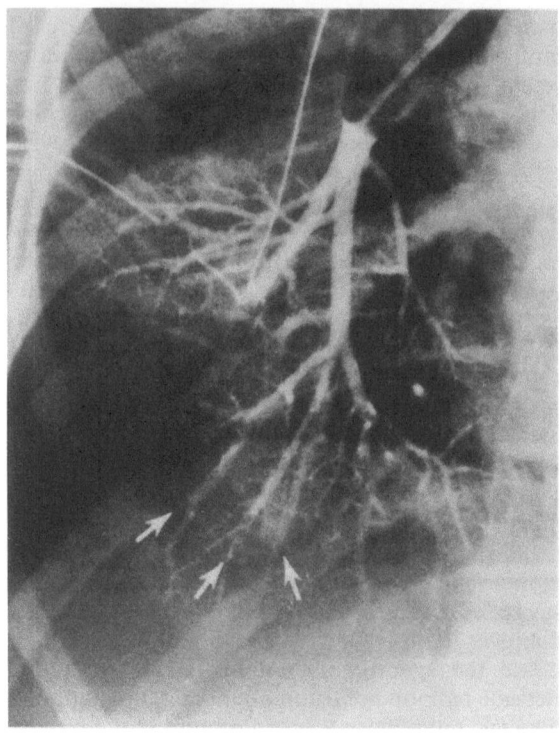

Fig. 5.7. Balloon occlusion pulmonary angiogram demonstrating multiple pulmonary artery defects (*arrows*) and decreased background opacification. By kind permission from Greene R, Boggis RM, Jantsch HS, Tomashefski JF (1985) Radiography and angiography of the pulmonary circulation in ARDS. In: Zapol W, Falke K (eds) Acute Respiratory Failure. Marcel Dekker Inc, New York, Basel.

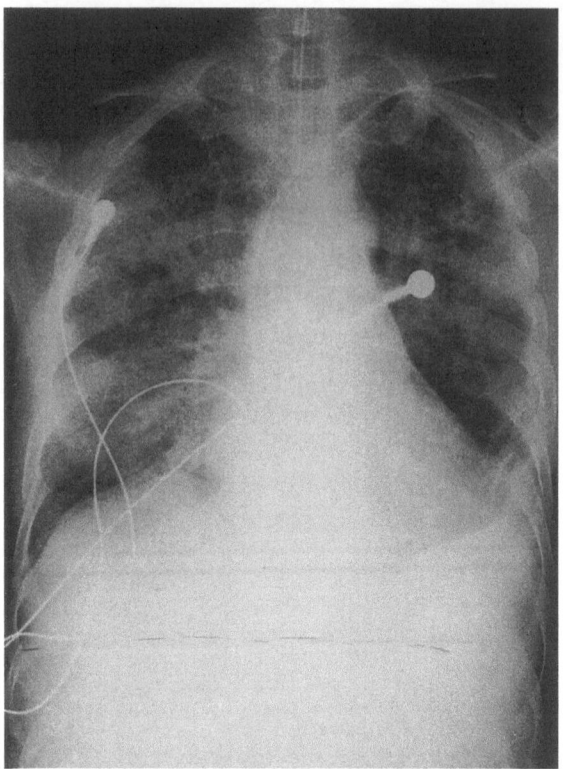

Fig. 5.8. Bilateral pulmonary infiltrates in a patient with active tuberculosis. There were large effusions present over 500 ml on both sides.

(Putman and Goodman 1983). Signs usually first occur between 12 and 36 h from onset in the form of peri-hilar haze, interstitial oedema and alveolar filling. There is little change in the primary disease after 36 h.

Other later-occurring radiological features of ARDS, such as cavitation, pulmonary interstitial emphysema (PIE), repeated pneumothoraces (PT) and scarring (Driedger et al. 1983) may in fact be the result of treatment and not part of the normal radiological features of ARDS. They occur as a result of barotrauma and lung damage due to high ventilatory pressures (Hillman 1985) (Fig. 5.21). Other conditions such as expansion of the interstitial space with crystalloid solutions may also be confused with ARDS (Twigley and Hillman 1985). When large amounts of crystalloid are used for resuscitation in conditions such as sepsis, multi-trauma and diabetic ketoacidosis, pulmonary oedema may result which invariably is clinically and radiologically identical with true ARDS.

Notable improvement in the radiological appearances of ARDS and many other types of paren-

chymal abnormalities can occur with positive-pressure ventilation and the application of positive and expiratory pressure (PEEP). This is not necessarily due to re-aeration of atelectatic alveoli, but may indicate overdistension of the smaller airways (Swischuk 1977) or alveolar rupture (Hillman 1985).

Pneumonia

Pneumonia is a clinico-pathological diagnosis. There is no definite radiological appearance which marks its presence in the critically ill and it is difficult to distinguish from other causes of intra-pulmonary shadowing (Figs. 5.8, 5.9, 5.10. 5.11). Furthermore, bacteria are often cultured in the sputum of seriously-ill patients in the presence of intrapulmonary shadows, but this does not mean the two are related. The association has resulted in gross over-prescribing of antibiotics in intensive care. In fact, there is a very poor correlation between sputum culture and the actual micro-

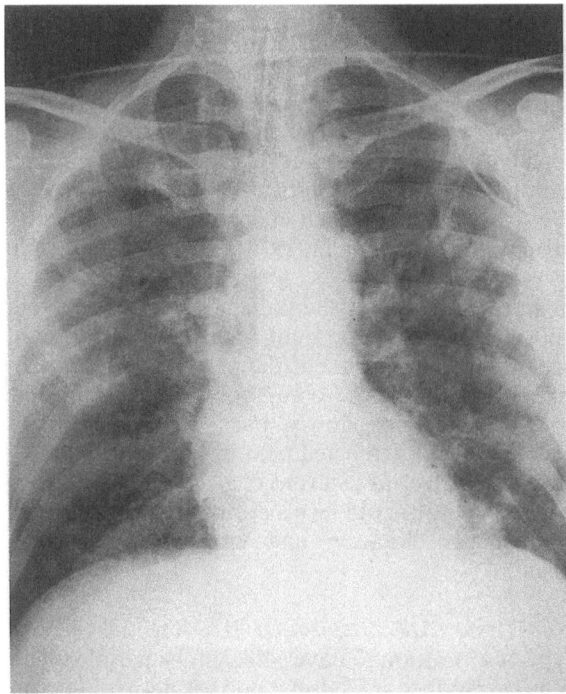

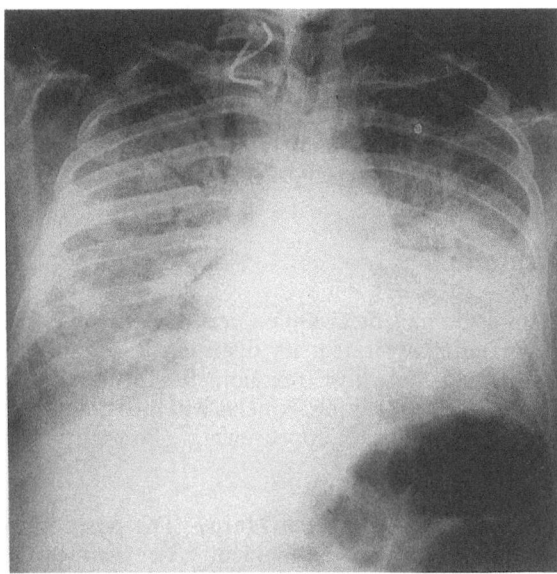

Fig. 5.10. Pneumocystis carinii: extensive shadowing, bilateral pulmonary infiltrates throughout both lungs.

Fig. 5.9. Psittacosis: non-specific patchy shadowing of left lung and right upper zone.

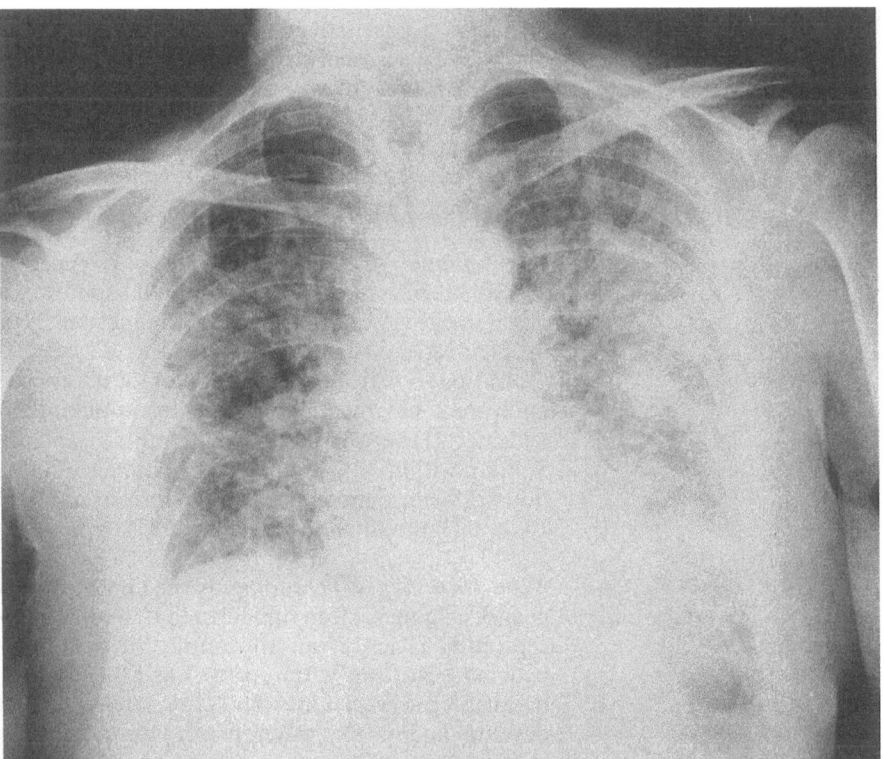

Fig. 5.11. Pneumonia: chicken pox pneumonia following chemotherapy for lymphoma. Significant bilateral pulmonary infiltrates are present in both lung fields.

biology of pneumonia (Berger and Arango 1985; French and Homi 1979). Apart from lobar consolidation, which is strongly indicative of bacterial pneumonia, the chest film is used as a tool to follow the course of treatment rather than as a specific diagnostic indicator (Fig. 5.12a, b).

Aspiration

Aspiration can be classified according to the type of material aspirated, its distribution within the lungs and the host reaction to the aspirated material. The resulting sequelae will then determine the radiological appearance (Putman and Goodman 1983):

Foreign Body-Particulate Matter. The position of the patient during the incident often dictates the

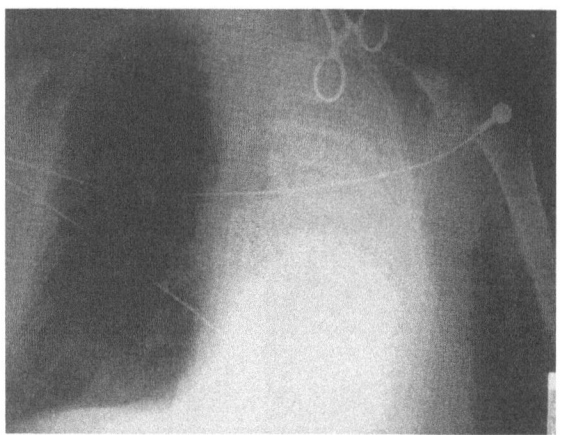

a

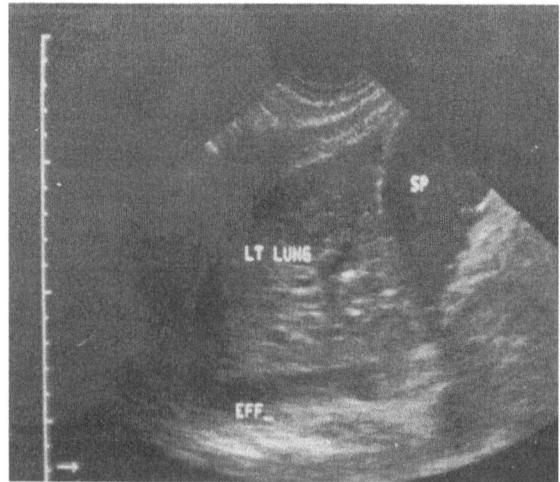

b

Fig. 5.12. a Consolidation of left lower lobe. **b** Ultrasound examination demonstrates transmission through the left lung and a small pleural effusion posteriorly (*EFF*).

area of lung affected. However, it is more common to aspirate into the right main bronchus. If radio-opaque, the material can be directly visualised. The effects of airway obstruction such as atelectasis, air trapping, mediastinal shift and lobar hyperinflation can be seen. An inflammatory response, particularly with plant matter and nuts, may be observed later. This can eventually result in fibrosis and granuloma formation (Bulmer et al. 1978).

Infected Material. If the patient is recumbent, the apical segments of the right upper and lower lobes are often affected while if the patient is sitting, the right lower lobe is commonly involved. Consolidation occurs slowly over 2–5 days, often accompanied by infected pleural exudate, and may take weeks to clear (Stevens et al. 1983). Cavitation with or without fluid levels occur within the parenchymal consolidation and empyema may also result.

Non-Toxic Liquid Aspiration. It is unusual for this type of aspiration to have sufficient bacterial inoculum to produce infection, nor specific volume or particulate size to produce significant airway blockage. Nothing more than a mild chemical pneumonitis usually results. There is a wide spectrum of radiological changes which may in their severest form lead to parenchymal (alveolar and interstitial) opacities, occasionally with atelectasis and effusions (Fig. 5.13). The distribution is usually bilateral, affecting the lower lobes more than the upper. Radiographic clearing occurs within 7–10 days if there is no complication from infection (Dooner and Sirbign 1966).

Toxic Liquid Aspiration. Mendelson is generally accredited with the first description of aspiration of gastric acid (1946). These days, Mendelson's syndrome is a term generally applied to all cases of aspiration of toxic liquid. The radiographic appearance may be indistinguishable from pulmonary oedema. However, the radiographic changes develop within 24–36 h and in the absence of infection (25% incidence), usually disappears within 7–10 days (Putman and Goodman 1983).

Near Drowning. The radiographic appearance in near drowning is often similar to that in toxic liquid aspiration. There is an appearance of pulmonary oedema occurring within 36 h (Fig. 5.14). If there has also been particulate inhalation, atelectasis can develop and if the water is contaminated, consolidation and/or even cavitation can occur. Despite claims that there is a different radiographic appearance with fresh- and salt-water drowning

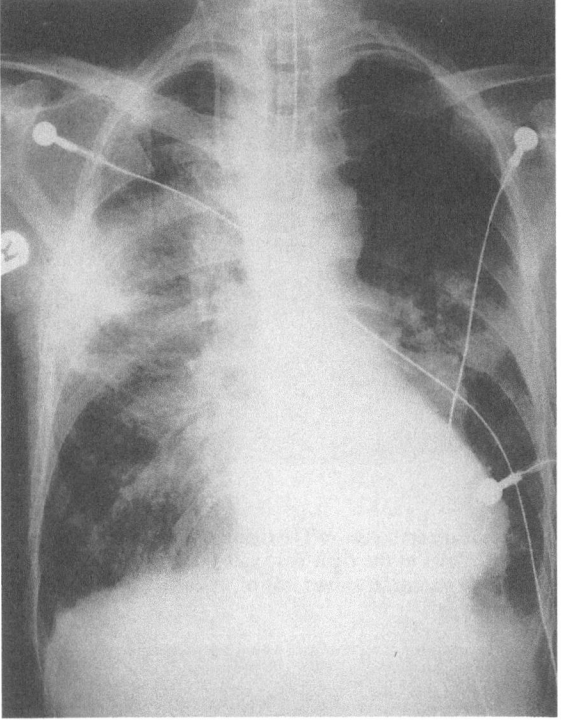

Fig. 5.13. Aspiration pneumonitis following inhalation of water-soluble contrast medium. There are bilateral peri-hilar densities with increased linear shadows. The endotracheal tube is in a satisfactory position.

(Putman et al. 1975), others suggest they are indistinguishable (Putman and Goodman 1983).

Smoke Inhalation

Inhalation of smoke and toxic gases can cause severe damage to the airways and lung parenchyma. Focal linear opacities may occur within 24 h after smoke inhalation and usually clear within three days (Putman and Goodman 1983). Focal or patchy alveolar filling can also occur within a few hours and up to three days. The standard chest radiograph is a relatively insensitive means of evaluating pulmonary abnormalities from smoke inhalation.

Pulmonary Embolism (Fig. 5.15a, b)

The portable chest film is not an accurate way to detect pulmonary emboli. The chest film can be normal or have a host of non-specific signs such as focal re-distribution of blood flow, pulmonary infarction, atelectasis, pleural effusions or a raised hemidiaphragm. In the presence of other intra-

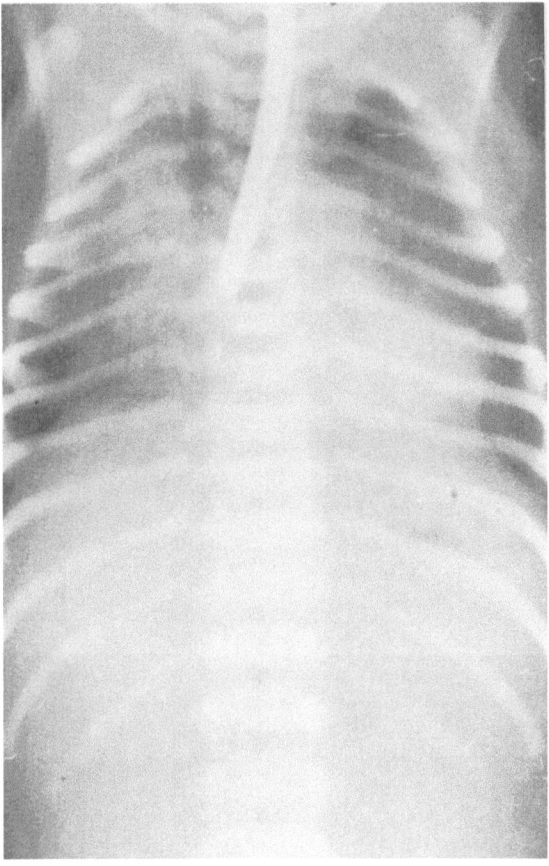

Fig. 5.14. Near drowning: non-specific shadows in both lung fields. Note that the tube is in the right main bronchus.

pulmonary pathology these signs are even less valuable. If a pulmonary embolus is suspected, perfusion lung scintigraphy or angiography should be performed. Intravenous digital angiography may be the investigation of the future.

Fat Embolism

Fat embolism is usually associated with equivocal chest radiographs sometimes progressing to an interstitial or alveolar pattern. Chan et al. (1984) described a typical "snow-storm" appearance of the chest radiograph in severe fat embolism, which may be indistinguishable from ARDS. These patients may also have a pulmonary angiogram with multiple subsegmental defects. The diagnosis may therefore rest on the history and biochemical investigations. Massive fat embolism with a large right to left shunt (Fig. 5.7) is usually associated with hypoxaemia as well as neurological changes and haemorrhagic petechi. Sudden death may occur

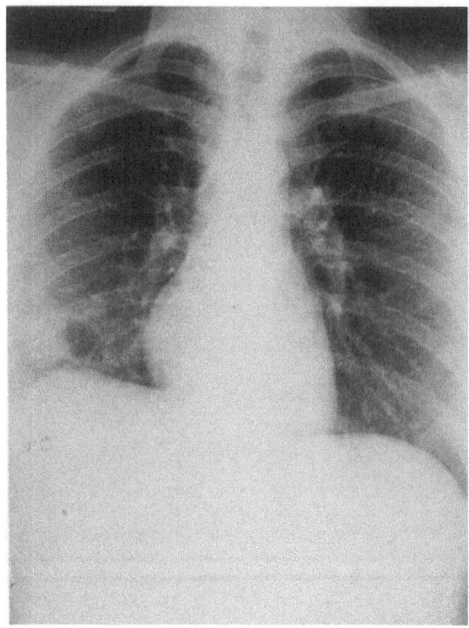

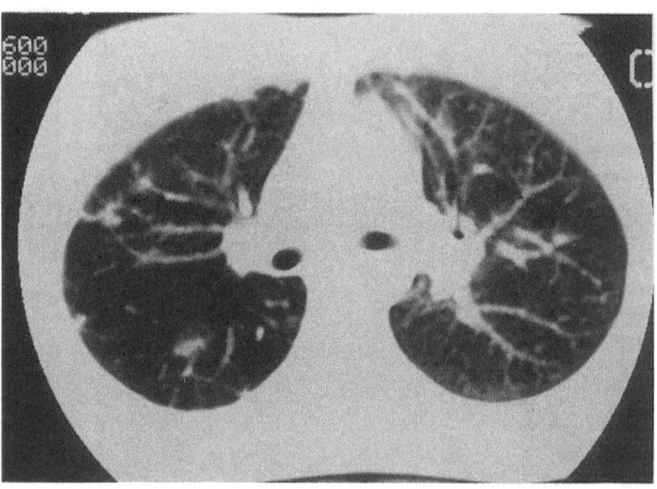

Fig. 5.15 a, b. Pulmonary embolism. **a** The right hemidiaphragm is raised. There are patchy shadows at the right base with some linear shadowing. **b** CT examination after contrast shows loss of vascularity posteriorly on the right.

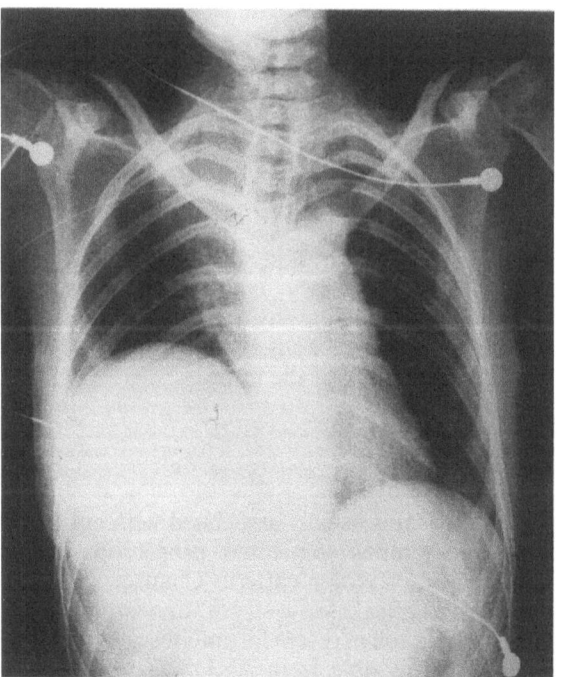

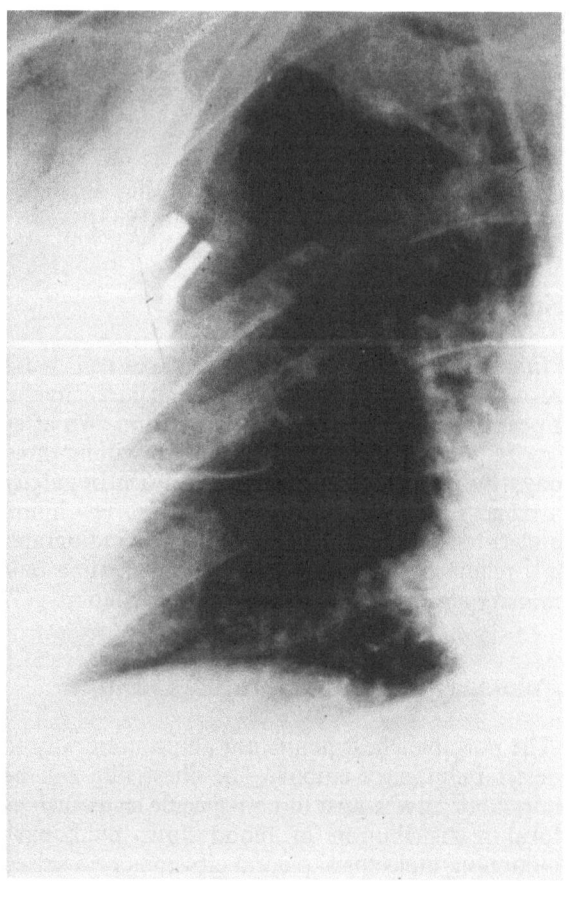

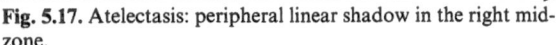

Fig. 5.16. Right upper lobe collapse following intubation of the right main bronchus. The right hemidiaphragm is raised, dense shadow obscures the upper right heart border, this is the collapsed lobe.

Fig. 5.17. Atelectasis: peripheral linear shadow in the right midzone.

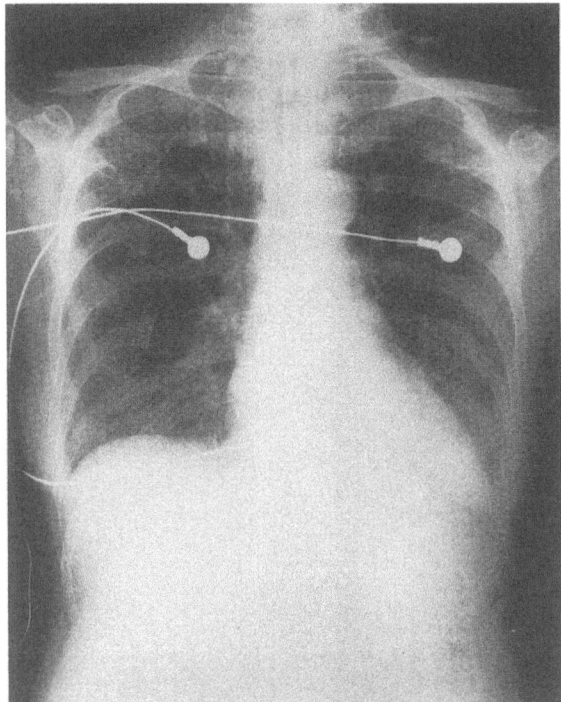

a

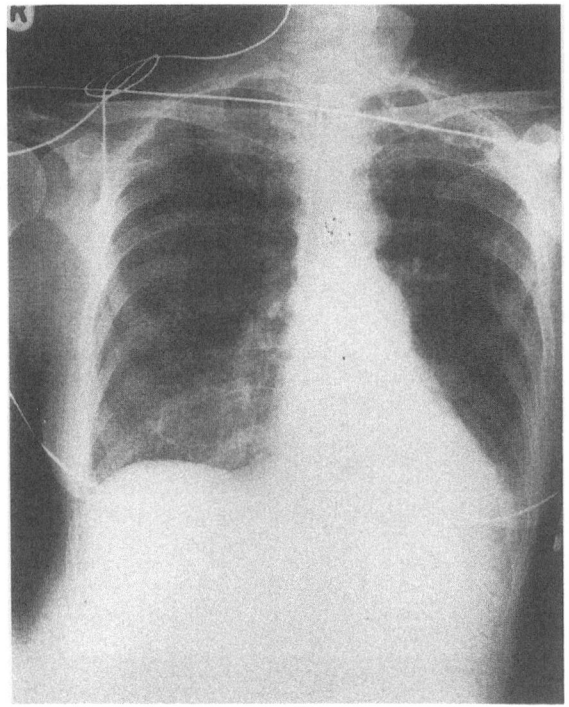

c

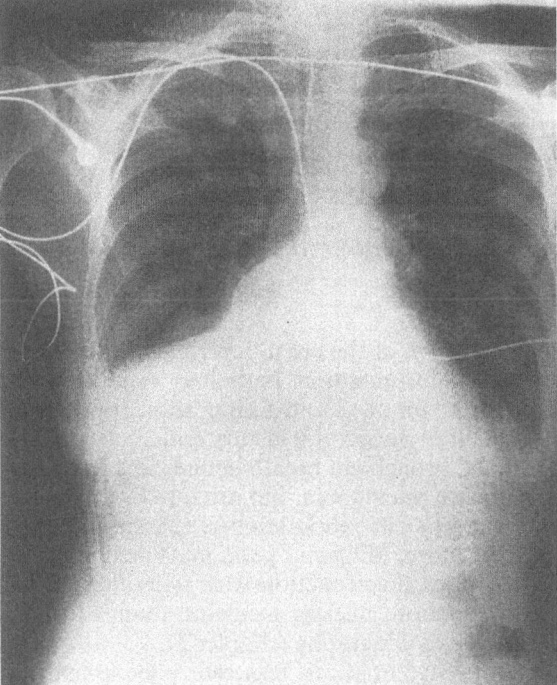

b

Fig. 5.18 a–c. Collapse of the right lower lobe. **a** Initial chest film taken 3 days before collapse of the right lower lobe. **b** Collapsed right lower lobe overlying the right heart border; the right hemidiaphragm is raised. **c** Film taken after bronchial lavage; some residual shadows present but the right hemidiaphragm and right heart border are now normal.

before any abnormalities can be demonstrated in the radiograph.

Atelectasis and Collapse

Consolidation and collapse often coexist. It is, however, convenient to consider the two phenomena separately (Fig. 5.12a). Pure consolidation shows no loss of volume, while collapse shows loss of volume of a lung or lobe. The most common cause of collapse in intensive care is intraluminal obstruction of the airways, particularly by mucous plugging. The radiological signs include the shadow of the collapsed lobe or lobes, the silhouette sign and displacement of structures to take up the space normally occupied by the collapsed lung. The signs of displacement include crowding of the lung markings, elevation of a hemidiaphragm, and mediastinal shift (Fig. 5.16).

Apart from collapse of a lobe or lung, there can also be collapse of smaller subunits of the lung – often referred to as atelectasis. These produce many types of shadows, and are often described as triangular, line or plate-shaped (Fig. 5.17). Following re-expansion of a collapsed lobe by either therapeutic bronchoscopy or application of PEEP, various shaped shadows often remain at the site of residual segmental collapse which are not totally resolved (Fig. 5.18a,b,c). Collapse and atelectasis

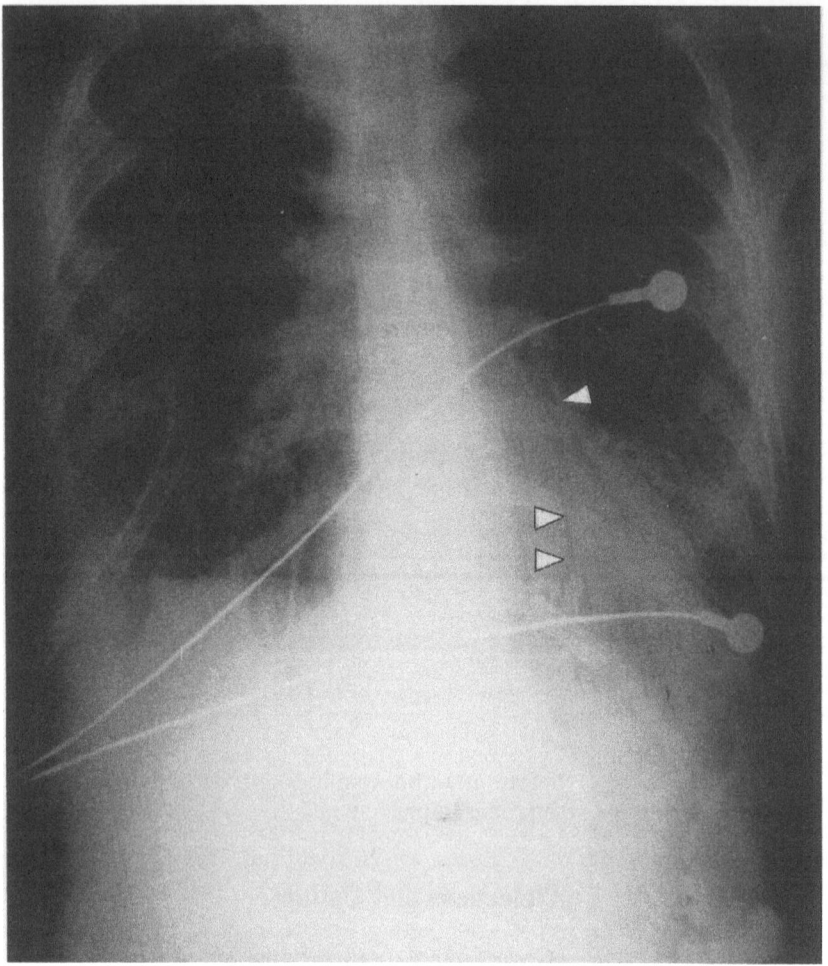

Fig. 5.19. Consolidation of the left lower lobe: There is significant air bronchogram (*arrows*). On the right side a large pleural effusion has been drained. There is still residual shadowing at the right costophrenic angle.

often respond rapidly to manoeuvres such as posturing, physiotherapy, suction and continuous positive airway pressure (CPAP) breathing (Fig. 5.19). The presence or absence of an air bronchogram in association with persistent collapse can give an indication as to whether fibreoptic bronchoscopy is indicated.

Differentiation between Lung Parenchymal Pathology

This is probably the greatest challenge in the interpretation of chest films in intensive care. As there are no absolute radiological differences between pathological processes such as ARDS, fat embolism, pneumonia, smoke inhalation, aspiration and cardiogenic pulmonary oedema, the interpretation of the chest film has to be tempered by clinical examination, pathology results and the time period for onset and disappearance of shadows as a result of the natural history and treatment. For example, bronchiole breath sounds are frequently found with pneumonia, but are rare in pulmonary oedema. The differentiation between the oedema in ARDS and cardiogenic pulmonary oedema is by assessing cardiac function with pulmonary artery catheterisation, nuclear medicine studies (chapter 9) or echocardiography (chapter 8).

The differentiation between pneumonia and ARDS remains difficult. Patients with pneumonia are often septic, and septic patients often develop ARDS. Conversely patients with ARDS may develop nosocomial infections. Both groups of patients are often febrile, have a leucocytosis and are hypoxic, with reduced lung volumes and compliance. The organisms causing pneumonia can often not be isolated, even with open lung biopsy. On histology, both ARDS and pneumonia can show hyaline membranes, interstitial fibrosis and changes in the epithelium (Esteban et al. 1983). In a recent comparison of the two diseases, pathogens were found in the sputum with equal frequency and only a minority of the patients with nosocomial pneumonia responded to antibiotics (Johanson 1984). It is not surprising, therefore, that the diagnosis and differentiation of ARDS and pneumonia remains one of the greatest challenges in critical care. The most reliable radiological guide remains the temporal relationship in the onset of ARDS. Unless patients are admitted to intensive care with primary pneumonia, it usually takes several days for it to develop, while ARDS occurs within hours of the initial insult.

Abdominal Pathology Affecting the Chest X-Ray

The chest X-ray film is sometimes a reflection of intra-abdominal pathology. The onset of ARDS or its persistence may be an indication of unresolved intra-abdominal sepsis. A generalised or localised intra-abdominal mass effect can often push the diaphragm upward, and thereby decrease lung volume as well as cause basal atelectasis and later infection or collapse. Basal effusions occur in approximately 50% of postoperative patients (Light and George 1976). Pneumoperitoneum can occur as a result of recent laparotomy, a ruptured intra-abdominal viscus or derived from pulmonary barotrauma. It is important to differentiate the cause, as definite treatment is urgently required for the latter two causes of pneumoperitoneum. Gastric dilatation is often seen as a result of recent resuscitation and positive pressure ventilation with a mask and airway (Fig. 5.20). It can also be encountered following abdominal surgery, sepsis or diabetic ketoacidosis.

Extra-Alveolar Air (EAA)

Extra-alveolar air should be looked for in all ventilated patients. With high intrapulmonary pressures alveoli are over-distended, and when alveolar

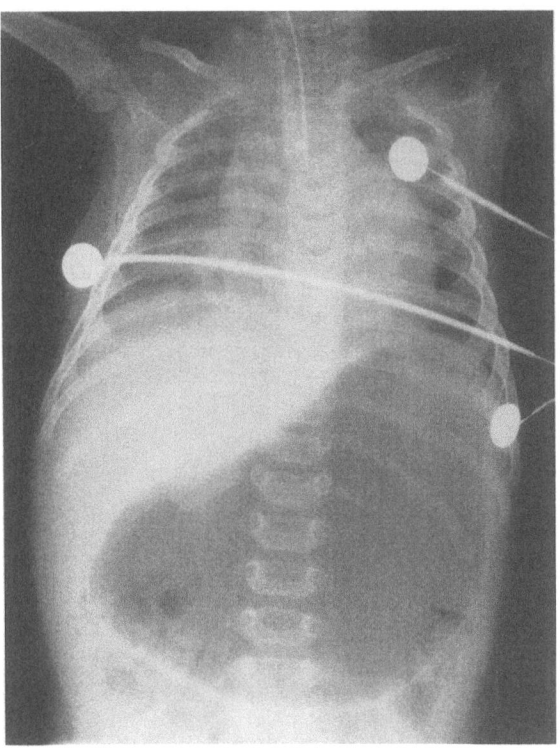

Fig. 5.20. Large gastric air bubble in a baby following resuscitation by ventilation via a face mask.

lining becomes damaged air migrates towards the lung hila and into the mediastinum to form mediastinal emphysema (Fig. 5.21). From there, with continued intrapulmonary pressure, the gas can form subcutaneous emphysema or burst through the thin mediastinal pleura to form pneumothoraces and under high pressures be forced along the aorta or oesophagus to form pneumoretroperitoneum and pneumoperitoneum (Hillman 1982, 1985). Each manifestation of EAA can cause serious adverse effects as well as being a marker of further manifestations of EAA. Mediastinal emphysema is important to recognise because as well as causing adverse cardiorespiratory effects, it is the precursor of air elsewhere, especially a pneumothorax. Unfortunately, unless it occurs laterally mediastinal emphysema may not always be obvious on an A–P film and may be mistaken for pneumopericardium, which is an extremely rare and usually a terminal event. Subcutaneous emphysema is usually obvious on a portable chest X-ray film and can be seen in the superior mediastinum before advancing into the

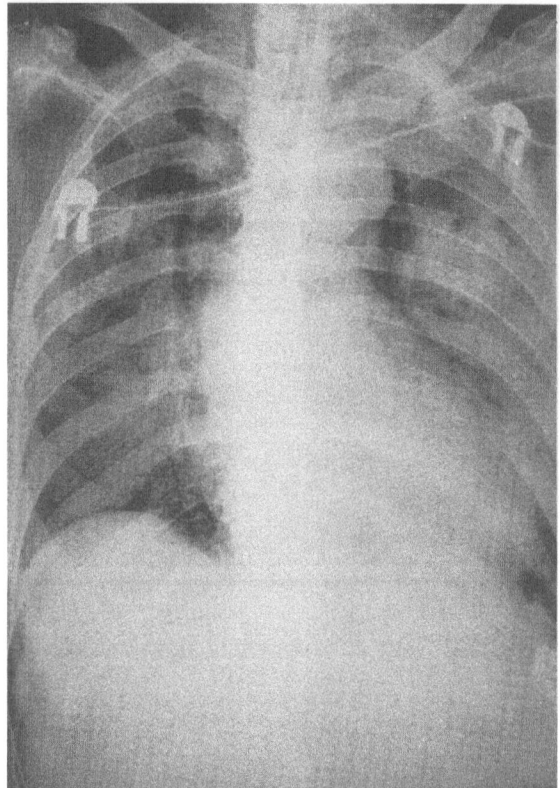

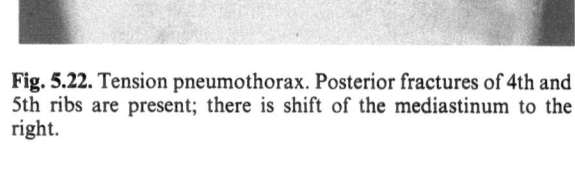

Fig. 5.22. Tension pneumothorax. Posterior fractures of 4th and 5th ribs are present; there is shift of the mediastinum to the right.

Fig. 5.21. Mediastinal air following barotrauma. Air has tracked into the right and left sides of the mediastinum.

neck and upper chest tissues. Pneumo-retroperitoneum is located more laterally than pneumoperitoneum.

Chest Trauma

Thoracic trauma are classified into two broad categories, penetrating trauma and blunt trauma. The term penetrating trauma encompasses a wide range of injuries in which the physical integrity of the thorax is violated by an object. The majority of injuries in this category are due to gunshot or knife wounds. Blunt chest trauma may be due to deceleration or shearing force, for example in a road traffic accident, but may also be due to sports or crush injuries.

The initial investigation must always be a chest radiograph with the availability of other techniques such as CT, ultrasound scan and angiography as the situation suggests. An urgent upright chest film is crucial in assessing chest trauma. The film must be taken with the patient upright so that effusions, parenchymal damage and pneumothoraces can be visualised. Pulmonary contusion is probably the commonest abnormality seen. It represents oedema or blood in the alveoli which may have resulted from direct impact or from a contra-coup injury. They are often seen immediately and usually are represented by maximum shadowing within 24 h. They begin clearing within 2–3 days and are usually completely cleared within 1–2 weeks (Goodman and Putman 1983). If not, one should suspect superimposed infection, concurrent aspiration or intra-pulmonary haematoma. Pulmonary haematoma presents as a round opacity that may become visible following clearing of an area of contusion.

The extent of fractured ribs and flail segments should be documented as a guideline for pain management and possible damage to other structures such as the spleen. Although fractured ribs can penetrate lung tissue and cause pneumothoraces, it is very common to have EAA formation, including pneumothoraces as a result of blunt lung trauma (Hillman 1985) (Fig. 5.22). Even in the presence of fractured ribs, there can be EAA in the form of subcutaneous emphysema and mediastinal emphysema as a result of blunt rather than penetrating injury. These patients may not have a pneumothorax and do not need an intercostal drain on the side of the fractured rib.

Fractures of the thoracic skeleton give some warning of the possibility of underlying soft-tissue injuries. In particular, the combination of clavicle and 1st rib or 1st and 2nd rib fractures raises the serious possibility of aortic rupture, and if associated with mediastinal widening then further investigations should take place (Fig. 5.23a,b). Similarly fractures of the lower ribs raise the possibility of damage to abdominal organs, notably the liver and spleen.

Most major injuries to the thoracic aorta occur just distal to the left subclavian artery and 80% are almost immediately fatal (Egan et al. 1980). The radiographic signs of aortic injury (widening of the mediastinum, a left apical pleural cap, and silhouetting of the descending aorta) are often difficult to evaluate on the usual supine portable chest radiograph. Angiography is certainly the diagnostic procedure of choice in the massively traumatised patient or where there is a strong clinical suspicion of aortic injury, as it can better define intimal injuries or small pseudoaneurysms (Egan et al. 1980). However, CT scanning may be useful in excluding aortic injury in a stable patient with mediastinal widening which may be due to other thoracic injuries.

De Bakey et al. (1965) described three types of dissection of the thoracic aorta. In type 1 the intimal tear originates near the root of the aorta and usually extends distal to the left subclavian artery, in type II it originates near the aortic root and extends to the origin of the innominate artery and in type III it develops immediately distal to the left subclavian artery and extends into the abdominal aorta. Diagnosis of aortic dissection requires demonstration of an intimal flap and both true and false lumina. For CT to replace aortography it would have to show not only the intimal flap but both the freeflow of contrast material in both lumina and if the false lumen is thrombosed or does not communicate with the true lumen only the latter will be enhanced.

Mediastinal widening on the initial chest radiograph may be due not only to vascular injury, but also to oesophageal and tracheo-bronchial disruption. Pneumomediastinum is an early diagnostic sign but may be missed due to the technical quality of the chest X-ray. The deep cervical fascia is in direct continuity with the mediastinum and lateral films of the neck may reveal deep cervical emphysema (Eijgelaar and Van der Heide 1970). Other important radiological signs include hyoid bone elevation indicating tracheal transection, pneumothorax, subcutaneous air, pneumopericardium, fractures limited to the upper rib

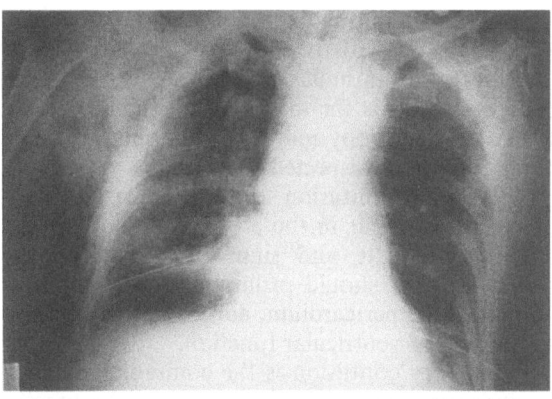

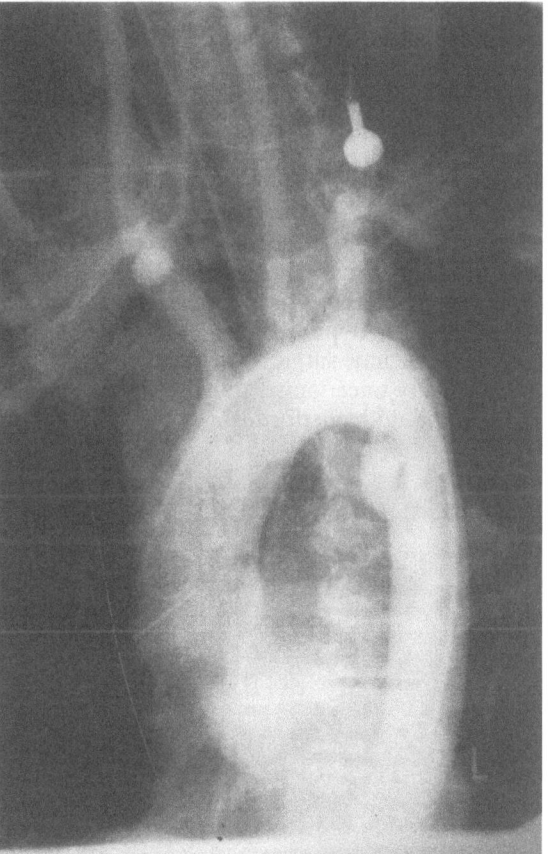

Fig. 5.23 a, b. Blunt chest trauma. **a** Chest radiograph. **b** Angiogram. Mediastinal widening caused by traumatic dissection of the descending part of the arch distal to the left subclavian artery.

cage or sternum, air surrounding the bronchus and obstruction in the course of an air-filled bronchus (Kirsh et al. 1976). When a main bronchus is transected within its pleural sheath, the characteristic appearance is that of the affected lung dropped down into the chest cavity; this is because it has lost the suspension normally provided by the bronchus. This contrasts with the finding in patients with pneumothorax without transection where the lung collapses towards the mediastinum (Kumpe et al. 1970). Laryngoscopy and/or bronchoscopy must be performed in all suspected cases of airway injury.

Myocardial contusion and acute cardiac tamponade may occur in the absence of an enlarged cardiac silhouette and signs of haemodynamic embarrassment should prompt ultrasound examination of the pericardium, aortic root, valves and assessment of ventricular function.

Pulmonary contusion is the commonest abnormality seen after chest injuries. It may be present initially, but if the patient is hypovolaemic it may only become apparent when blood volume is restored. A pulmonary haematoma usually presents as a visual opacity on the chest radiograph following clearing of an area of contusion, and CT scanning should reveal the nature of the lesion if there is doubt. Pulmonary contusion may also lead to pneumothorax and/or tear of the pulmonary artery. A tear of the artery is best diagnosed on the chest film by loss of the vascular pattern in the dependent areas as well as the clinical signs of hypovolaemia and hypoxaemia, and these should warrant immediate surgical intervention (Fig. 5.24). If there is any uncertainty, pulmonary artery angiography should be performed.

Diaphragmatic rupture may be apparent immediately, or may be masked by other injuries to the mediastinum, pulmonary parenchyma, chest wall or abdomen. It may be associated with visual herniation on the plain chest radiograph or there may be non-specific signs such as pleural effusion, lower lobe atelectasis, loss of hemidiaphragm contour and contra-lateral mediastinal shift. Phrenic nerve injury may be indistinguishable (Fig. 5.25). CT scanning is of value in this situation to identify the hemidiaphragm and the lower extent of the lung.

Identifying Cardiorespiratory Support and Monitoring Equipment

It is important to verify the proper placement of the various types of monitoring and support equipment used in seriously ill patients.

Endo or Nasotracheal Tube and Tracheostomies

Every tracheal intubation should be followed immediately by a chest film in order to check the

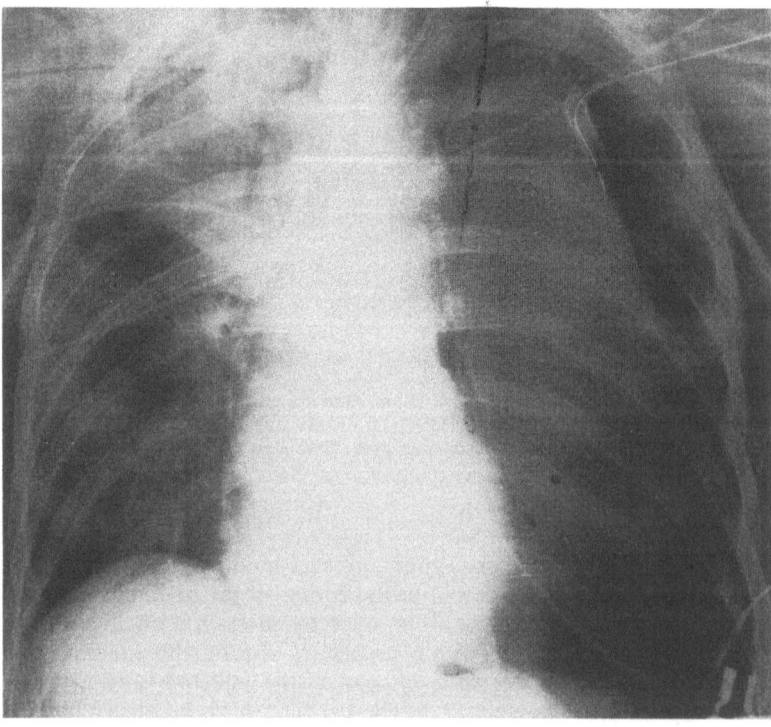

Fig. 5.24. Chest injury after a road traffic accident: There is a fracture to the left 8th rib posteriorly. No lung vascular markings are present in the left lung field. The patient's left main pulmonary artery is ruptured. The patient also has a pneumothorax and surgical emphysema.

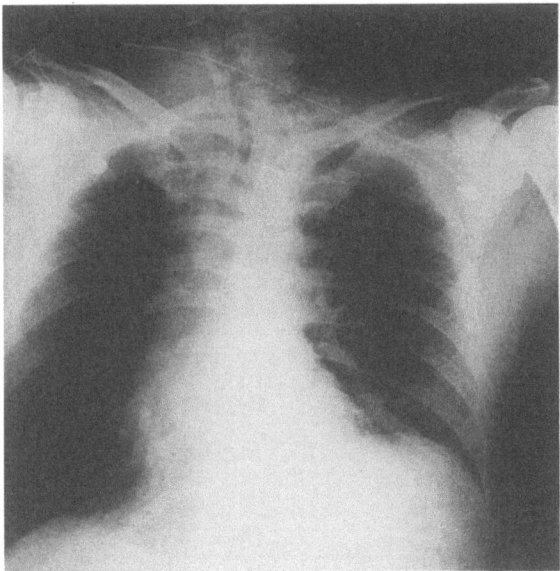

Fig. 5.25. Phrenic nerve injury. Raised left hemidiaphragm after injury to the phrenic nerve.

proper position of the tube. It is important that the tip of the tube is more than 2 cm proximal to the carina and that the cuff is 2 cm distal to the vocal cords to allow for the considerable variation in tube movement with flexing and extension of the head. Approximately 10% of endotracheal tubes are initially situated in the right main stem bronchus (Fig. 5.26). Following tracheostomy, the chest film should be checked for evidence of EAA and to ensure that the tip of the tube is at least 2 cm proximal to the carina.

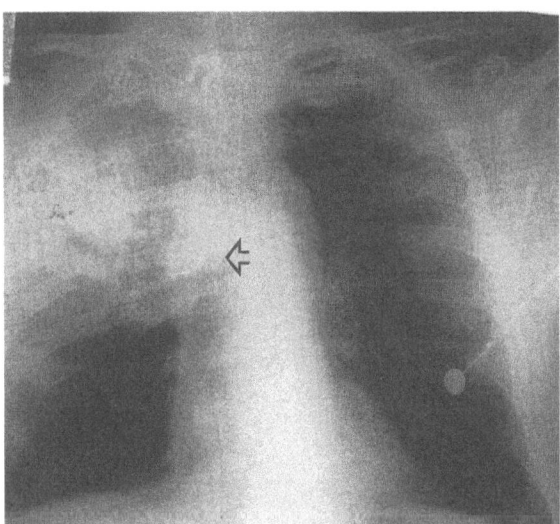

Fig. 5.26. Right upper lobe consolidation with the endotracheal tube in the right main bronchus (*arrow*).

Central Venous Catheters

Central venous catheters are commonly employed for monitoring pressure and delivering drugs. A chest film should be taken immediately after placement to confirm correct positioning and to look for iatrogenic complications such as bleeding, ectopic fluid collection or pneumothoraces (Fig. 5.27 a, b). The tip should be located beyond all peripheral valves but not necessarily within the right atrium.

Infusion of fluid into the mediastinal or pleural space is suggestive of the radiological appearance of intrathoracic bleeding and may even mimic aortic rupture. A common complication of the use of drum catheters is the shearing off of parts of the catheter (Fig. 5.28). Should this incidence occur interventional radiological techniques have to be employed to recover the broken part of the catheter (chapter 14). If these fail, thoracotomy has to be considered for removal of the catheter.

Pulmonary Artery Catheter

Pulmonary artery catheters are associated with the same complications as central venous lines as well as other, often more dangerous ones, such as pulmonary embolism or infarction distal to the catheter tip and even pulmonary artery rupture with bleeding. The knowledge of the position of the tip of the catheter may help in the interpretation of wedge pressures. Excessive coiling in the heart can predispose to migration and undesired wedging of the catheter (Fig. 5.29).

Intra-Aortic Counter Pulsation Balloon (IACB)

The tip of the IACB should be placed just distal to the left subclavian artery. If it is inserted any further, it may obstruct the bracheo-cephalic arteries or increase the risk of cerebral embolism. The tip should be at the level of the aortic knob on an upright A–P chest film.

Transvenous Pacemakers (PM)

Depending on where the catheter is inserted, complications similar to central line placement can occur. The tip of the PM should be positioned at the apex of the right ventricle to ensure contact with the endocardium. Abberant locations include the coronary sinus, right atrium, pulmonary airflow tract and pulmonary artery. Rarely, perforation of the myocardium can occur (Fig. 5.30).

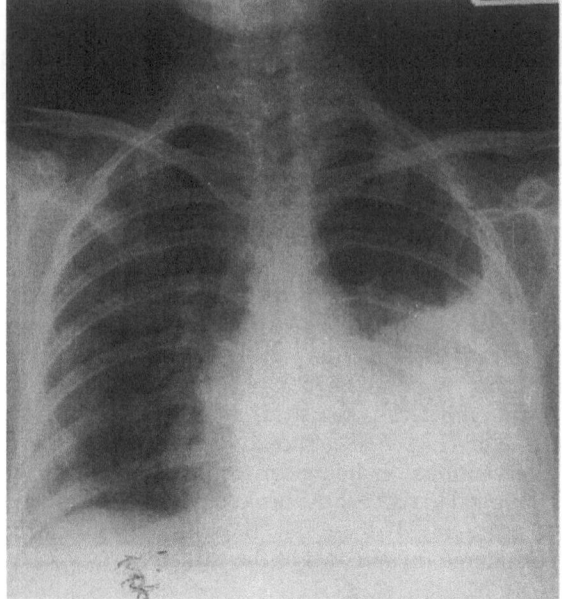

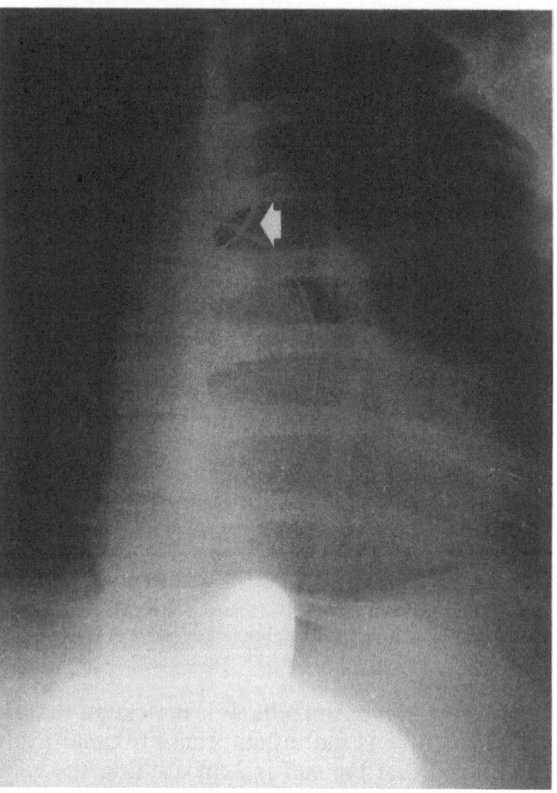

Fig. 5.28. Broken drum catheter in the right ventricle with tip curled in the main pulmonary artery trunk (*arrow*).

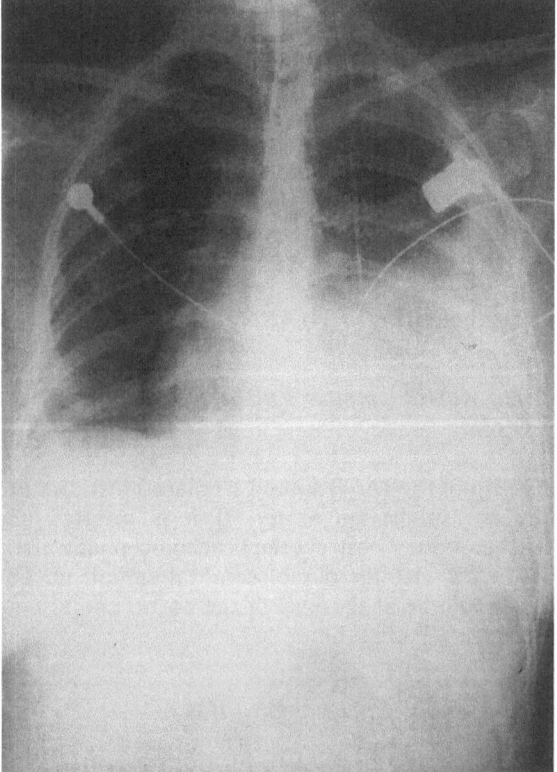

Fig. 5.27. a Patient with a large pleural effusion. **b** Central venous line inserted through left internal jugular vein, perforating the jugular vein and entering the pleural space. Unfortunately blood was freely withdrawn from the catheter, causing a delay in the decision to remove it.

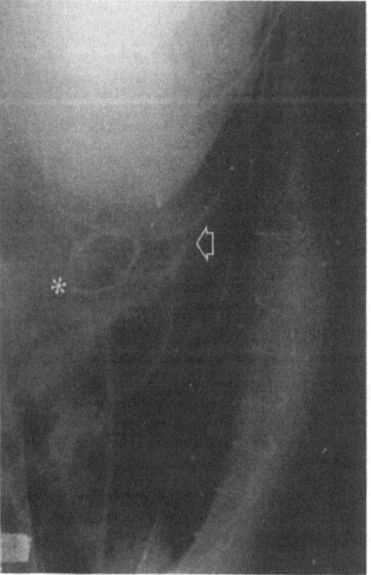

Fig. 5.29. Swan–Ganz catheter inserted after mitral valve replacement (*star*) which curled up in the right ventricle forming a knot (*arrow*).

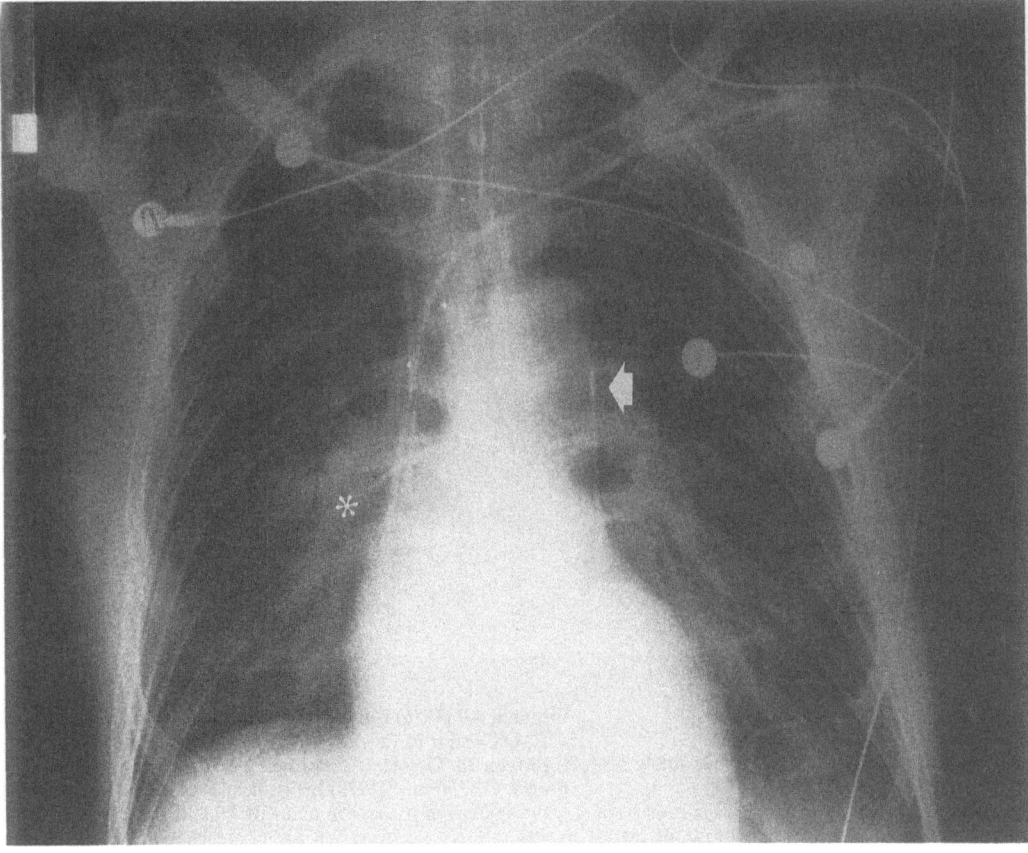

Fig. 5.30. Perforation through the myocardium by a transvenous pacemaker (*arrow*). The star indicates the tip of the Swan–Ganz catheter.

Nasogastric Tubes (NG)

The position of the NG tube should be checked, particularly when tubes with oesophageal balloons for the measurement of oesophageal pressures are used. The top of the NG tube itself should follow the anatomical structure of the oesophagus. If the line follows one of the main bronchi (Fig. 5.31 a, b), the NG tube should be taken out and replaced despite the tip of the NG tube deceptively coinciding with gastric air bubbles.

Conclusions

Portable chest films are an essential complement to clinical and pathological information in intensive care. Interested intensivists and radiologists can gain invaluable information from these films and develop their own skills by constantly discussing the films together. Not only are the films essential for the assessment of pulmonary pathology but they often provide clues to other aspects of the patient such as chronic mediastinal and cardiac abnormalities. Even information about more distant sites of pathology such as the abdomen can be gleaned from a portable chest film. In addition, Slasky et al. (1983) analysed the value of portable real-time ultrasonography in 107 intensive care patients and concluded that ultrasound was underused. We feel that a continuous presence of ultrasound in intensive care would be justified in the same way as portable radiography; these two techniques are sufficiently complementary to give a high yield of information. Where there is still doubt or the examinations have been unsatisfactory a CT scan examination of the chest is fully justified, particularly where there is suspected major vessel injury.

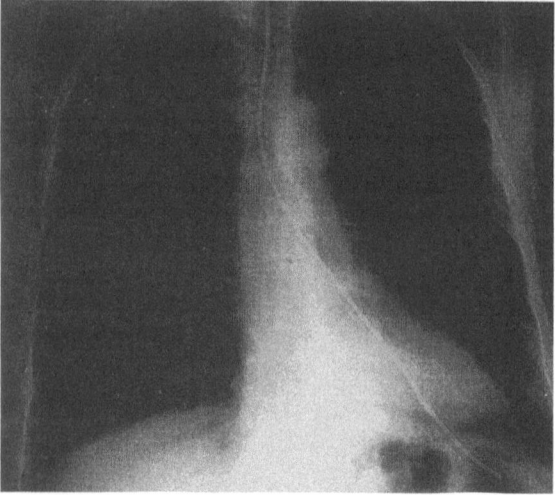

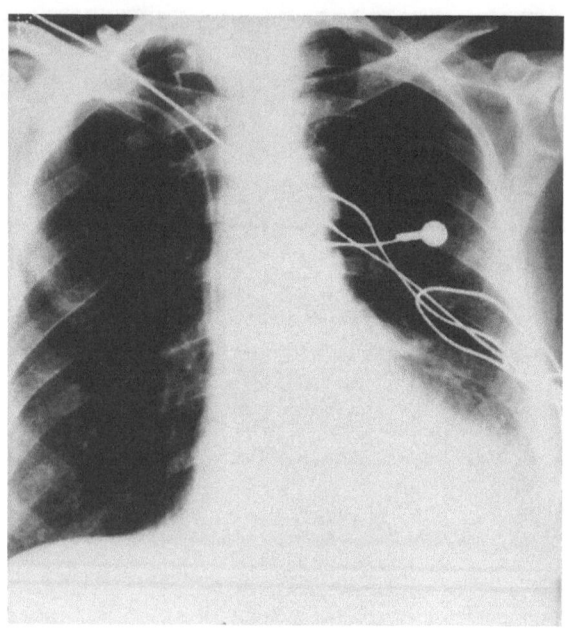

Fig. 5.31. a NG tube in the left main bronchus. The tube has perforated the lung and the tip of the catheter coincides deceptively with colonic gas shadows. **b** Left lower lobe opacity after NG feeding was commenced despite the control chest film (**a**).

References

Ashbaugh D, Bigelow D, Petty T, Levine B (1967) Acute respiratory distress in adults. Lancet I: 319–323

Baudendistel L, Shields JB, Kamiski DL (1982) Comparison of double indicator thermodilution measurements of extravascular lung water (EVLW) with radiographic estimation of lung water in trauma patients. J Trauma 22: 983–988

Berger R, Arango L (1985) Etiological diagnosis of bacterial nosocomial pneumonia in seriously ill patients. Crit Care Med 13: 833–836

Bulmer SR, Lamb D, McCormack RJM, Walbarum PR (1978) The aetiology of unresolved pneumonia. Thorax 33: 307–314

Chan KM, Tham KT, Chiu HS et al. (1984) Post-traumatic fat embolism – its clinical and subclinical presentations. J Trauma 24: 45–49

De Bakey ME, Henly WS, Cooly DA, Morris GC, Cranford ES, Beall AC (1965) Surgical management of dissecting aneurysms of the aorta. J Thorac Cardiovasc Surg 49: 130–148

Don C, Johnson R (1977) The nature and significance of peribronchial cuffing in pulmonary oedema. Radiology 125: 577–582

Dooner MW, Sirbign ML (1966) Cinefluorographic analysis of pharyngeal swallowing in neuromuscular disorders. Am J Med Sci 251: 600–609

Driedger AA, Sibbald WJ, Lefcoe M, McCallum LJ (1983) Diagnostic imaging in the critically ill. In: Ledingham IMcA, Hanning CD, (eds) Recent advances in critical care medicine. Churchill Livingstone, Edinburgh, pp 211–287

Egan TJ, Neiman HL, Herman RJ, Malave SR, Sanderj JH (1980) CT diagnosis of aortic aneurysm dissection of traumatic injury. Radiology 136: 141–146

Eijgelaar V, Homan van Der Heide JN (1970) A reliable early symptom of bronchial or tracheal rupture. Thorax 25; 120–125

Esteban A, Fernanades-Segoviano P, Oliete S, Ruiz-Santana S, Castello J. Cal A de la (1983) Radiographic findings for the adult respiratory distress syndrome in patients with peritonitis. Crit Care Med 11: 880–882

Fishman AP (1976) Clinical disorders of lung liquids. In Porter R, O'Connor M (eds) Lung Liquids. Ciba Foundation Symposium 38. Elsevier, Amsterdam p. 312

French GL, Homi J (1979) Insignificance of colonic bacteria in the sputum of patients in a new ICU. Crit Care Med 7: 487–491

Goodman LR, Putman CE (eds) (1983) Intensive Care Radiology: Imaging of the critically ill. WB Saunders, Philadelphia

Harrison MO, Conte PJ, Heitzman ER (1971) Radiological detection of clinically occult cardiac failure following myocardial infarction. Br J Radiol 44: 265–272

Hillman KM (1982) Pneumoperitoneum – a review. Crit Care Med 10: 476–481

Hillman K. (1985) Pulmonary barotrauma. In: Dobb G, (ed) Clinics in Anaesthesiology. WB Saunders, London, pp 877–898

Hublitz VF. Shapiro JH (1969) A typical pulmonary pattern of congestive failure in chronic lung disease. The influence of pre-existing diseases on the appearance and distribution of pulmonary oedema. Radiology 93: 995–1006

Johanson Jnr WG (1984) Bacterial infection in ARDS: Pathogenic mechanisms and consequences. In: Shoemaker WC (ed) Critical Care: State of the Art. Fullerton: The Society of Critical Care Medicine 5(H): 1–43

Kirsh MM, Orringer MB, Berhrendt DMS, Sloan ME (1976) Management of tracheobronchial disruption secondary to non-penetrating trauma. Ann Thorac Surg 22: 93–101

Kumpe DH, Kook Sang Oh, Wyman SM (1970) A characteristic pulmonary finding – unilateral complete bronchial transection. Am J Koentgenol 110; 704–706

Laggner A, Kleinberger G, Haller J, Lenz K, Sommer G, Druml W (1984) Bedside estimation of extravascular lung water in critically ill patients: comparison of the chest radiograph and the thermal dye technique. Intensive Care Med 10: 309–313

Laing FC, Filly RA (1978) Problems in the application of ultrasonography for the evaluation of pleural opacities. Radiology 126: 211–214

Lawler PG (1986) Pulmonary occlusion (wedge) angiography in adult respiratory distress syndrome. Anaesthesia 41: 605–610

Light RW, George RB (1976) Incidence and significance of pleural effusion after abdominal surgery. Chest 69: 621–627

Mendelson CL (1946) The aspiration of stomach contents into the lungs during obstetric anaesthesia. Am J Obstet Gynaecol 52: 191–199

McHugh TJ, Forrester JS, Adler L et al. (1972) Pulmonary vascular congestion in acute myocardial infarction: Haemodynamic and radiological considerations. Ann Intern Med 76: 29–36

Milne ENC (1978) Some new concepts of pulmonary blood flow and volume. Radiol Clin North Am 16: 515–536

Putman CE, Tummillo A, Myerson D et al. (1975) Drowning: another plunge. AJR 125: 543–536

Putman CE, Goodman L (1983) Imaging in the critically ill or injured. In: Shoemaker WC, Thompson WL, (eds) Critical care: State of the Art. Fullerton: The Society of Critical Care Medicine 4(A): 1–63

Sibbald WJ, Warshawski FJ, Shork AK, Harris J, Lefcoe MS, Holliday RL (1983) Clinical studies of measuring extravascular lung water by the thermal dye technique in critically ill patients. Chest 83: 725–731

Snashall PD, Keyes SJ, Morgan BM, McAnulty RJ, Mitchell-Heggs PF, McIvor JM, Howlett FA (1981) The radiographic detection of acute pulmonary oedema. A comparison of radiographic appearances, densitometry and lung water in dogs. Br J Radiol 54: 277–288

Starling EH (1886) On the absorption of fluids from the connective tissue spaces. J Physiol 19: 312–328

Slasky BS, Auerbach D, Skolnick ML (1983) Value of portable real-time ultrasound in the ICU. Crit Care Med 11: 160–164

Staub NC (1974) Pulmonary oedema. Physiol Rev 54: 674–811

Stevens JM, Lees WR, Mason RR (1983) Radiology. In: Tinker J, Rapin M (eds) Care of the critically ill patient. Berlin: Springer-Verlag. pp 963–983

Strain DS, Kinasewitz GT, Vereen LE, George RB (1985) Value of routine daily chest X-rays in the medical intensive unit. Crit Care Med 13: 534–536

Swischuk LE (1977) Bubbles in hyaline membrane disease. Differentiation of three types. Radiology 122: 417–426

Twigley AJ, Hillman KM (1985) The end of the crystalloid era? Anaesthesia 40: 860–871

Chapter 6

Computed Tomography in Acute Respiratory Failure

L. Gattinoni, A. Pesenti, A. Torresin, S. Vesconi, G. P. Rossi, R. Fumagalli,
R. Marcolin, D. Mascheroni, M. Langer, G. Iapichino, F. Rossi and S. Baglioni

Introduction

The Adult Respiratory Distress Syndrome (ARDS) is characterised by increased permeability of the lung capillaries with consequent pulmonary oedema and increased extravascular lung water. This leads to an increase in the density $(g\,cm^{-3})$ of the lungs. Computed tomography (CT) may detect the density changes in the lung parenchyma without interference from overlying and underlying structures. CT scanning has only rarely been used in the study of ARDS patients (Rommelsheim et al. 1983; Gattinoni et al. 1986 a, b), probably because of the difficulties in transporting critically ill patients with life-threatening conditions which necessitate some form of respiratory assistance. We describe in this chapter our approach to the CT scanning of patients with ARDS and, in particular:

1. The diagnostic value
2. The morphological pattern of ARDS as visualised by CT scan
3. The morphological response to changes in positive end expiratory pressure (PEEP), mode of ventilation and body position
4. The "quantitative" profiles of ARDS in terms of density distribution and the quantitative estimation of lung weight by CT scan.

Methods: Computed Tomography, Methodological Approach

A Pfizer AS/EO 450 CT scanner was used. The exposures were taken at 120 KV, 50 mm A, 5 s.

The slice thickness was 9 mm, the dimensions of the pixel of the reconstruction matrix were 1.5×1.5 mm.

The technical characteristics of the CT scanner used have been described in detail elsewhere (Borasi et al. 1984). The spatial resolution was 0.31 p/mm at 50% of modulation transfer function with a standard deviation of 4.5 Hounsfield units (H). The system was calibrated using an appropriate phantom.

Diagnostic Studies

In diagnostic studies of patients with ARDS the main indications were for the detection of a lung abscess or a localised tension pneumothorax in anterior or posterior regions of the lungs. In these circumstances the patients underwent a normal CT scan and the ventilatory treatment was the same as that normally undertaken in an intensive therapy unit (ITU) such as continuous positive pressure ventilation (CPPV) or continuous positive airway pressure (CPAP).

Functional Studies

A series of studies was made to detect the morphological changes induced during CPPV by variations of positive and expiratory pressure (PEEP). The aim was to determine the extent of recruitment. In another series of patients with ARDS the morphological pattern during spontaneous breathing with CPAP was investigated.

Finally, a third series of patients was studied in different positions (from supine to prone) with fixed ventilator settings. The functional studies were performed by scanning three lung levels (apex, hilum and base above the diaphragm) after the acquisition of a frontal tomogram of the chest as described by Hedenstierna et al. (1985) for normal anaesthetised and paralysed subjects.

Imaging Analysis

The transverse areas of the thorax were obtained planimetrically. In the case of each lung the boundary was drawn manually along the inside of the ribs and the edge of the mediastinal organs. The total cross-sectional lung surface area was then obtained from the scan of each of the 6 individual areas (2 apex, 2 hilum, 2 base).

The surfaces of the contoured areas (in cm) were computed by the PDP 11/23 Digital computer (RT II operative sytem).

The planimetric method used was checked by scanning a model of different materials of known area. The coefficient of variation was in the range 0.3% to 1%.

In the planimetry of the real images with areas of different size and shape the coefficient of variation ranged from 1% and 7% (the higher the area, the lower the error).

CT Number and Physical Density

Every pixel of the CT scan image was characterised by a CT number. The CT number was defined as the difference between the attenuation coefficient of the X-ray in a defined volume of the studied material and the water attenuation coefficient. The CT numbers, expressed as Hounsfield units (H), lie on a scale of 0 to 1000 (water $= 0$ H, air $= 1000$ H).

The relationship between the CT number and the density is quite complex and is dependent on the incident energy, the atomic number of the lung tissue, the mass electron density and the density itself. However, in a given isolated lung, we found, as expected, that a reduction in density (ie increase of air in the lung) was linearly related to the mean CT number of the whole lung. The CT number was thus strictly related to the gas/tissue ratio.

Frequency Distribution of CT Numbers

The frequency distribution of the CT numbers of the total cross-sectional lung surface area (nor-

malised to units) was computed using eleven equally spaced intervals from -900 h to $+100$ h in steps of 100 H. Pixels showing a CT number below -400 H were considered to be indicative of areas of pathology. The percentage of pathological surface was then computed as the cumulative frequency from $+100$ H to -400 H inclusive.

Lung Weight Computation

We considered the lung to be made up only of a mixture of water and air. Additionally we assumed that the three CT sections obtained (apex, hilum and base) were a representative sample of the total cross-sectional lung surface area and would provide a valid estimate of the mean CT number of the whole lung.

To compute the fraction of the lung that was occupied by air, we used the relationship:

$$\text{Fraction of air} = \frac{\text{Mean CT number of the whole lung}}{(\text{CT number of the air}) - (\text{CT number of the water})}$$

where the fraction of air was the ratio of the volume of air to the volume of air plus the volume of the lung tissue. Determination of the total amount of air in the lung by an independent procedure (FRC by helium dilution) enabled us to compute lung weight.

The validity of this computation procedure was tested in isolated pig lungs of known weight scanned at different states of inflation.

Results

Diagnostic Value

Figure 6.1 shows an example of the difference between a conventional X-ray and the CT scan, taken 1 h apart. The end expiratory pressure level, the clinical condition of the patient, the ventilator settings and the gas exchange were constant. The CT scan shows pneumothoraces on both sides that were not clearly detectable on the conventional X-ray. We have in the last few years seen several such cases suggesting that the incidence of anterior and posterior pneumothorax without complete lung collapse is probably higher than has been suspected.

Morphological Pattern in ARDS

The morphological pattern of ARDS, in patients treated with muscle relaxants, anaesthesia and

Fig. 6.1. Example of the diagnostic value of the CT scan during ARDS (from bacterial pneumonia). The CT scan shows a right pneumothorax (less readily detectable on the chest X-ray films). A tension pneumothorax in the left lung is questionable on the X-ray film but evident on the CT scan.

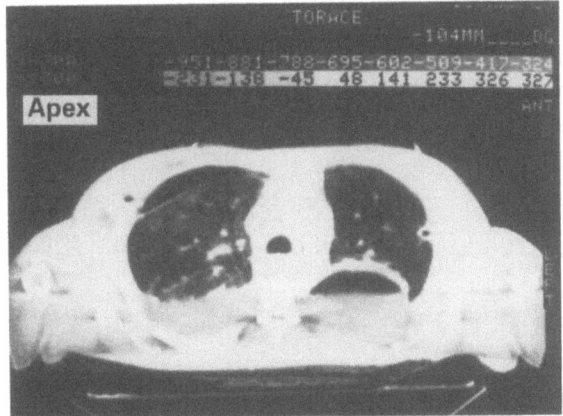

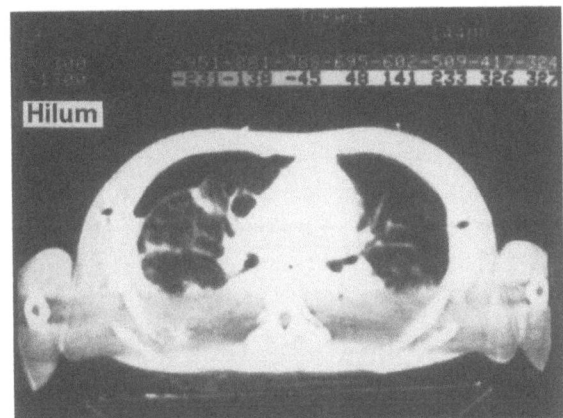

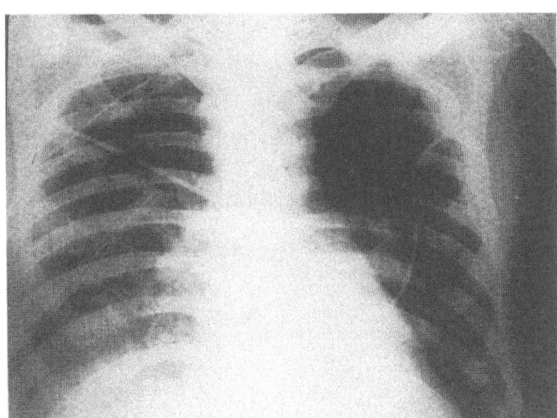

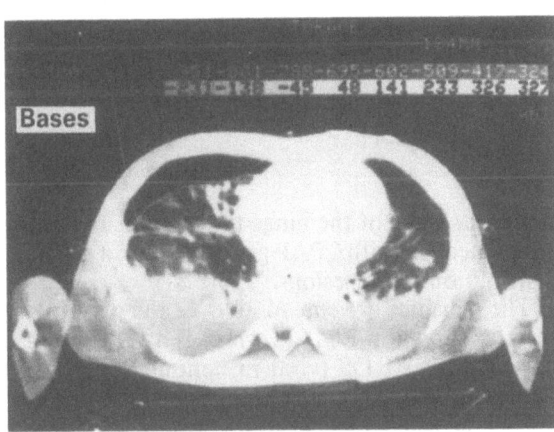

mechanical ventilation, typically shows the lower parts of both lungs to be more affected than the upper. Thus the hila and bases are generally more affected than the apices. Figure 6.2 shows a representative example of the lungs of a patient with ARDS as seen by the CT scan. The parenchyma appears as a patchwork of dense and ventilated areas, mostly with well-defined boundaries.

Morphological Response to PEEP

Sixteen patients with ARDS of various origins were subjected to CT scanning at three levels of Peep (5, 10 and 15 cm H_2O) with all the other ventilatory parameters unchanged. Most of the patients showed a decrease in density highly correlated with the changes in oxygenation. Figure 6.3 shows a typical response to an increase in PEEP in a patient with ARDS (bacterial pneumonia). The effects of PEEP are generally more evident at the hila and

bases and no significant changes are found at the apices (Gattinoni et al. 1986 a).

ARDS Morphology during Spontaneous Breathing

While during mechanical ventilation patients with ARDS show more accumulation of dense areas in

Fig. 6.2. Example of ARDS pattern on the CT scan during CPPV (ARDS from bacterial pneumonia). Both CT scan and X-ray films were taken at $15\,cmH_2O$ PEEP, at the end of the expiration. $PaO_2 = 48$ mmHg, shunt fraction 60%, FiO_2 1.0.

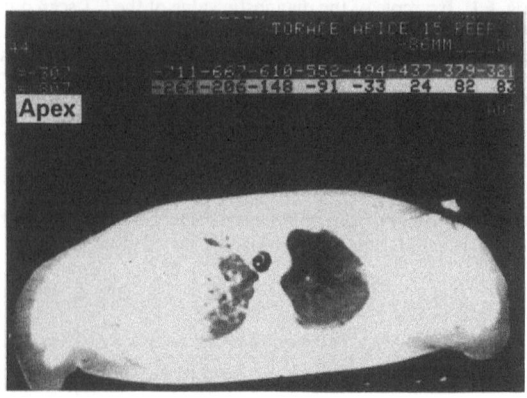

PEEP = 15 cmH₂0

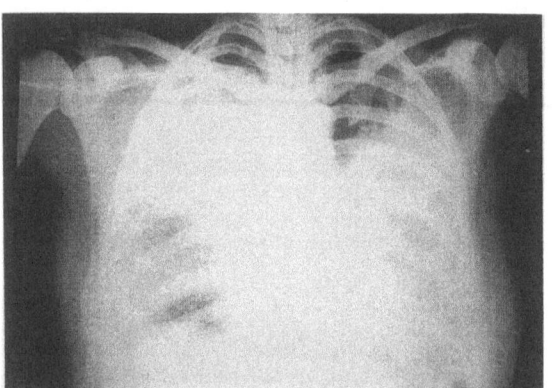

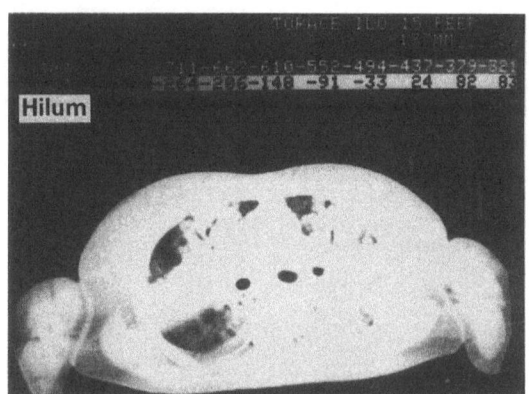

PEEP= 15 cmH₂0

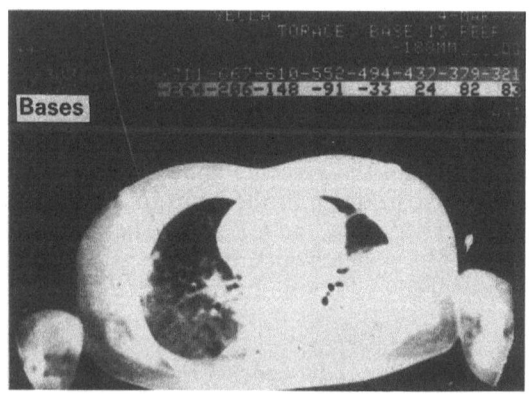

PEEP = 15 cmH₂0

the lower parts of the lungs the patients breathing spontaneously with CPAP generally have a different distribution of the lesions.

The densities are spread all over the pulmonary field, as shown in Fig. 6.4, which is a CT scan of a patient with ARDS (viral pneumonia). The same patient for clinical reasons had to be anaesthetised and paralysed. The anaesthesia was started in the CT scanner suite and Fig. 6.5 shows the effect of changing from CPAP tp CPPV (plus paralysis and anaesthesia) after 30 min. The densities appear to be concentrated in the lower parts of the lungs as is usually found in patients treated in this way.

Dense areas, however, as shown by Hedenstierna et al. (1985) are a common finding during anaesthesia even in normal subjects. Unfortunately it is not possible to "quantitate" the individual contributions of mechanical ventilation, anaesthesia and paralysis to the modification of the dis-

tributions when the change is made from CPAP to CPPV. Although very few observations have been made in patients with ARDS treated with CPAP, our preliminary findings suggest that the mode of ventilatory treatment may alter the topography of the densities very markedly.

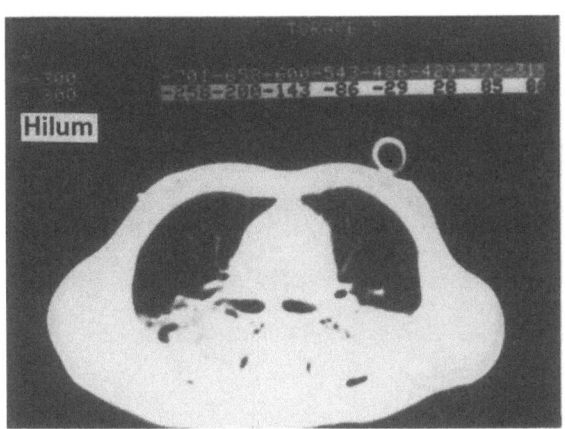

PEEP = 5 cmH₂0

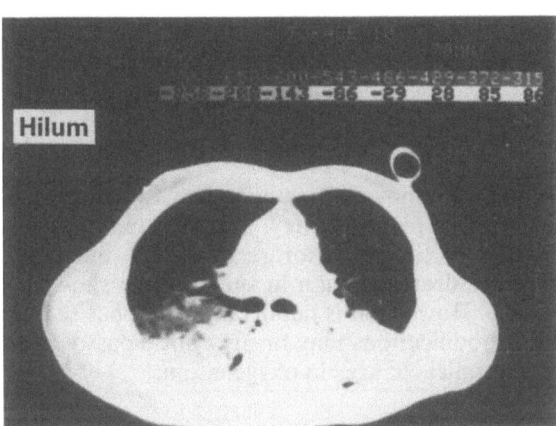

PEEP = 10 cmH₂0

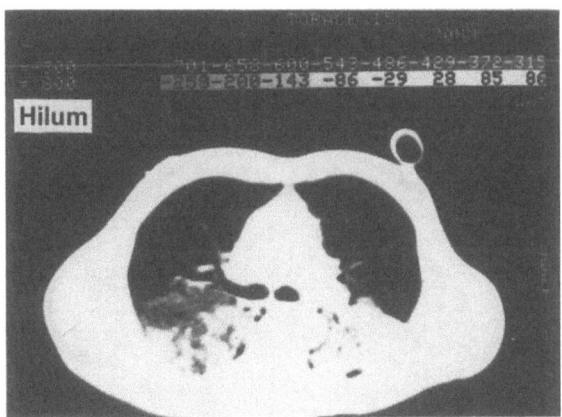

PEEP = 15 cmH₂0

Fig. 6.3. Effect of PEEP (from 5 to 15 cm H₂O) on CT scan morphology during CPPV (ARDS from bacterial pneumonia). Substantial clearing of the right lung can be seen. Shunt fraction 43% at 5 cmH₂O PEEP, 42% at 10 cmH₂O PEEP, 30% at 15 cmH₂O PEEP.

CPAP = 10 cmH₂0

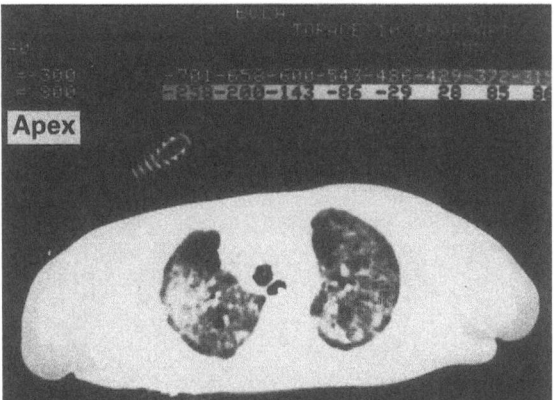

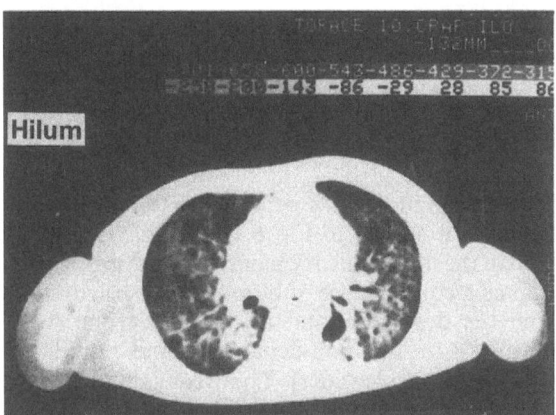

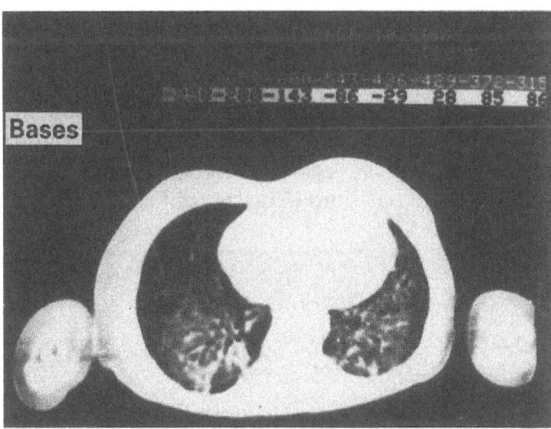

Fig. 6.4. Example of ARDS pattern on the CT scan during spontaneous breathing (viral pneumonia). PEEP = 10 cmH₂O.

Effects of Positioning on the Topography of the Densities

Douglas et al. (1977) and Langer et al. (1986) reported a beneficial effect of the prone position on

CPAP

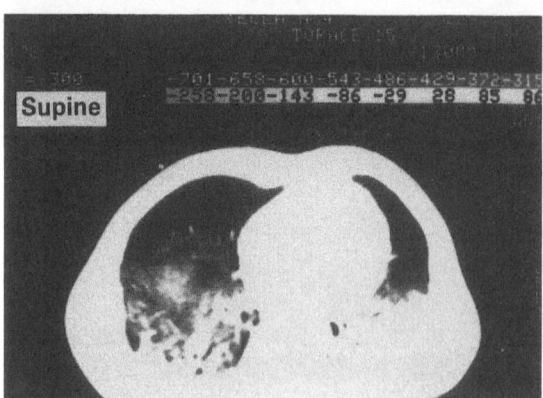

CPPV

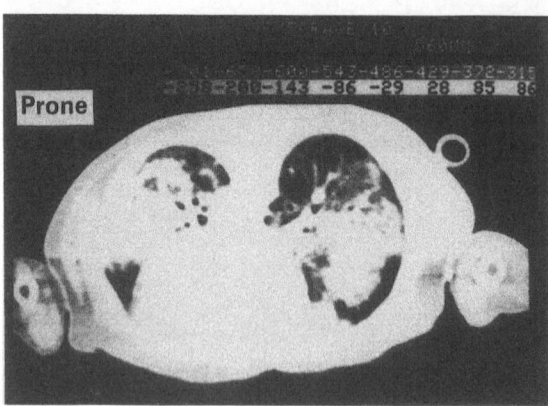

PEEP = 15 cmH₂0

Fig. 6.5. Changes of density distribution, as detected by CT scan, when changing from CPAP to CPPV at the same PEEP level (15 cmH₂O).

oxygenation in patients with ARDS. In the light of the pattern shown in Fig. 6.1, it seems logical to explain the improved oxygenation in the prone position as a consequence of blood flow redistribution from the dependent and unventilated zone (with densities) to the non-dependent and ventilated zones (without densities). To investigate this effect we studied patients with ARDS in both the supine and the prone position while maintaining the same PEEP and identical ventilatory conditions.

Surprisingly we consistently found that, with or without improved oxygenation, the densities migrated from the previously dependent regions (posterior regions of the lung in supine position) to the new dependent regions (anterior regions of the lung in prone position) (Mascheroni et al. 1986).

Figure 6.6 shows an example of this phenomenon which takes place in a few minutes (15 min). The clearing of the posterior regions was sometimes far more dramatic than in the example shown in Fig. 6.6. However it is important to emphasise that these modifications may or may not be associated with parallel changes in oxygenation.

ARDS Profiles by CT Number Distribution

The CT scan picture provides information about the topography of the lesions and, in some cases, about the nature of the lesions (abscess, pneumothorax, effusions etc). However, information about the numbers of densities is equally important.

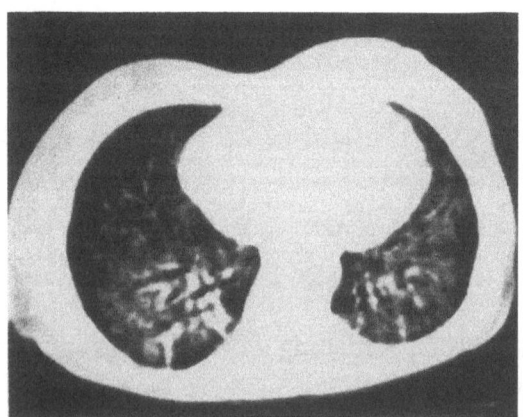

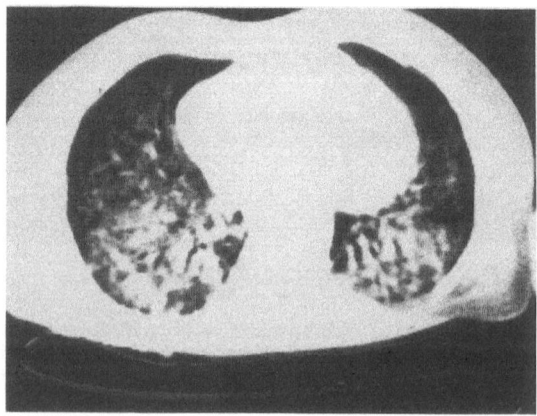

Fig. 6.6. Effect of change from the supine to the prone position on the distribution of densities. Evident clearing of the posterior regions of the lungs can be seen.

At the first attempt we had to establish a definite CT number to distinguish between normality and "pathology" of the lung parenchyma. We chose a CT = −400 H as the discriminant value following Rosenblum et al. (1980) who had found, in normal subjects, lung parenchyma CT numbers ranging from −400 H to −900 H, −400 H being the highest "normal" CT number observed in healthy adult lungs. Using a CT = −400 H as the discriminant value we found that densities (ie, areas of lung with CT ⩽ −400 H) in patients with ARDS ranged from 20% to 90% of the total cross-sectional area (ie, the sum of areas of apex, hilum and base). These densities were negatively correlated with arterial oxygenation. The CT value of −400 H appears to be a reasonable rough discriminant value between normal and dense areas. However, to describe the ARDS lung rather better we used a CT scan distribution employing a model of 11 equally spaced compartments (from −1000 H to +100 H in steps of 100 H). Using this approach (Pesenti et al. 1986) normal lungs showed a unimodal narrow distribution with the mode in the −800 H, −700 H compartment.

In patients with ARDS we found three patterns of distribution (types 1, 2 and 3) as shown in Fig. 6.7. Type 1 patients had a bimodal distribution (one mode in almost the normal range (−700 H) and a second mode near to the water compartment (0 H)). Type 2 patients had a unimodal narrow distribution with the mode close to the water compartment (0 H), while type 3 patients had a broad CT distribution in the abnormal CT range. The physiological significance of these different distribution patterns is not clear. It is possible that the different types reflect different pathologies or degrees of pathology. Moreover, the different types may show a different response to the application of PEEP. Type 1 patients, for example, seem to respond less effectively to PEEP than do type 2 and type 3 patients.

Lung Weight Computation

Using isolated pig lungs we were able to establish the relationship:

$$\frac{\text{Air Volume}}{\text{Air volume} + \text{tissue volume}} =$$

$$\frac{\text{Mean CT number of the whole lung}}{(\text{CT number of the air}) - (\text{CT number of the water})}$$

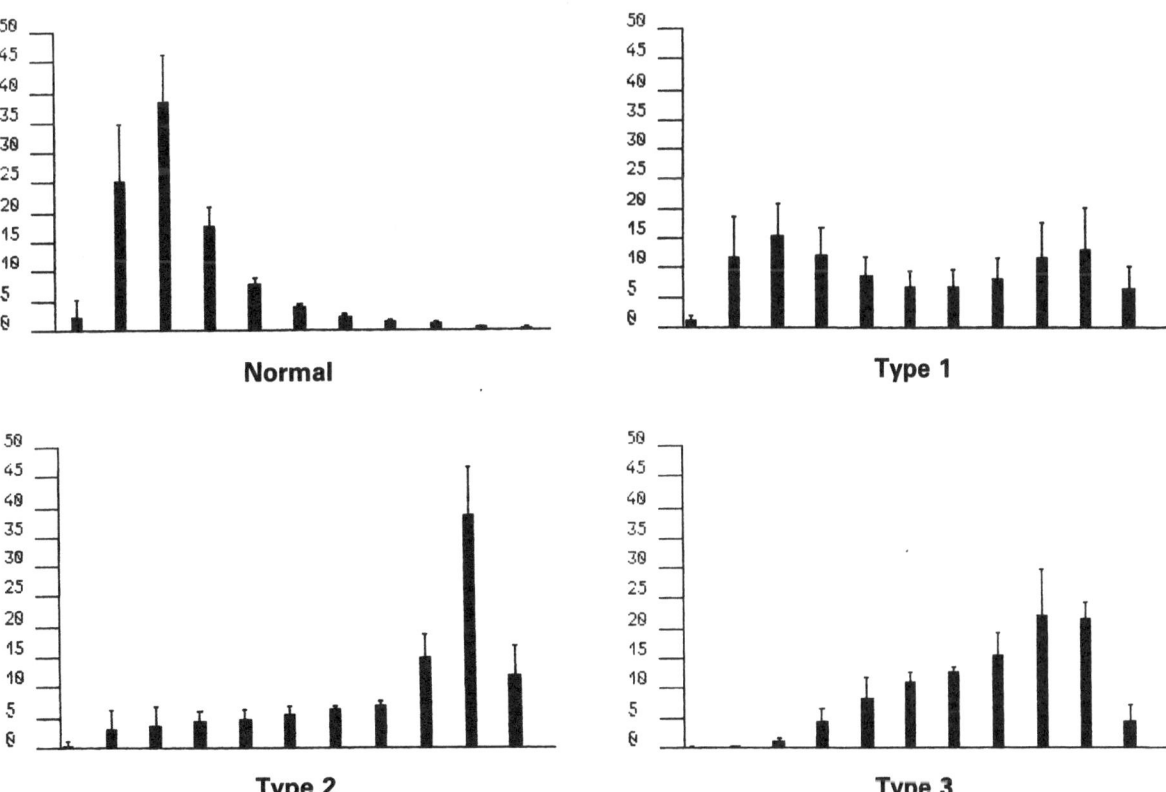

Fig. 6.7. CT number distribution in normal subjects and in types 1, 2 and 3 patients. In each panel the 11 bars refer to 11 compartments equally spaced in steps of 100 from −1000 H to −900 H, (first compartment, left) to 0 H, to 100 H (11th, right).

The correlation coefficient was greater than 0.9 (Gattinoni et al. 1986b). It appears that the mean CT number closely reflects the amount of air in the lungs. Having determined the volume of air by independent measurement (we used the helium dilution method) and by assuming the specific weight of the tissue to be equal to 1, the lung weight was easily calculated.

In the isolated lung, in controlled conditions, the difference between the measured lung weight and the computed lung weight was 3%. However, to compute the lung weight "in vivo" (after measuring the lung volume by the helium dilution method) we had to assume that the mean CT number of the total cross-sectional lung surface (which was measured) is a reasonable estimate of the mean CT number of the whole lung.

In normal subjects, due to the substantial uniformity of the lung parenchyma, this could be easily accepted. In normal volunteers, in whom the CT scan was performed as in patients with ARDS and where FRC was measured by the same method, the average lung weight (including blood) was 19.00 ± 2 g/kg body weight. This value is close to the average weight of healthy lungs measured at autopsy (International Commission on Radiological Protection 1975).

It is questionable whether, in particular ARDS patients, three slices (apex, hilum and base) are a representative estimate of the whole lung. However, when we computed the lung weight in these patients we found an average of 40 g/kg body weight. This value fits very well with the values observed at autopsy in patients with ARDS (Teplitz 1976).

The net increase in lung weight in comparison to normal controls is definitely higher than the increase in extravascular lung water (EVLW) measured in patients with ARDS by the double indicator technique (Sibbald et al. 1985). However, it is important to recall that the thermodilution measures only the EVLW of the perfused regions while the CT scan detects the non-perfused regions also. Both PaO_2 and shunt fraction were highly correlated with the lung weight.

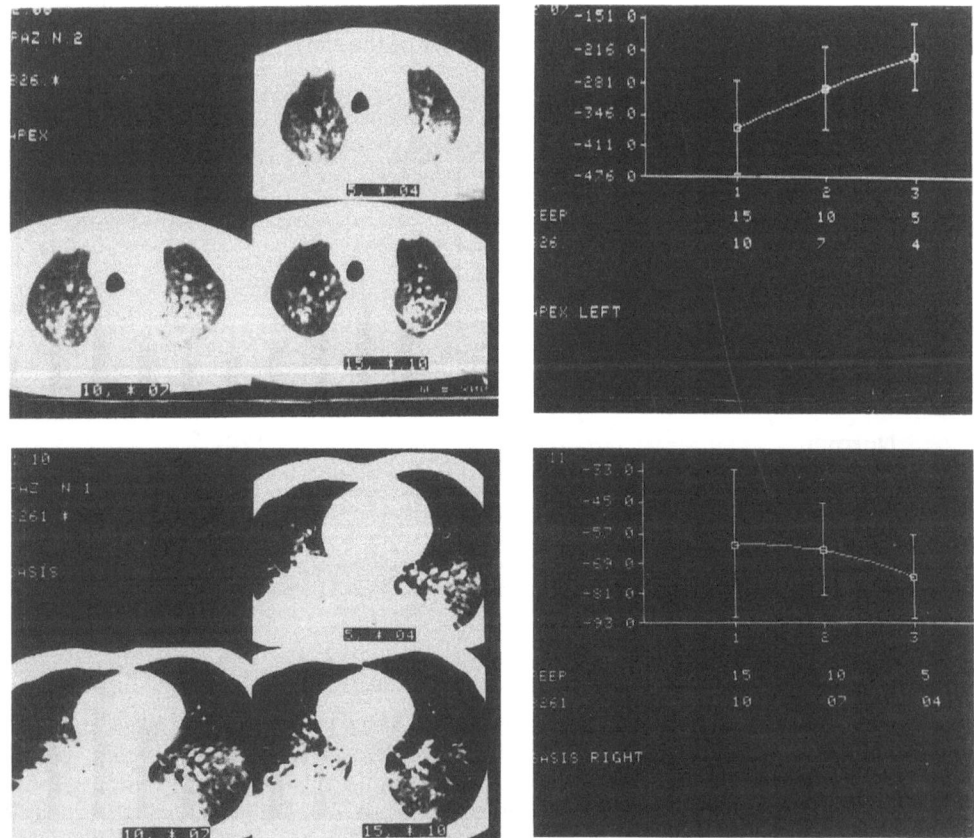

Fig. 6.8. Upper panel. Clearing of the left apex from 5 to 15 cmH$_2$O. The mean CT number of the dense area became more negative (increase in gas/tissue ratio). Lower panel, right lung. From 5 to 15 cmH$_2$O PEEP the mean CT number of the dense area became less negative (decrease in gas/tissue ratio). The left lung, on the contrary, showed a reduction in density.

Nature of the Densities

Consolidation, oedema and atelectasis are generally considered to be the pathological substrate of the lung in ARDS. Unfortunately, with the CT scan we cannot discriminate between these conditions which all appear as densities. However, some inferences about the nature of the densities may be made when we consider the morphological response to changes in PEEP, positioning, etc to which the patients were subjected.

While the oedema and atelectasis may change with PEEP (reabsorption, opening pressure etc) consolidation will persist. Moreover, the effect of PEEP on the lung regions around the consolidation could compress the consolidation, thus increasing the density. On the other hand, a sudden and complete clearing of one lung region when PEEP is applied could be due to the opening of atelectasis. Figure 6.8 shows an example of this phenomenon. The same region of the lung was examined at three different levels of PEEP. The PEEP-induced clearing of the density in the right lung (upper panel) is shown by the reduction in the CT number (ie, increased air/tissue ratio); in the left lung (lower panel) increasing levels of PEEP led to an increase in density (compression of a consolidated region?) as shown by the increase in the CT number. In this patient the increase in PEEP reduced arterial oxygenation.

Conclusion

At the moment the distinction between oedema and atelectasis remains difficult. However, the response to PEEP or to changes in position occur very rapidly. This supports the hypothesis that the changes in densities observed are caused by resolving atelectasis.

Acknowledgement. This work has been supported in part by CNR grants nos. 840209887 and 850148758, Rome "Special projects in biomedical engineering".

References

Borasi G, Castellani G, Domenichini R et al. (1984) Image quality and dose in computerized tomography: evaluation of four CT scanners. Med Phys 11: 321

Douglas W, Rehder K, Beynen FM et al. (1977) Improved oxygenation in patients with acute respiratory failure: the prone position. Am Rev Respir dis 115: 559–566.

Gattinoni L, Mascheroni D, Torresin A et al. (1986 a) Morphological response to positive end expiratory pressure in acute respiratory failure. Computerized tomography study. Intensive Care Med 12: 137–142.

Gattinoni L, Pesenti A, Torresin A et al. (1986 b) ARDS profiles by computerized tomography. J Thorac Imaging, 3: 25–30.

Hedenstierna G, Strandberg A, Brismar B et al. (1985) Functional Residual Capacity, thoraco-abdominal dimensions and central blood volume, during general anesthesia with muscle paralysis and mechanical ventilation. Anesthesiology 62: 247–254.

International Commission on Radiological Protection (ICRP) (1975) Report of the Task Group on reference man. 1: 8.

Langer M, Mascheroni D, Beck E et al. (1986) The effects of prone position in ARDS patients. 3rd Europ. Congr. on Intensive Care Medicine, 125: 168.

Mascheroni D. Marcolin R, Fumagalli R et al. (1986) Effects of positioning in ARF. CT scan study. 3rd Europ. Congr. on Intensive Care Medicine, 125: 222.

Pesenti A, Gattinoni L, Torresin A, et al. (1986) Quantitative morphometric evaluation of lung CT scan in Arf. 3rd Europ. Congr. on Intensive Care Medicine, 125: 220.

Rommelsheim K, Lackner K, Westhofen P et al. (1983) Dan respiratorische Distress-Syndrom des Erwachsenen (ARDS) im computertomogramm. Anaesth. Intensivither Noftallmed 18: 59.

Rosenblum LJ, Mauceri RA, Wellenstein DE, et al. (1980) Density patterns in the normal lung as determined by computed tomography. Radiology 137: 409–416.

Sibbald WJ, Short AK, Warshawski FJ, et al. (1985) Thermal dye measurements of extravascular lung water in critically ill patients. Chest 87: 585–592.

Teplitz C (1976) The core pathobiology and integrated medical science of adult acute respiratory insufficiency. Surg Clin North Am 56: 1091–1133.

Chapter 7

Radionuclide Imaging of the Lungs

R. F. Jewkes

Disorders of the respiratory tract are very common in the intensive therapy unit (ITU) probably affecting the majority of patients. Even if such patients do not originally present with lung disease, immobility, severe illness with infection, prolonged assisted ventilation and embolism may result in life-threatening respiratory disorders. Sometimes the patient's condition is clear-cut and may be allocated to a definite diagnostic category, specific or non-specific pneumonia, pulmonary embolism or chronic obstructive airways disease, but often the causes are multiple and difficult to define and the best that can be done is a statement of the physiological deficit to suggest what remedies are required. For instance hypoxia to some degree is almost universal after major surgery and has various causes (Cooper 1972). Apart from the depressant effect of anaesthesia and analgesia, abdominal pain may severely affect ventilation. Functional residual capacity is reduced and closing volume affected adversely. Spontaneous tidal breathing of such patients occurs from a lower total lung volume, with impaired expiration from early small airways closure, particularly at the lung bases. Against this picture it may be difficult to recognise focal pulmonary atelectasis, pneumonic consolidation and major bronchial obstruction. In some of the very ill, the cause of severe respiratory failure may be quite obscure. Some of these difficult cases may seem to merge into typical adult respiratory distress syndrome (ARDS) with obvious widespread lung damage.

Periodic assessment of the state of the lungs and the efficacy of respiration is an essential part of the care of such patients. After clinical examination, the chest radiograph and analysis of blood gases are probably the commonest investigations. Analysis of blood gases may show the total effectiveness of respiration, but gives only a hint of the nature of the patho-physiology and no regional information concerning the lungs. It has long been recognised that there may be no relationship between the degree of post-operative hypoxia and clinical and radiological chest findings (Hamilton et al. 1964). This is not really surprising. The chest radiograph shows where the air is in the thorax, not where effective ventilation is occurring. It provides virtually no information about the distribution of lung perfusion.

Scintigraphic radionuclide studies are relatively simple techniques which can show vividly the distribution of both ventilation and perfusion. Gamma-camera images can often be analysed adequately by simple inspection, though modern gamma cameras frequently have computer facilities which allow more complex analyses to be carried out. Moving a sick patient, perhaps with a ventilator, to a nuclear medicine facility may be a major undertaking, but will be well rewarded by the quality of information which is obtainable. In the best equipped units a portable gamma camera may be available in the ITU. These cameras are mainly intended for cardiac imaging, but those with a larger field of view may make adequate pictures of ventilation and perfusion without the patient having to be moved from his treatment room. This may be a great help in managing very ill patients but such bed-side investigations are not ideal as a full series of views is difficult to obtain. However, for the demonstration of gross patho-physiological changes such a limited study may be adequate.

Lung scintigraphy has two aspects, the depiction of the pattern of pulmonary arterial flow to the lungs (perfusion imaging) and the demonstration of the distribution of ventilation.

Perfusion Imaging

Perfusion imaging is initiated by the intravenous injection of Technetium-99m-labelled particles of denatured human serum albumin. These may be either macro-aggregates or microspheres which are available commercially and seem equally satisfactory. The distribution of radioactive particles to each region of the lung is proportional to the fraction of pulmonary arterial blood flow which the region receives. Conventional doses $(2–5\,mC^{99m}Tc)$ represent 50000 to 150000 particles of $5–100\,\mu m$ in diameter which in the normal subject represents plugging of one in a thousand arterioles (Harding et al. 1983). They have a half-life of 2–9 h before being broken down in situ. This gives a wide margin of safety even in patients with a restricted volume of functioning lung. Special preparation of high specific radioactivity particles is only required in patients with severe pulmonary hypertension.

Images of the perfusion patterns can be made immediately from various angles, each view taking 0.5 to 1.5 min. The most important views are the posterior, allowing comparison of the two lungs, and the posterior oblique views of regional assessment. Lateral views may be easier to produce in a patient who must remain supine, if allowance is made for any "shine-through" from the more distant lung. Anterior and anterior oblique views are easiest to produce but unfortunately less helpful.

Occasionally it may be distressing for a patient to cooperate for more than a short period. In such cases it may be desirable to increase the dose of administered radioactivity, if necessary by a factor of 2 or 3. A more desirable alternative is the use of a high-sensitivity collimator on the gamma camera if one is available. This can achieve the same effect at the expense of lower resolution of the images. However this can usually be tolerated as the test compares relatively large lung areas imaged against the inevitable motion of tidal breathing.

When the injection is given to an upright or semi-recumbent normal subject, distribution is homogeneous but there is a gradation of distribution with relatively less radioactivity in the upper zones than at the lung bases. The lung outlines correspond to those of the chest radiograph. In the ITU, patients are nearly always injected supine. When an injection is given to a supine healthy subject, the gradation disappears and there is an even distribution of radioactivity from base to apex. The primary factor determining the distribution in a patient is the distribution of *ventilation* which is usually abnormal in some way.

Regions of lung with reduced ventilation are usually associated with reduced regional pulmonary perfusion, similarly distributed though often of lesser extent. This relationship renders an isolated perfusion scan often difficult to interpret without some demonstration of regional ventilation. The supine patient who is ill or has undergone recent surgery virtually always has reduced ventilation of the lower lobes compared with the upper lobes, and perfusion will be similarly affected (Fig. 7.5a, b).

Ventilation Imaging

Ventilation patterns are not quite so readily demonstrated as perfusion patterns. Either the radioactive substance is only periodically available (radiokrypton) or the demonstration requires some ingenuity and practice (radioxenon or technetium aerosols). Though pulmonary embolism is the most commonly suspected pulmonary complication, in practice ventilation abnormalities are much more frequent and ventilation images are essential for a complete statement concerning the distribution of pulmonary function. The effort involved is well worthwhile.

Use of Radiokrypton (81-Kr)

The radioactive agent that best demonstrates ventilation is krypton-81m (Fazlo and Jones 1976). The most striking characteristic of radiokrypton is its transience (half-life 13 s). The practical importance of this (besides eliminating any hazard from exhaled radioactivity!) is that though the radioactivity readily penetrates well-ventilated regions, it cannot build up in poorly ventilated regions. However long it may be breathed any penetration of radioactive krypton molecules into such areas is more than matched by the rate of physical decay. Images of radioactive krypton therefore demonstrate effective ventilation (or more correctly ventilation per unit lung volume) and not total lung volume.

Radiokrypton has to be produced on the spot where the ventilation imaging is being carried out. This is achieved by a 'krypton generator', a small quantity of radioactive rubidium in a convenient lead-shielded container. The radioactive decay of the rubidium atoms produces radioactive krypton gas which can be removed by a gentle air stream and breathed by the subject through a simple face mask. Images can be made from any chosen angle, each view usually taking 1–3 min to complete.

Gamma rays emitted by radiokrypton have a slightly higher energy than those from technetium-99m and this difference can be distinguished by appropriate adjustment of the gamma camera. Radiokrypton distribution can therefore be imaged even in the presence of injected technetium particles. Conversely, technetium imaging is simply done as the krypton is rapidly eliminated when the airstream is turned off. Sequential ventilation and perfusion images can be made from each chosen angle, permitting precise comparison of any defects. All illustrations of ventilation patterns in this chapter are of radiokrypton studies unless otherwise stated.

The disadvantage of radiokrypton is its limited availability. Rubidium generators are only productive on the day of manufacture. Most centres can only obtain krypton for ventilation imaging on one or at most two days each week. Since respiratory problems will often not await the availability of radiokrypton, especially in the ITU, other agents are still in use or are being developed.

Use of radioxenon (^{133}Xe)

The original agent for ventilation studies was radioxenon (^{133}Xe), another inert gas (Alderson et al. 1976). With a half-life of about 5 days, it can be kept constantly available. Its disadvantages are, however, numerous. It emits a very low energy gamma ray which gives poor picture quality. The persistence of the radioactivity gives it a conveniently long shelf-life but limits its availability to show ventilation. If it is breathed for some minutes it will gradually penetrate ill-ventilated areas until they are indistinguishable from well-ventilated areas. To show effective ventilation therefore the gas should be administered as a bolus at a single inhalation, and an image made as rapidly as possible thereafter. In an acutely ill patient, such an image, if it can be obtained at all, is likely to be unrepresentative of tidal breathing. The alternative is for the air/radioxenon mixture to be administered from a spirometer or other rebreathing device. Usually a wash-in period of 3–4 min (if the patient can tolerate it) will suffice to achieve an equilibrium between the radioactive gas in the spirometer and the gas in the patient's lungs. Very poorly ventilated regions will fail to achieve equilibrium and will appear as defects in the lung image. The spirometer is then turned off and the patient allowed to respire room air for 5–10 min. Further images are made during this time and areas of poor ventilation can be identified if an uneven or irregular pattern develops as the gas is cleared from the lungs. Normally-ventilated lung will become indistinguishable from background in about 3 min. This technique can usually only be used to produce images from one view, usually posterior, and does not produce a complete set of images which are directly comparable to the perfusion series.

Use of Technetium aerosols

The most readily available form of radioactivity in a nuclear medicine department is technetium-99m. Ways of using this in aerosol form have been developed and have found favour despite certain disadvantages (Alderson et al. 1984; Agnew et al. 1982). The use of technetium aerosols is not new, but in recent years simpler and more effective nebulisers have become available (Adischan 1982). Deposition of aerosol particles depends on many factors, size, shape, density, and electrostatic charge, interacting with both lung geometry and the pattern of ventilation. Large particles (10 μm in diameter and larger) are deposited chiefly by impaction whilst smaller ones (1–5 μm in diameter) are deposited by sedimentation. The very small particles (those less than 1 μm in diameter) are spread by diffusion. Polydisperse aerosols (with a wide range of particle size) may produce a very uneven distribution of deposition in the respiratory tract, particularly if there is any obstruction of airways. Modern nebulising systems are more effective at filtering out the larger droplets, improving image quality and consistency. The nebuliser is charged with some technetium compound of which technetium DTPA (diethylene triamine penta acetic acid) seems the simplest and most popular. Following a period of inhalation lasting 0.5–2 min, pictures of pulmonary ventilation can be made from any desired angle.

In the absence of gross obstructive airways disease, the images are usually remarkably similar to those provided by radiokrypton, though there is some tendency for aerosols to deposit preferentially in the dependent parts. Obstruction of airways produces local turbulence which may lead to selective deposition of aerosol particles, producing disfiguring hot-spots along the major bronchi and giving the lung images a "lumpy" appearance. However, only in severe cases does this render the study useless. Concentrations of technetium in the oropharynx or swallowed in the oesophagus or stomach are easily identified.

At first sight there would seem to be a difficulty in the use of the aerosols in that they employ the same radionuclide as is used for perfusion imaging. In practice this difficulty can be easily overcome. The various views of the lungs have to be made sequentially. First of all the ventilation images and then the perfusion images (or occasionally the other way round). Though losing the elegant correspondence of ventilation and perfusion images possible with technetium and krypton, this is in practice a minor inconvenience. The second series

of pictures have to be made with 3–5 times as much radioactivity as is employed in the first series of pictures, to swamp the effects of the first dose of technetium. This is easier to manage if the injected perfusion scanning agent is given second.

Use of Technetium "Pseudogas"

Recently a new approach to the production of technetium aerosols, "pseudogas", has been used successfully (Burch et al. 1982). An ultra-fine mono disperse aerosol can be produce when an inflamm-

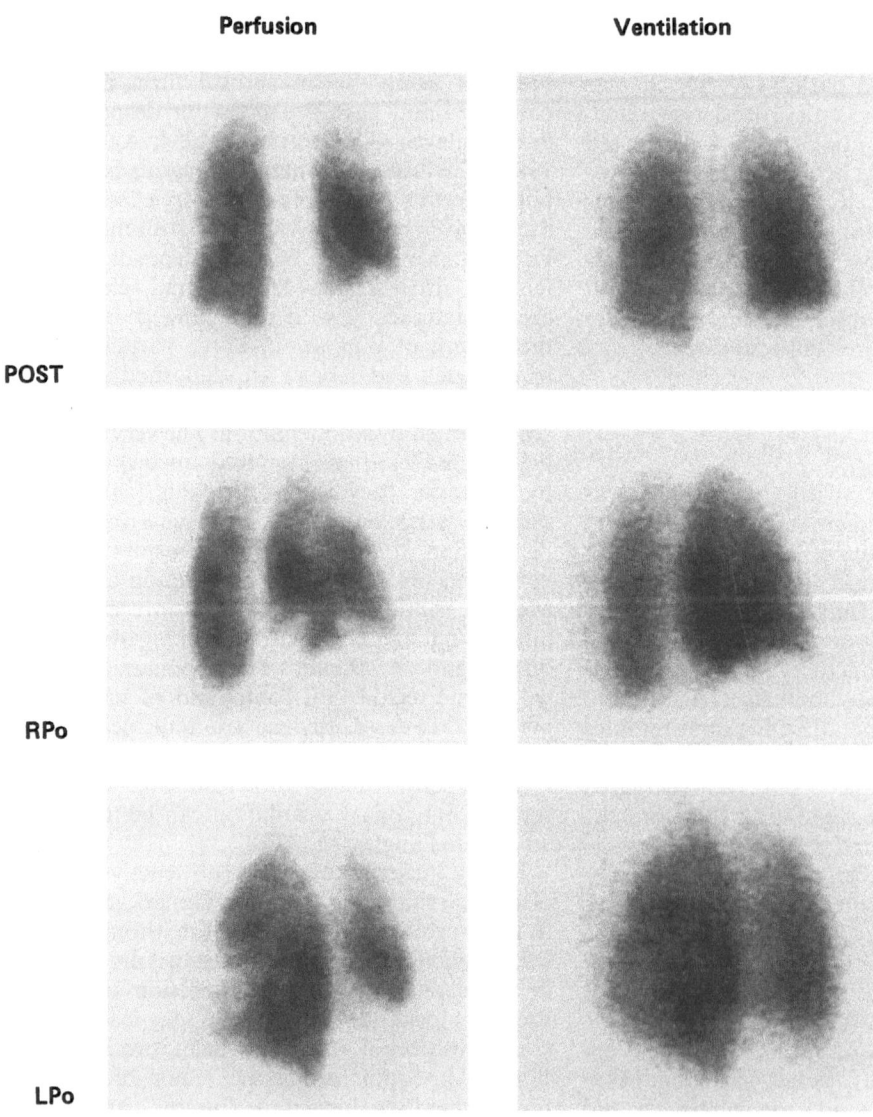

Perfusion   **Ventilation**

POST

RPo

LPo

Fig. 7.1. Scintigraphic diagnosis of pulmonary embolism: a typical presentation. The ventilation pattern (right) is normal but the perfusion pattern (left) shows abnormalities. *POST*, posterior view. *RPO*, right posterior oblique. *LPO*, left posterior oblique.

able spray (technetium in ethanol) is burned. The products of combustion are collected in an anaesthetic rebreathing bag and, after a few minutes to allow cooling, can be inhaled through a standard anaesthetic mask. Clearance from the alveoli into the blood stream gives a disappearance half-time between 10 and 100 min depending on the subject and the state of the lungs. This is sufficient time for as many views of the lungs as necessary, while the relatively rapid disappearance assists the subsequent imaging of perfusion. The quality of images seems rather better than with aerosols from conventional nebulisers and it is less likely to produce unhelpful images in cases of severe chronic obstructive airways disease.

The ventilation techniques can be used to assess patients receiving positive pressure ventilation. This is most easily done with radiokrypton, but methods have been described using 133-xenon (Vieras et al. 1982) and technetium aerosols (Vezing et al. 1985).

Imaging for Pulmonary Embolism

Pulmonary emboli are usually detached thrombi from the larger veins of the legs or the veins of the pelvis, less frequently from thrombosis in the inferior vena cava, the arms, the right side of the heart or intra-vascular indwelling catheters. Other causes of embolism include fat, air, liquor amnii or fragments of tumour. Immediately following an embolus, pulmonary blood flow is diverted to the rest of the lungs, pulmonary artery pressure rises but cardiac output is often little altered. This hyperperfusion of the unaffected lung appears to cause inefficient oxygenation of the pulmonary arterial blood with consequent clinical hypoxia. Clinical suspicion of pulmonary embolism must be the starting point, but it is notoriously inaccurate (Sasahara 1974). In the ITU setting, only a minority of cases where it is suspected show any confirmatory

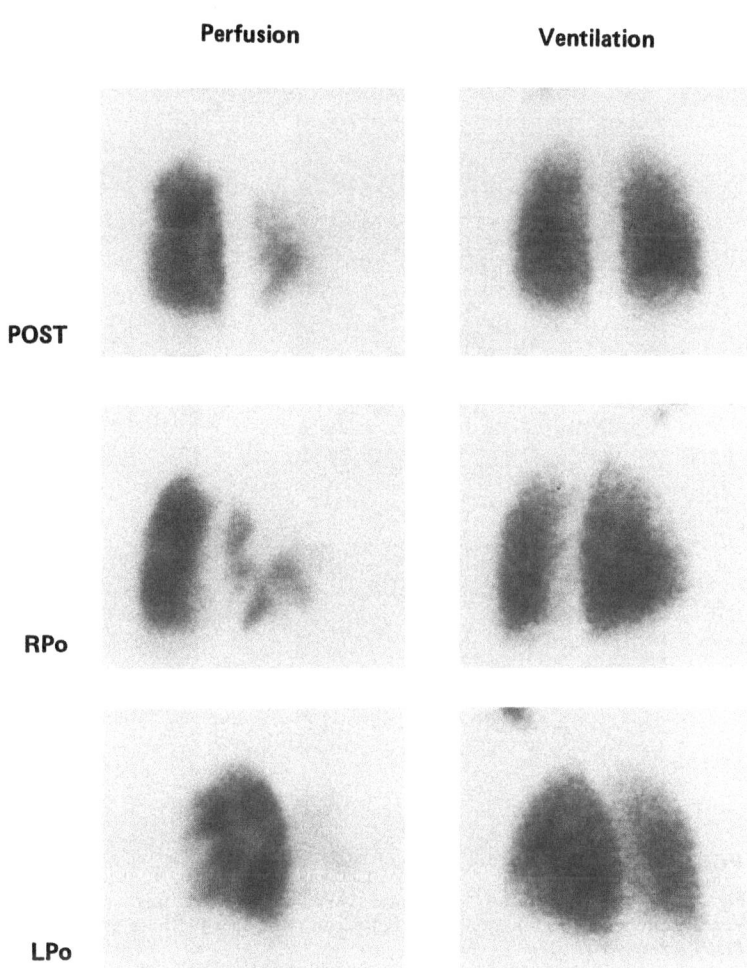

Perfusion   **Ventilation**

POST

RPo

LPo

Fig. 7.2. Scintigraphic diagnosis of pulmonary embolism; extensive pulmonary embolism. The ventilation pattern (right) is normal but perfusion images are abnormal. The posterior perfusion image (*POST*) shows gross asymmetry. *RPO*, right posterior oblique *LPO*, left posterior oblique.

evidence. Perfusion imaging is the easiest approach to the verification or refutation of this clinical suspicion.

Perhaps scans are most reliable when they are relatively "normal" as this makes pulmonary embolism extremely unlikely. In the ITU this means that though the distribution apex to base or between the lobes may not be quite that of a healthy subject, the distribution is relatively homogeneous and the whole outline of each lung can be seen to be intact. This can usually be best appreciated on posterior oblique views, but a posterior view is very desirable for direct comparison of the two lungs in case of gross inequality of total perfusion between the two sides. If the patient cannot easily be moved, other views may have to suffice. Unfortunately an anterior view rarely shows the left lung well because of the heart, and neither does it show the lung bases. Anterior oblique views are a second best to posterior oblique views, though they are obviously required if clinical suspicion makes an anterior lesion likely.

Pulmonary embolism is usually not associated with any change in ventilation. In fact pulmonary broncho-constriction of brief duration has been produced in experimental animals and has very rarely been recognised in ventilation studies on patients. However the normal delays in carrying out the test seem to prevent this being commonly recognised and it is not a likely cause of diagnostic confusion. Later, small areas of pulmonary atelectasis may develop, apparently due to deficient surfactant production in embolised regions. These may produce linear shadows on the chest radiograph but are usually too small to show up on the ventilation images which have much poorer resolution. Occasionally a region of lung may be consolidated (infarcted), with or without pleural effusion. Such a region will produce a ventilation defect indistinguishable from any other pathological cause of pulmonary consolidation, and may cause diagnostic difficulty especially if other causes of consolidation are present in the lungs.

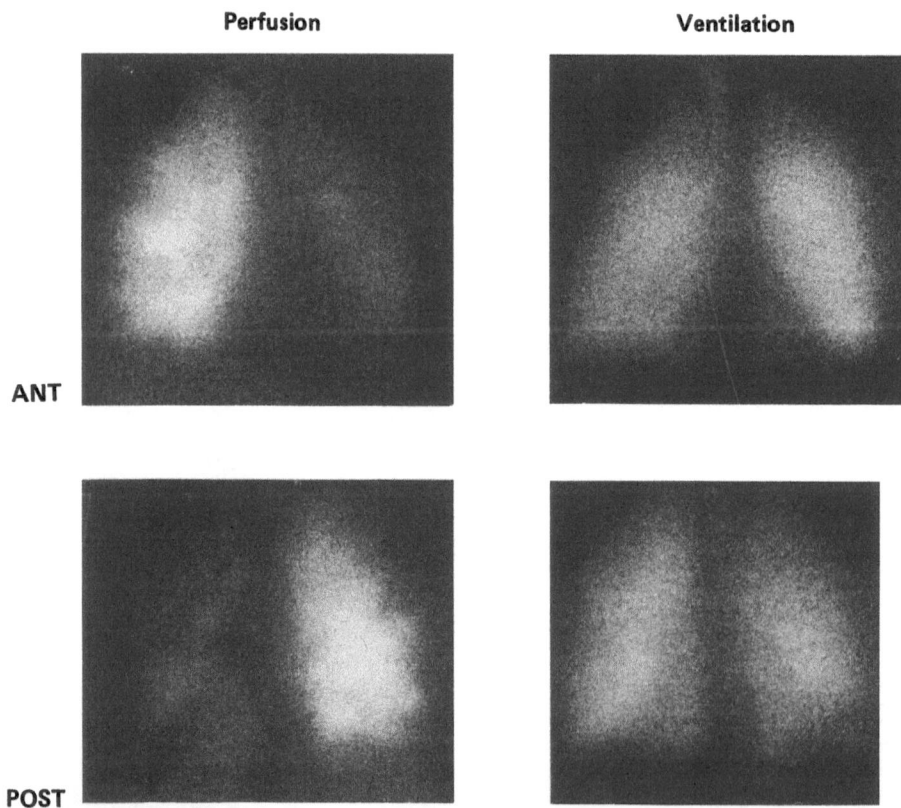

Fig. 7.3. Scintigraphic diagnosis of pulmonary embolism: images made within 1 h of life-threatening massive pulmonary embolism. Ventilation images (right) are normal, but perfusion images (left) are abnormal (see text for further details). *ANT*, anterior view; *POST*, posterior view.

Criteria for the Scintigraphic Diagnosis of Pulmonary Embolism

It is generally agreed the scintigraphic lung perfusion image is a very sensitive technique for detecting pulmonary embolism (Wagner et al. 1975). It is however very non-specific and much work has been carried out to define more exact criteria for the diagnosis of pulmonary embolism. Unfortunately, many published studies were carried out using technology inferior to that commonly available today, but the conclusions are likely to be still valid. The

pulmonary angiogram is the only available standard against which to access the accuracy of diagnosis, and for obvious reasons has never been applied across the board to an unselected series of patients suspected of pulmonary embolism. However some quite large series of angiograms have been analysed and compared with scintigraphs. Useful criteria have emerged based on the probability of scintigraphic findings correlating with angiographically proven pulmonary emboli.

A relatively simple yet comprehensive account has been given by Biello et al. (1979). They found both the number and size of perfusion defects important, as well as the presence of corresponding

Perfusion **Ventilation**

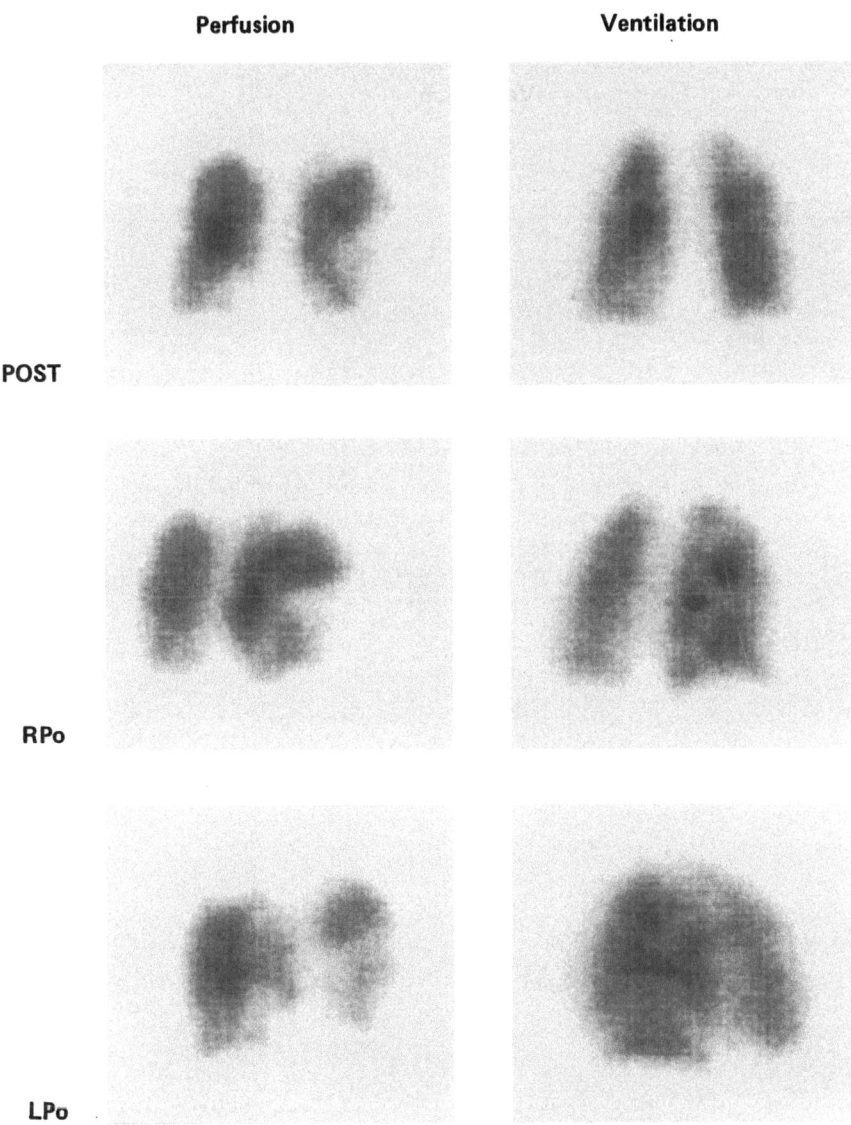

POST

RPo

LPo

Fig. 7.4. Scintigraphic diagnosis of pulmonary embolism: a case of chronic obstructive airways disease (see test for further details). *POST*, posterior view; *RPO*, right posterior oblique *LPO*, left posterior oblique.

ventilation defects or radiographic abnormalities. Using their system, cases were initially divided into those without significant chest radiographic abnormalities and those in whom these were present. They also divided perfusion defects (regions in which perfusion is virtually absent) into the small (less than 25% of anatomical lung segment), medium (25%–75% of a segment), and large (virtually a whole segment).

No Radiographic Abnormality Present. Small perfusion defects were not associated with confirmable pulmonary emboli, whether associated with ventilation defects or not. Moderate-size or large perfusion defects were rarely positive if the defects were matched with ventilation defects. If not matched,

however, one moderate-sized perfusion defect was occasionally due to pulmonary embolism (33% of cases), while more than one moderate sized defect, or any unmatched large defect, was usually associated with pulmonary embolism (more than 90%).

Radiographic Abnormality Present. These are expected to be associated with perfusion and ventilation defects and these cases were more of a problem. The best guide was the relative size of the defect. If the perfusion defect was larger than the ventilation defect or radiographic opacity, then Biello et al. found confirmable pulmonary embolism to be common (nearly 90%). If the perfusion defect was smaller than the ventilation defect or radiographic abnormality, pulmonary embolism

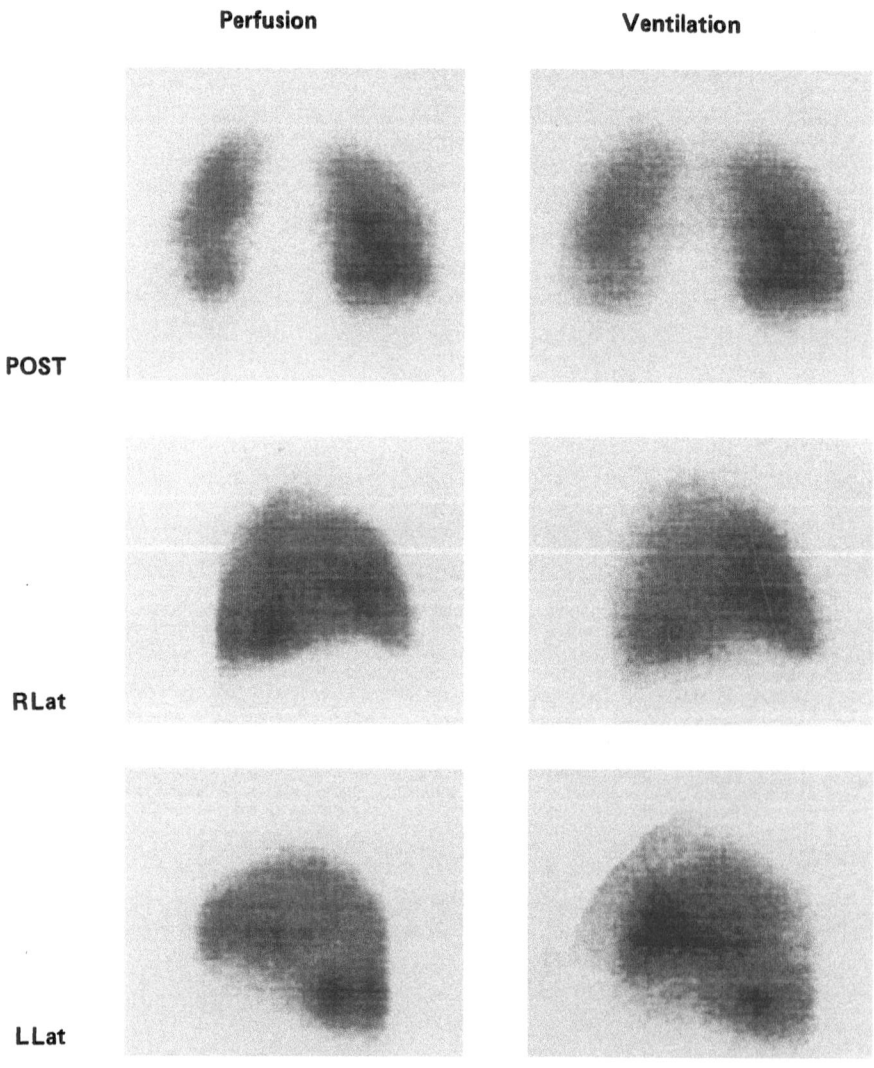

Fig. 7.5 a, b. Scintigraphic images from a patient undergoing total hip replacement surgery. **a** Pre-surgery images. **b** Post-surgery images.

was rarely found (less than 10%). If the perfusion, ventilation and radiographic defects matched each other closely then the result was inconclusive and diagnosis had to be made by other means.

The degree of abnormality shown in cases of pulmonary embolism is very variable and depends on the size and number (or fragmentation) of the emboli. The sensitivity of the test depends to a large extent on the fact that emboli are so often multiple. Alderson et al. (1976) reported 4 to 19 fragments per pulmonary angiogram, average 11, in one series. Clearly some of these will produce defects too small to be resolved scintigraphically, and emboli which incompletely occlude vessels are known to be frequently missed (Alderson et al. 1977), but it is clearly rare for no fragment to be resolved sufficiently to permit a diagnosis. A further problem is posed by resolution of emboli if there should be some delay in referring the patient for study. This is less likely to be a problem in the ITU than in the out patient department or general ward.

The range of abnormalities may be illustrated by a few cases:

Patient A.M. (*Fig. 7.1*). This represents a fairly typical presentation of pulmonary embolism. The ventilation pattern is normal but the perfusion pattern shows two moderate sized defects in the right lower lobe, and an ill defined defect in the right upper lobe. On the left side there is a large perfusion defect affecting virtually the whole of the lingula.

Patient M.J. (*Fig. 7.2*). This case shows more extensive pulmonary embolism. The ventilation images are completely normal but the posterior perfusion image shows gross asymmetry. Perfusion

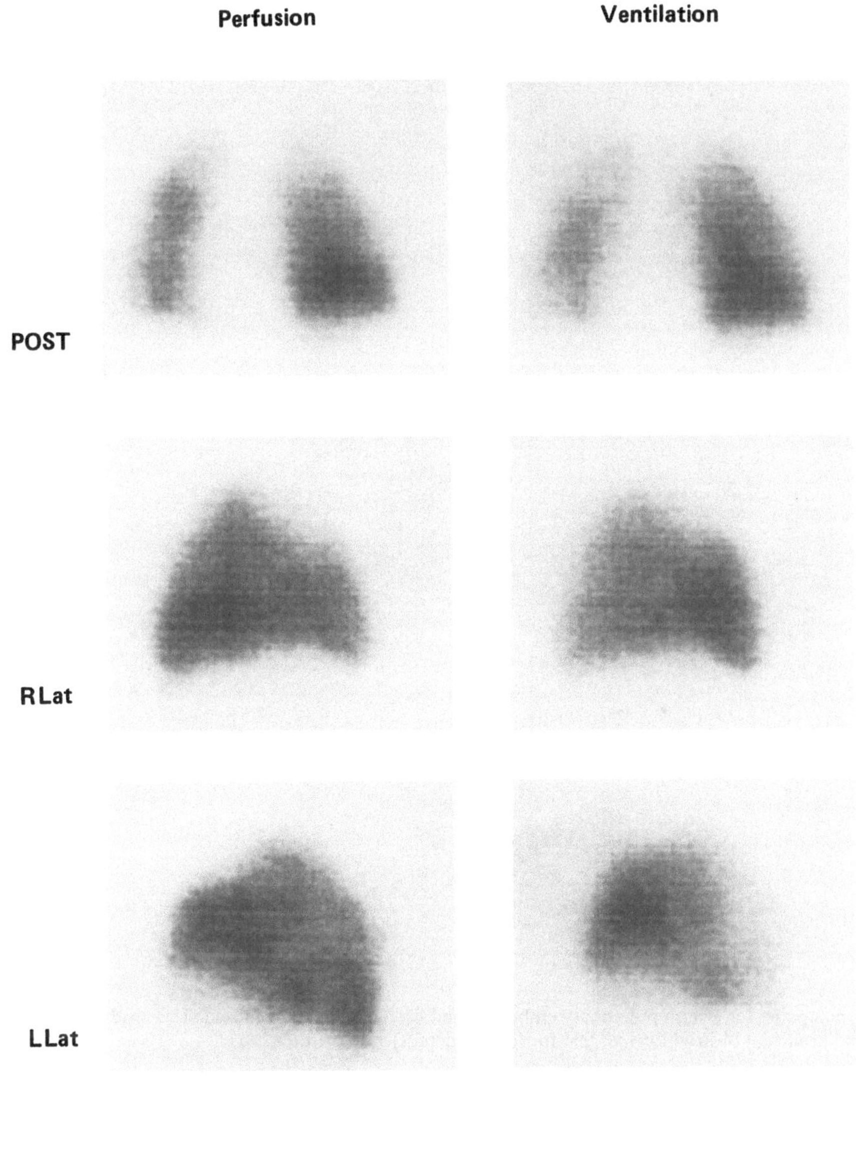

Fig. 7.5b

in the right lung is only present in a few sub-segmental areas. The perfusion pattern of the left lung is relatively intact but there is a coarse irregularity of pattern and a moderate sized perfusion defect of the lingula. It therefore seems certain that the left side has also been affected by embolic fragments.

Patient D.D. (*Fig. 7.3*). These images were made within an hour of a life-threatening massive pulmonary embolism. The ventilation images were entirely normal. The perfusion images show only faint traces of perfusion remaining in the left lung. The perfusion pattern of the right lung is also very abnormal for though there are no well-defined moderate or large-sized perfusion defects, the outline of the lung has a scalloped appearance indicating very irregular perfusion. It is interesting that far from showing broncho-constriction in the most affected lung, the radiokrypton image of the left lung seems if anything slightly brighter than that of the right indicating slightly greater ventilation.

When the scan was repeated 48 h after strep-tokinase therapy, the perfusion abnormalities had almost completely resolved and the perfusion patterns of the two lungs were very similar to the ventilation patterns

Patient C.V. (*Fig. 7.4*). This represents a case which could not possibly be assessed without some form of ventilation imaging, in this case a tech-

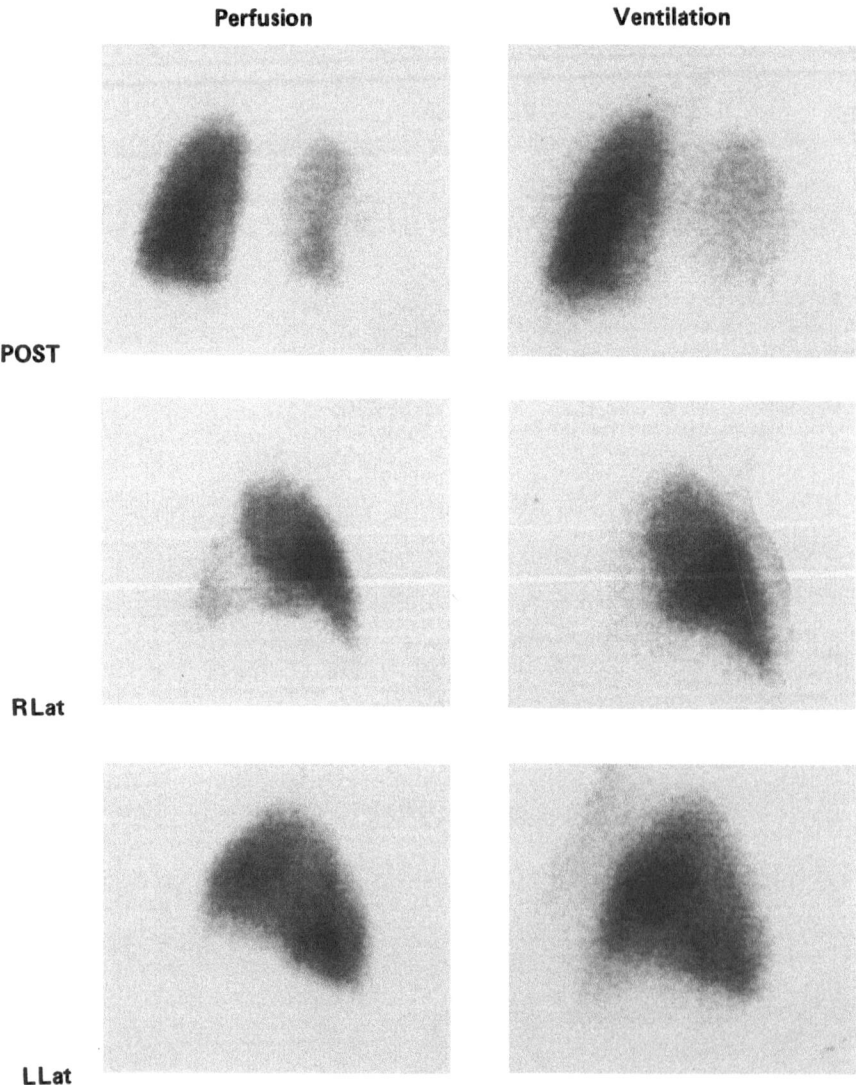

Perfusion   **Ventilation**

POST

R Lat

L Lat

Fig. 7.6. Scintigraphic images from a patient in whom pulmonary embolism had been clinically diagnosed. This study indicates that the condition is likely to be partial bronchial obstruction (see text for further details).

Perfusion   **Ventilation**

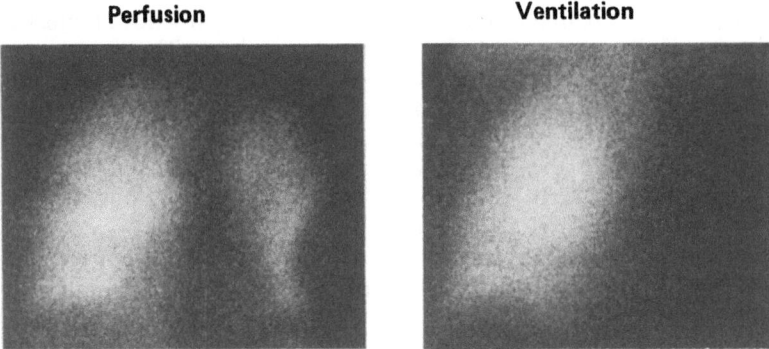

ANT

Fig. 7.7. Scintigraphic image of case of lobar pneumonia (see text for further details). Anterior view.

netium aerosol. The patient was known to have chronic obstructive airways disease but the extent of the lung disorder was not known. The ventilation images are moderately irregular with patchy concentration of radioactivity on both sides, particularly in the mid zones, typical of deposition of aerosol in the larger air passages. Though the outline of both lungs can be fairly well discerned on the ventilation pictures there is some loss of outline in the left lower lobe posteriorly. Corresponding perfusion images show much more abnormality, particularly in the right, middle and lower zones. There is a large perfusion defect in the lower part of the right upper lobe, possibly also involving the middle lobe. On the left side there is considerable perfusion irregularity which seems more marked than the corresponding ventilation irregularity, though it is difficult to define any moderately large or large un-matched defects. Overall however the defects of perfusion are clearly much greater than the ventilation irregularities. It is therefore highly likely that this patient has pulmonary emboli.

Regional Ventilation Problems

Defects of ventilation may pre-exist or be acquired in the ITU. As stated earlier hypoxia to some degree is almost universal after major surgery and additional complications such as pulmonary atelectasis with or without infection, and partial major bronchial obstruction may be difficult to recognise. Countering these threats is a major concern to the ITU staff. The role of lung scintigraphy is confined to the demonstration of major defects and attempting to show which of these factors may be present. The demonstration of poor ventilation or absence of ventilation in quite extensive areas of lung may explain vividly the reason for a patient's condition. Comparison with the chest radiograph may show defects to coincide with opacities or to be associated with very little abnormality. The place of ventilation imaging is probably best shown by the consideration of a number of individual cases.

Patient G.F. (*Figs. 7.5a, b*). This shows pre- and post-surgery lung images from a patient undergoing

Perfusion   **Ventilation**

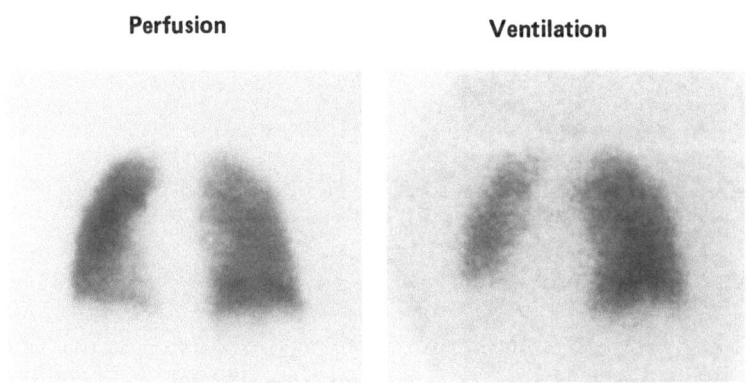

POST

Fig. 7.8. Limited scintigraphic images in case of severe cardiac arrythmia, which excludes massive pulmonary embolism as the precipitating factor. Posterior view.

total hip replacement, part of a series of such paired studies done to assess the incidence of silent post-operative pulmonary embolism. Both sets of images were carried out with the patient supine. The pictures are essentially normal. The pre-surgery study shows a slight reduction in perfusion along the posterior aspect of each lung, and a more marked reduction in ventilation. The post-surgery study is similar, but the ventilation changes are more marked. This is likely to be the "normal" pattern for ICU patients who are usually imaged supine.

Patient P.L. (*Fig. 7.6*). These images are from a patient who suffered multiple lower limb fractures from a road traffic accident. Two weeks later he developed haemoptysis and chest radiograph showed faint shadowing in the right lower zone. A clinical diagnosis of pulmonary embolism was made. The lung images, however, showed a quite different picture. The images on the left are normal with the slight relative loss of ventilation in the left lower lobe common-in supine patients. On the right, the upper and middle-lobe ventilation images are

normal, but there is total absence of effective ventilation in the lower lobe. The perfusion image reveals a faint but clear outline of the right lower lobe which is smaller than normal but contains no focal defect. This study virtually excludes pulmonary embolism and indicates that the condition is likely to be partial bronchial obstruction probably associated with infection.

Patient F.G. (*Fig. 7.7*). This elderly man was admitted with a fairly classical presentation of lobar pneumonia. Chest radiograph showed dense shadowing in the lower half of the left lung field, but an apparently normal upper half. After initial improvement on antibiotic therapy he was noted to be increasingly hypoxic though the chest radiograph did not change. Perfusion imaging showed an image which corresponded well with the chest radiograph, showing a normal outline on the right and a reduced but still substantial perfusion of the left lung (and a suspicion of an encysted effusion). The ventilation image however showed no effective ventilation occurring in the left lung. Bronchoscopy

Perfusion   **Ventilation**

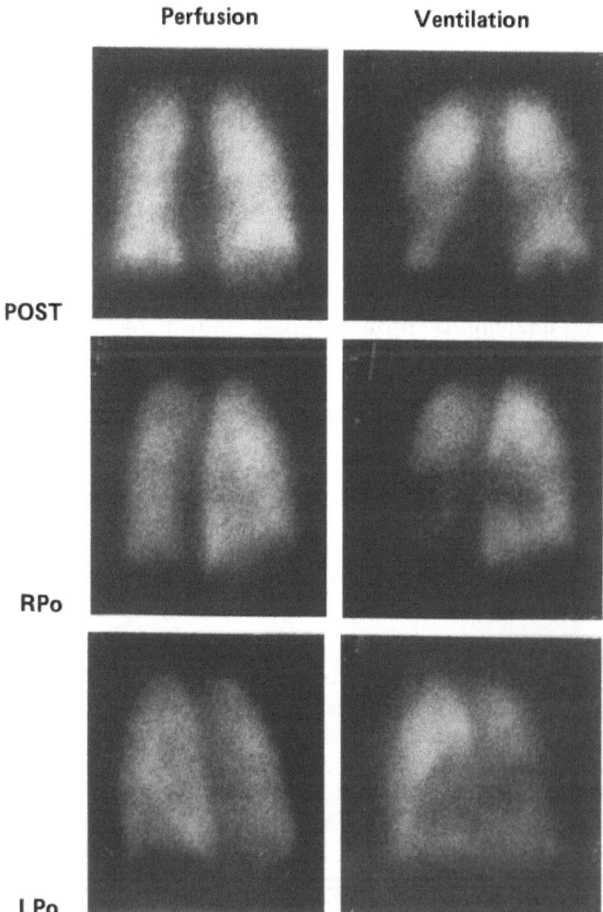

POST

RPo

LPo

Fig. 7.9. Scintigraphic image of patient recovering from myocardial infarction and left ventricular failure. Posterior view.

subsequently showed blockage of the left main bronchus. Aspiration of secretions was followed by immediate improvement.

Patient K.B. (Fig. 7.8). This patient presented with a sudden onset of a severe cardiac arrythmia which proved initially resistant to treatment and precipitated apparent left ventricular failure. This responded eventually only to be followed by an episode of cardiorespiratory arrest. Subsequently he remained intermittently hypoxic on a ventilator. The chest radiograph report suggested an abnormal hilar shadow and queried massive pulmonary embolism as the precipitating factor. The perfusion image instantly virtually excluded this showing a surprisingly normal perfusion pattern on both sides, but the ventilation image showed gross asymmetry which proved to be due to an ill-secured endo-

tracheal tube. He subsequently recovered completely.

Patient J.K. (Fig. 7.9). A patient with myocardial infarction and left ventricular failure recovered from the initial crisis but some days later developed chest pain, possibly pleuritic, and pulmonary embolism was feared. The perfusion image however was completely normal. Ventilation images showed gross reduction of ventilation in those parts of the lungs which are dependent when supine. Pulmonary embolism was excluded and the non-anatomical ventilation defects were presumably an unusual residue of pulmonary oedema.

Patient J.R. (Fig. 7.10). This heroin addict suffered head injury and multiple fractures in a road traffic accident. He remained unconscious and intubated but hypoxic and pulmonary embolism

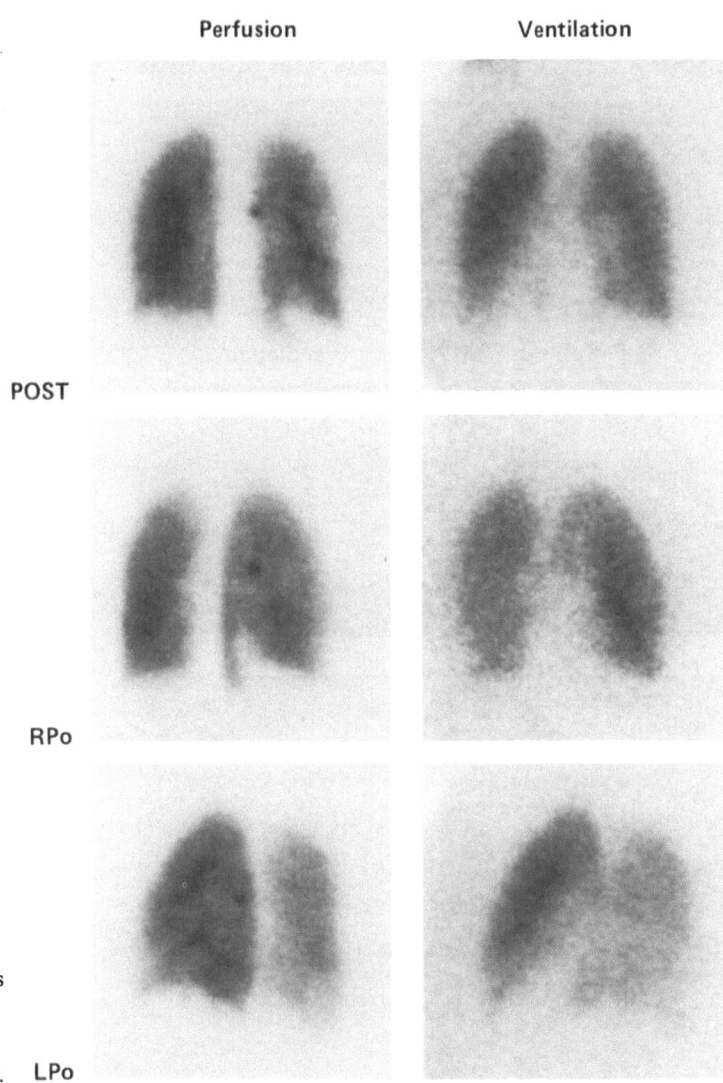

Perfusion   Ventilation

POST

RPo

LPo

Fig. 7.10. Scintigraphic images of unconscious and intubated patient with suspected pulmonary embolism (see text for further details). *POST*, posterior view; *RPO*, right posterior oblique *LPO*, left posterior oblique.

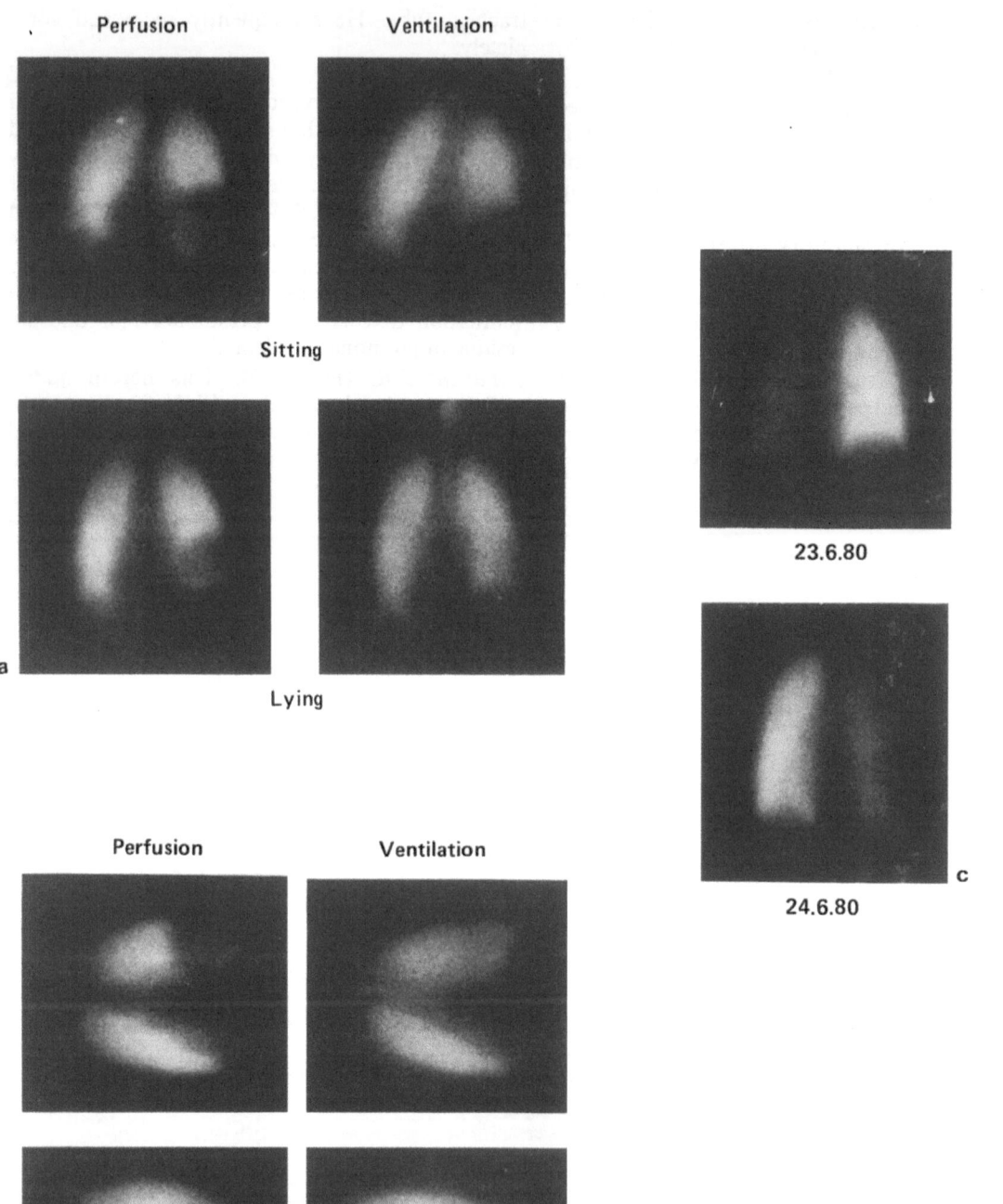

Fig. 7.11 a–c. A series of studies on a quadriplegic patient
a Ventilation is absent in lower half of right lung with
patient upright (upper pictures) but is restored when
patient is supine (lower right picture). b Ventilation
images when patient is on his side, with right lung
uppermost (top) and with left lung uppermost (lower
pictures). c Perfusion studies on two occasions with
patient supine, which show the inconstancy of the effect
of posture (see text for further details).

was suspected. The perfusion images showed surprisingly intact perfusion patterns with one subsegmental defect on the right. The ventilation images showed gross hypoventilation at both lower lobes which was clearly his main problem. The solitary right basal perfusion defect could be due to a small pulmonary embolism, particularly suggested by the sharp outline, but in view of the gross ventilation defect, this must be considered low probability.

Patient P.L. (Fig. 7.11a-c). A series of studies on this quadriplegic patient not only explained a clinical problem, but also vividly demonstrated the effectiveness of the normal reflexes which match perfusion to ventilation. The patient experienced recurrent respiratory distress whose cause was uncertain. The initial study done upright (Fig. 7.11a, upper pictures) showed absent ventilation in the lower half of the right lung, and an appropriate perfusion image with barely detectable perfusion in the same region. When the patient was placed supine (Fig. 7.11a, lower pictures), ventilation was restored throughout the right lung (the perfusion pattern was unchanged having been determined by the state of regional perfusion at the time of the injection of radioactive particles). The subsequent pictures were carried out with the patient horizontal, lying on his side, first with the left side underneath (Fig. 7.11b, top) and then with the right side underneath (Fig. 7.11b, bottom). The perfusion images remained as before, but in the first position ventilation of the right lung is fully restored. In the second position ventilation of the right lung (now underneath) has virtually ceased.

The inconstancy of the effect of posture was shown by subsequent studies when radiokrypton was unfortunately not available. Three days later a perfusion study carried out with the patient supine showed nearly total absence of perfusion of the left lung, presumably secondary to temporary obstruction to the left main bronchus. The study repeated 24 h later showed the complete reverse, intact perfusion of the left lung and near total absence of

perfusion of the right, presumably secondary to obstruction of the right main bronchus (Fig. 7.11c).

The study indicated the most unusual vulnerability of this patient's major airways to closure and explained his episodic breathlessness.

References

Adischan N (1982) An improved technique for inhalation imaging. Clin Nucl Med 7: 180–186

Agnew JE, Francis RA, Pavia D, Clarke SW (1982) Quantitative comparison of ^{99m}Tc aerosol and ^{81m}Kr ventilation images. Clin Phys Physiol Meas 3: 21–30

Alderson PO, Rujanavech N, Secker Walker RH, McKnight RC (1976) The role of ^{133}Xe ventilation studies in the scintigraphic detection of pulmonary embolism. Radiology 120: 633–640

Alderson PO, Doppman JL, Diamond SS, Mendenhall KG (1977) Ventilation-perfusion lung imaging and selective pulmonary angiography in animals with experimental pulmonary embolism. J Nucl Med 18: 605

Alderson PO, Biello DR, Gottschalf A et al. (1984) ^{99m}Tc-DTPA aerosols and radioactive gases compared as adjuncts to perfusion scintigraphy in patients with suspected pulmonary embolism. Radiology 153: 515–521

Biello DR, Mattar AG, McKnight RC, Siegel BA (1979) Ventilation – perfusion studies in suspected pulmonary embolism. Amer J Roent 133: 1033–1037

Burch WM, Sullivan PJ, Lomas FE et al. (1986) Lung ventilation studies with technetium-99m pseudogas. J Nucl Med 27: 842–846

Cooper AE (1972) Postoperative lung dysfunction. Proc Roy Soc Med 65: 10–14

Fazio F, Jones T (1975) Assessment of regional ventilation by continuous inhalation of Radioactive krypton-81 m. Br Med J 3: 673–676

Hamilton WK, McDonald JS, Fischer HW, Bethards R (1964) Postoperative respiratory complications. Anesthesiology 25: 607

Harding LK, Horsfield K, Singhal SS et al. (1983) The proportion of lung vessels blocked by albumin microspheres. J Nucl Med 14: 579–581

Sasahara AA (1974) Current problems in pulmonary embolism: introduction. Prog. Cardiovasc Dis 17: 161–165

Vezina W, Chamberlain M, Vinitski S. et al. (1985) Radioaerosol ventilation imaging in ventilator-dependent patients – technical considerations. Clin Nucl Med 10: 759–766

Vieras F, Jacobus JP, Grisson MP (1982) The technique for the performance of xenon-133 ventilation studies during artificial ventilation. J Nucl Med 23: 540–542

Wagner HN Jnr, Strauss HW (1975) Radioactive tracers in the differential diagnosis of pulmonary embolism. Prog Cardiovasc Dis 17: 271–282

Cardiovascular Assessment

Chapter 8

Cardiac Ultrasound

R. Donaldson

Introduction

Ultrasonic imaging of the heart or "echo-cardiography" based on pulsed echo techniques, allows the movements of intracardiac structures to be studied noninvasively with ease and reproducibility. The echo signal indicates the presence and location of a structure along the sound beam. Ultrasound technology has advanced substantially in the past few years. It is a safe, cost-effective, powerful tool for the assessment of cardiac anatomy and pathology.

There are two methods of cardiac ultrasound; the *"M" mode* and the *two-dimensional cross-sectional mode*. The *Doppler* shift of ultrasound can be combined with both methods to provide information about the velocity and direction of blood flow. *Contrast enhancement* by the injection of microbubbles (*contrast echocardiography*) provides additional information in congenital cardiac lesions. Techniques are also available for the extraction of information on tissue characterisation from ultrasonic images.

M Mode Echocardiography

The echoes reflected from different interfaces are converted into spots which fall on light-sensitive paper moving at constant speed. A graph of the position of the reflecting structures of the heart relative to the transducer against time is produced (Fig. 8.1). The "M"-mode or time motion echo is effectively a high fidelity graph of depth (down a particular direction) against time. By altering the direction of the "M"-mode path it is possible to examine most intracardiac structures and make precise measurements of dimensions of velocity of motion.

Two-Dimensional or Cross-Sectional Echocardiography

By making the ultrasound beam oscillate very rapidly back and forth through an arc of 90° (or by adding a number of beams together) the information from a larger number of "M"-mode scans is combined. The series of images will produce an accurate moving picture of the structures within the heart (Fig. 8.1).

Thus, lateral as well as axial distances between structures can be appreciated, and the images obtained resemble heart morphology. Cross-section echocardiography (CSE) allows complete visualisation of all intracardiac structures and regional differences in cardiac function can be evaluated. The structures shown on CSE depend on both the transducer position and the direction of oscillation. The cross-sectional or two-dimensional echocardiograms are effectively tomograms, showing morphology as a slice of the heart in several cross-sectional planes (Figs. 8.2–8.4).

Resolution Within an Ultrasound System

Resolution is the ultimate performance measure of an ultrasound system. Axial resolution is the ability of the device to resolve a structure from the one behind it and most ultrasound instruments functioning at 3.5 to 5 MHz have axial resolution capa-

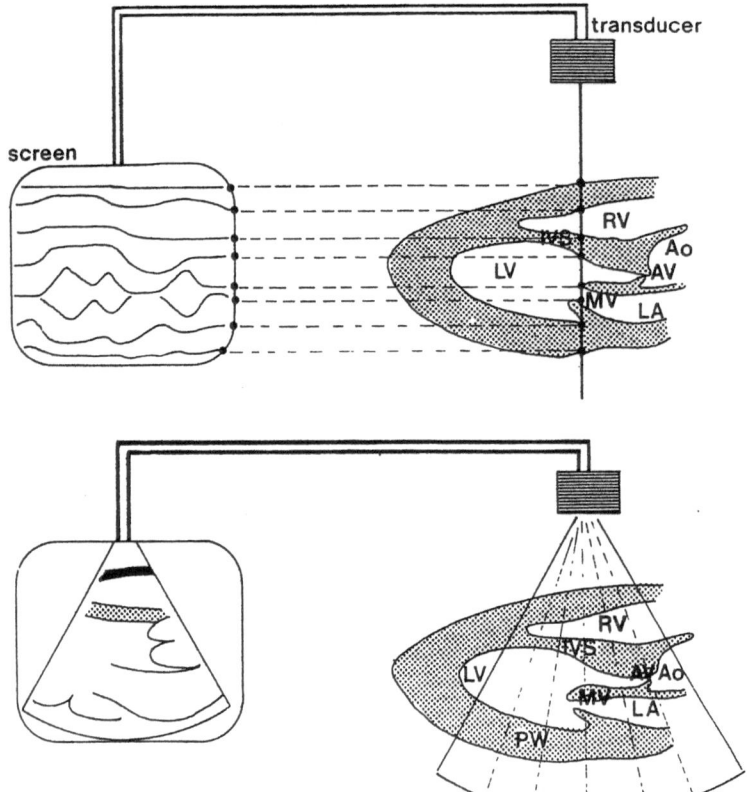

Fig. 8.1a. M-mode line crossing the left ventricle at mitral valve level. Echoes generated from this line are displayed as dots; these dots are swept across the screen to form a graph of depth against time in the M-mode recording. **b** The CSE echo is created from a fan of many individual echo lines and displayed on the video screen in real time. RV, right ventricle; IVS, interventricular septum; LV, left ventricle; Ao, aorta; MV, mitral valve; LA, left atrium; AV, aortic valve; RA, right atrium.

bilities in the submillimetre range. Lateral resolution refers to the ability of the ultrasound beam to resolve structures lying next to each other, and is usually about 1.5 mm.

Doppler Echocardiography

All Doppler instruments work on the Doppler principle which is the property of any moving structure to back-scatter energy at a frequency different from the frequency transmitted. In cardiac applications, circulating red blood cells back-scatter ultrasonic waves emitted from a piezoelectric transducer so that the returning sound energy differs from the transmitted frequency by a function of the vector red cell motion along the direction of interrogation.

Continuous Wave (CW) Doppler Mode (Figs. 8.8–8.11)

This mode requires separate transmit and receive elements. Velocities are recorded all along the ultrasonic beam and there is no selection of the depth of

the Doppler processing in this mode. Nonetheless, this technique is capable of resolving very high flow velocities, even those arising from stenotic valves producing a flow velocity up to 8 msec^{-1}.

Pulsed (PD) or Range-Gated Doppler Mode

In this mode, a temporal gate is established during the returning echo signals so that the returning information is analysed for Doppler shift only during the selected period. The position of the sample volume is guided by simultaneous CSE.

The signal can thus be localised in depth but the velocity resolution of pulsed Doppler is limited to around 1–1.5 msec^{-1}: thus the very high velocities of pathologic flow cannot be resolved by this mode. If the velocities exceed this maximum limit, the velocities beyond this point appear to reverse direction. This reversal is called "aliasing": the peak velocity appears to wrap around the velocity record so that initially it is moving in the correct direction but the peak appears in the wrong part of the graph. With CW and PRF Doppler which have range ambiguity, there are no limitations within the

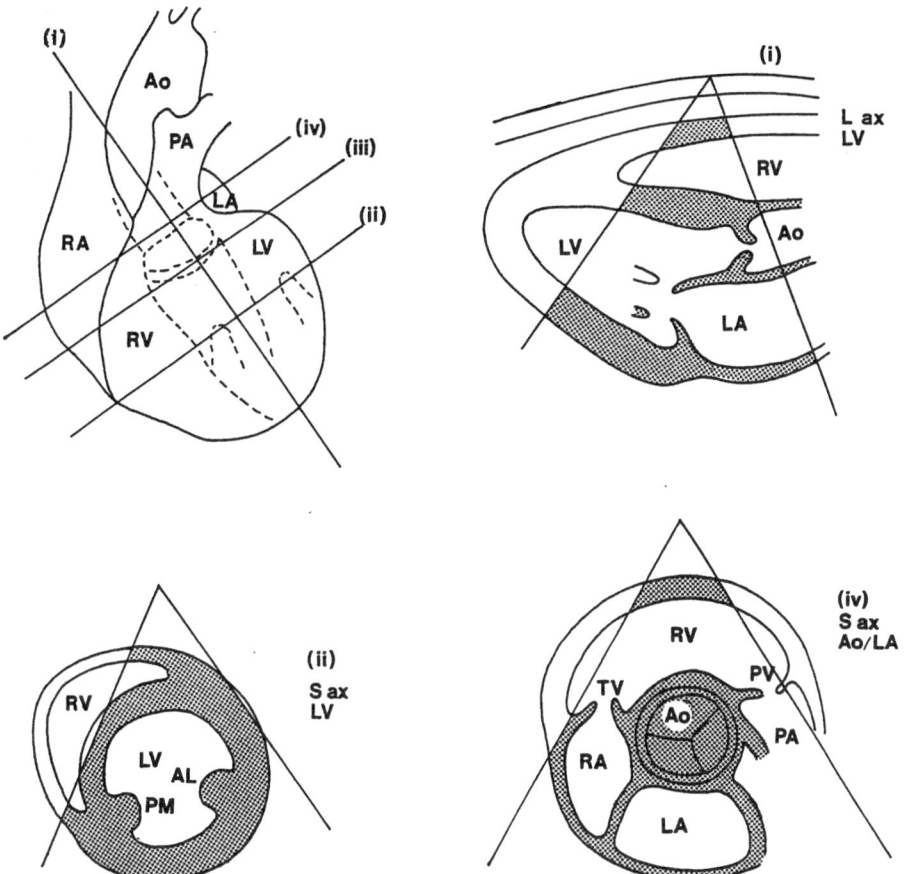

Fig. 8.2. Drawing of the heart demonstrating 4 ultrasonic phases. Line (i) represents the phase of the long axis of the left ventricle (see Fig. 8.3); lines (i), (iii), (iv) represent short axis planes of the heart at the level of the papillary muscles, mitral valve (see Fig. 8.4) and great arteries.

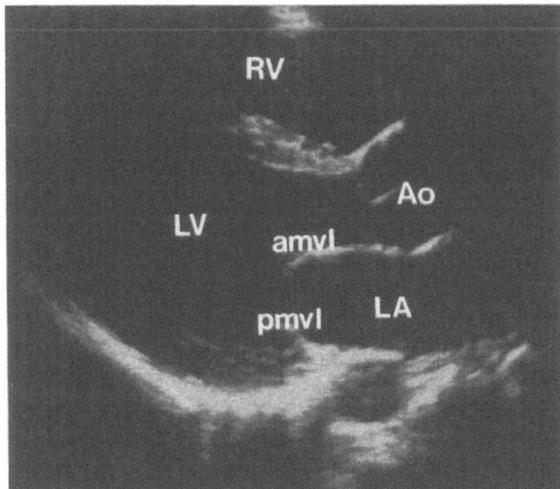

Fig. 8.3. Parasternal long axis view of the left ventricle. RV, right ventricle; LV, left ventricle; LA, left atrium; Ao, aorta; amvl, anterior mitral valve leaflet; pmvl, posterior mitral valve leaflet.

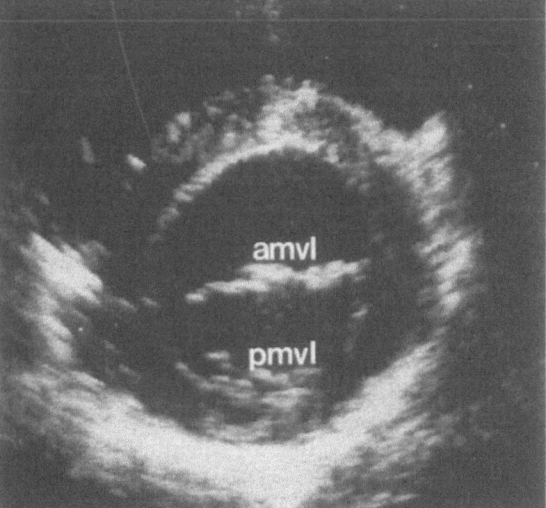

Fig. 8.4. CSE Parasternal short axis view at the level of the anterior (amvl) and posterior (pmvl) mitral valve leaflets.

physiological range and therefore aliasing occurs only with pulsed Doppler.

High Pulsed Repetition (PRF) Range-Gated Doppler Mode

This utilises the principle of range ambiguity to place a number of sample volumes of fixed intervals which are multiples of a base-line depth of interrogation.

Resolution Within a Doppler System

Doppler sample widths are wider than echocardiographic beam width, often ± 2 mm at a depth of 4.6 cm.

Doppler Displays

The spectral output display contains information as to the arithmetic mode of velocity shift, the shift most commonly present within the Doppler sample volume and also information on the spectral width or dispersion. A grey-scale pattern of component velocities within the signal is displayed. Velocities are obtained by aligning the Doppler cursor with the expected direction of flow, searching for the signal with the highest velocity and least spectral dispersion. Flow directed towards the transducer is shown as positive and upward; flow away from the transducer downward and negative. Calibration for velocity is in m (or cm) msec^{-1}.

Contrast Echocardiography

Ultrasonic contrast agents rely on the injection of microbubbles or gas to produce enhancement. They appear as a cloud of echoes on the echo-cardiogram. This is conveniently accomplished by the rapid manual injection of fluids such as 5% dextrose in water, or saline. Hydrogen peroxide will give a strong contrast effect by producing tiny intravascular bubbles of oxygen. The microbubbles are contained in the fluid or are flushed from the walls of syringes or tubing.

At present the clinical applications of contrast echocardiography fall into two general categories: the verification of cardiac anatomy and the evaluation of cardiac blood flow. The use of contrast echo-cardiography in the assessment of blood-flow patterns has primarily involved the detection of right to left intracardiac shunts and valvular regurgitation. More recently, contrast echocardiography has been used to produce hard-copy records reflecting cardiac output and function.

Equipment

Three general types of ultrasound scanner configuration are currently in use for echocardiography: mechanical sector scanners (with either oscillating or rotating transducer devices); electronic sector scanners (phased array devices); and the mechanical scanners with annular arrays. The functioning of instrumentation should be reviewed in the standard ultrasound texts (see Bibliography). A solid-state video display converts the sector scan raster into a rectilinear raster ("scan conversion") assigning each of the positions within the polar coordinates of the sector scan and shows up on the video screen. Most devices have at least 64 levels of grey for scale resolution. Such scanners can be combined with Doppler systems. Because a phased array device contains many crystals, it can image and record Doppler simultaneously and can usually switch from pulsed to continuous wave Doppler. One major problem is that some phased array devices do not permit the movement of the cursor line, and the operator has to find a way to put the cardiac area of interest on the cursor line. Simultaneous imaging and Doppler is not available from a mechanical scanner. A separate "stand-alone" continuous wave Doppler system can also be used for cardiac studies.

Clinical Application

The clinical applications are listed in Table 8.1. Cardiac ultrasound is currently the method of

Table 8.1. Clinical applications of cardiac ultrasound investigation.

Echocardiography (M-mode and CSE)

1 Valve structure and motion
2 Congenital heart disease
3 Cardiac shunts
4 Abnormalities of the great arteries
5 Global and regional wall motion
6 Complications of myocardial infarction
7 Chamber size and wall thickness
8 Pericardial effusion
9 Intracardial masses

Doppler ultrasound

1 Intracardiac pressures estimates
2 Short detection and quantifications
3 Valvular stenosis and regurgitation
4 Ventricular performance (cardiac output)
5 Visualisation of abnormal blood flow

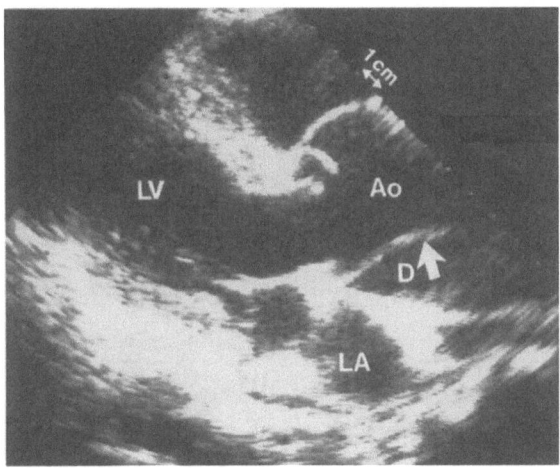

Fig. 8.5. Dissecting aneurysm of the aorta. CSE, long axis view. LV, left ventricle; LA, left atrium; Ao, aorta. Arrow points to the spiral aortic tear of dissection (D).

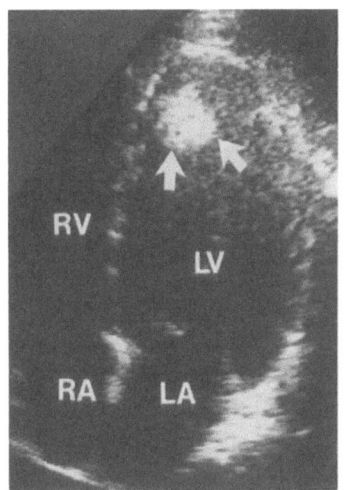

Fig. 8.6. CSE, apical four chamber view. Antero-apical infarct and mural thrombus (arrows). RV, right ventricle; LV, left ventricle; RA, right atrium; LA, left atrium.

choice for noninvasive anatomical assessment of the heart. Although magnetic resonance imaging and X-ray computed tomography will offer more consistent images than echocardiography, the latter technique is of superior value in the identification of morphologic abnormalities, particularly at the bedside of the severely ill patient.

Acquired valvular heart disease (mitral stenosis, mitral prolapse or rupture, aortic stenosis and regurgitation, tricuspid valve disease) can be visualised by cardiac ultrasound. "Deductive echocardiography" is useful in the diagnosis of congenital heart disease by means of the accurate identification of the atria, atrioventricular valve, ventricles, semilunar valves and great vessels and their inter-relationships. Cardiac ultrasound is also helpful in the diagnosis of cardiac shunts by detecting the actual defect between the two sides of the heart, by evaluating the haemodynamic consequences of the shunted blood and by visualising the shunted blood with contrast and Doppler echocardiography. Congenital and acquired abnormalities of the great arteries can also be detected by ultrasound. It is possible to examine the entire aorta using echocardiography and thus aortic dilatation, aneurysm formation and dissection (Fig. 8.5) can be visualised.

Cardiac ultrasound also offers substantial insight into the global and regional systolic wall motion of the heart. The diagnosis of ventricular aneurysm and pseudoaneurysm is possible and echocardiography is particularly useful in detecting other complications of myocardial infarctions such as mural thrombus (Fig. 8.6), ventricular septal rupture, papillary muscle dysfunction, myocardial scarring.

Accurate evaluation of chamber size and wall thickness is obtained by ultrasound, and the hypertrophic, dilated (Fig. 8.7) restrictive cardiomyopathic have characteristic echocardiographic features. The detection of pericardial effusion has been one of the most useful applications of echocardiography (Fig. 8.7).

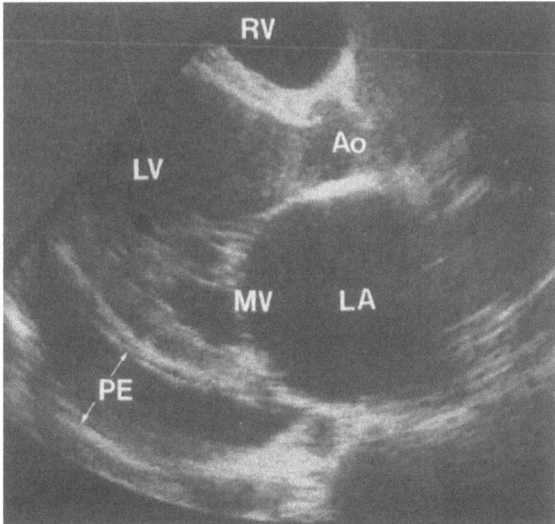

Fig. 8.7. Dilated (congestive) cardiomyopathy and posterior pericardial effusion (PE). CSE, long axis view. RV, right ventricle; LV, left ventricle; LA, left atrium; Ao, aorta; MV, mitral valve.

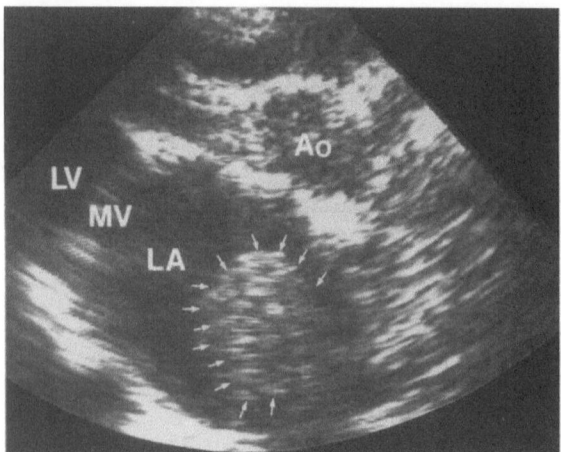

Fig. 8.8. Left atrial thrombus (arrows). LV, left ventricle; LA, left atrium; Ao, aorta; MV, mitral valve.

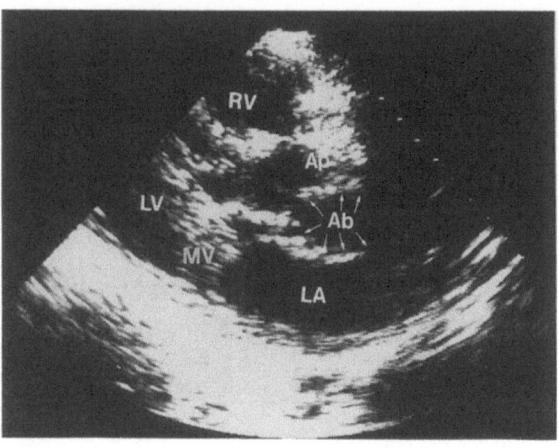

Fig. 8.9. Aortic root abscess (Ab, arrows). Complicating prosthetic valve endocarditis. Ap, aortic prosthesis; LV, left ventricle, RV, right ventricle; LA, left atrium; MV, mitral valve.

Intra-cardiac masses (tumours, thrombus) (Fig. 8.8), as well as the complications resulting from infective endocarditis (vegetations, abscess formation (Fig. 8.9)) can also be identified.

Doppler echocardiography has become a valuable adjunct to CSE by providing information about the flow of blood within cardiac chambers and great vessels. By utilising certain principles, Doppler technique provides information assessing intracardiac pressures and shunts and allows the assessment of valvular stenosis (Fig. 8.10), regurgitation (Fig. 8.11) and cardiac output. By utilising colour-encoded, multi-graded digital Doppler flow analysis, noninvasive visualisation of blood flow is

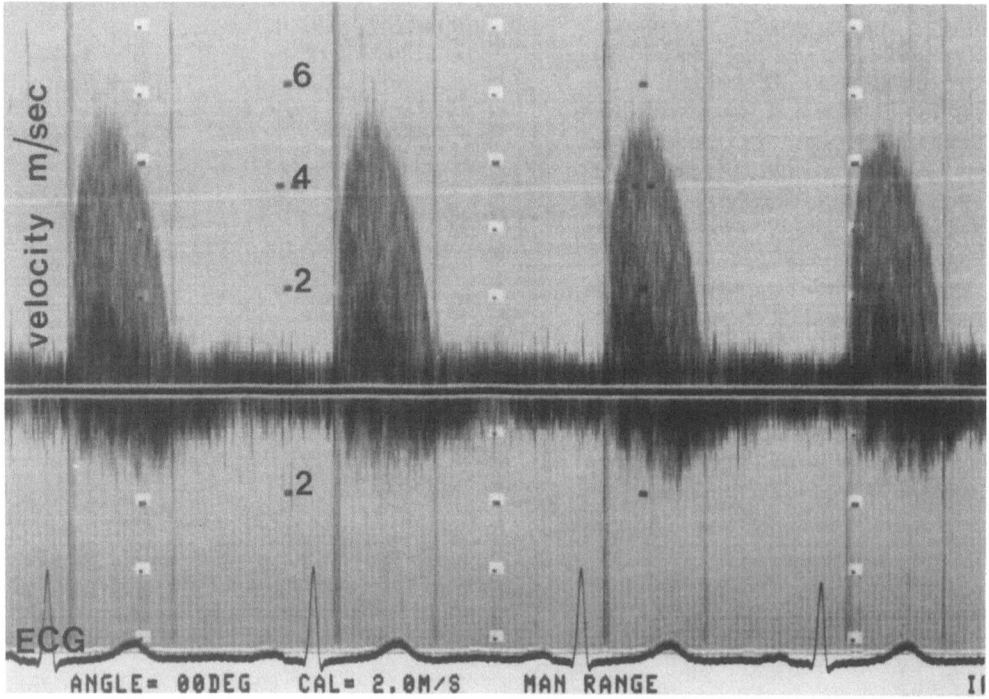

Fig. 8.10. Severe aortic stenosis. Continuous wave Doppler echocardiographic study. From the maximal aortic flow velocity (5.7 msec^{-1}) a mean pressure drop across the valve of 125 mmHg is calculated. $P = 4V^2$, where V is the maximum velocity msec^{-1}.

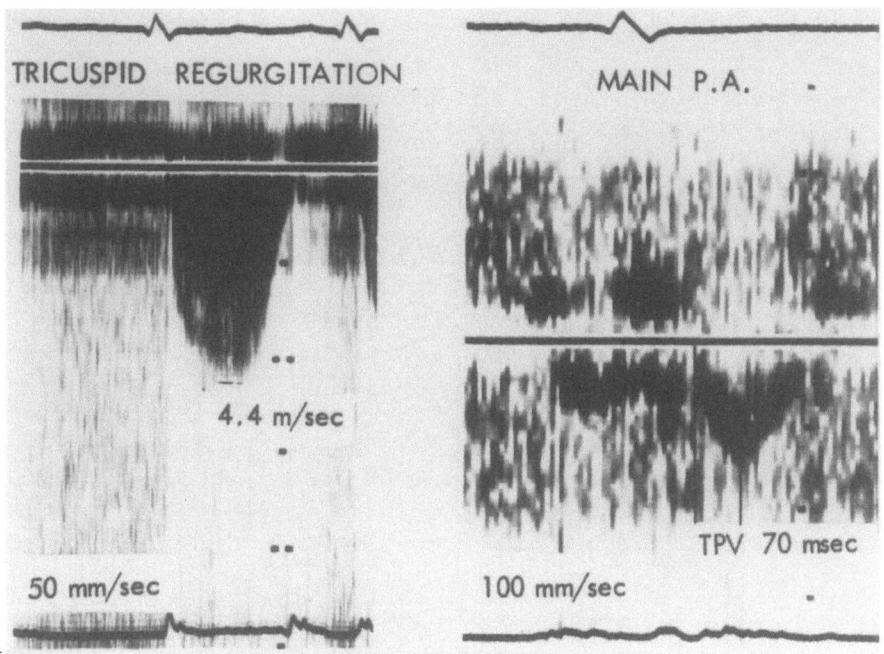

Fig. 8.11. Pulmonary hypertension. CW Doppler recordings of retrograde high velocity flow into the right atrium in systole due to tricuspid regurgitation (left). Estimated pressure derived = 87 mmHg. An abnormally short time to peak velocity (TPV) (<100 msec^{-1}); abnormal pulmonary-artery (PA) pressure (right).

possible. This colour flow mapping has thus the ability to display visually the spatial extent of abnormal velocities caused by regurgitant lesions.

Bibliography

Arvan S (1984) Echocardiography. Churchill Livingstone, New York

Donaldson RM, Westgate C (1985) A guide to Cardiac Ultrasound. King & Wirth, London

Feigenbaum H (1986) Echocardiography. 4th Edn. Lea and Febiger, Philadelphia

Hagan A, Di Sessa T, Bloor C, Calleja MB (1983) Two dimensional echocardiography. Clinical pathological correlations. Little Brown & Co, Boston

Hatle K, Angelsen B (1985) Doppler ultrasound in Cardiology. Physical principles and clinical application. Lea and Febiger, Philadelphia

Nanda NC (ed) (1985) Doppler Echocardiography. Igaku-Shoin, New York

Sahn DJ, Anderson C (1982) Two dimensional anatomy of the heart. J Wiley & Son, New York

Chapter 9

Radionuclide Imaging of the Cardiovascular System

S. R. Underwood

Introduction

Nuclear cardiology involves the use of radio-pharmaceuticals to obtain information about the heart. It differs from the majority of other investigative techniques in that it provides functional information, and although structure can be deduced, spatial resolution is poor and anatomy is not always well demonstrated. This does not limit its value, however, since cardiac function is not easily assessed by other noninvasive techniques. Most district general hospitals are now able to perform nuclear investigations, although not all have a mobile camera to study patients on the intensive care unit, and transfer to the nuclear medicine department may be necessary. Information is usually obtained during dynamic exercise as well as at rest, and although this may not always be possible with sick patients, a knowledge of the wide range of information that can be obtained is important in order to select investigations appropriately.

Techniques

Radiopharmaceuticals

The handling of a radiopharmaceutical by the body depends upon its chemical properties and dictates the type of information that is obtained. A wide range of radiopharmaceuticals can be used for the heart and Table 9.1 lists the more important ones, although it is by no means exhaustive.

Table 9.1. Some of the radiopharmaceuticals in more common use in nuclear cardiology.

Radio-nuclide	Bound to	Uses
$99m_{Tc}$	Erythrocytes	First-pass and equilibrium angiocardiography (ventricular function)
$99m_{Tc}$	Pyrophosphate	Acute infarct imaging
$195m_{Au}$	Ionic	First-pass angiocardiography
201_{Tl}	Ionic	Myocardial perfusion imaging
123_{I}	Fatty acids	Myocardial metabolism
111_{In}	Platelets	Detection of thrombus
111_{In}	White cells	Detection of inflammation or infection

Technetium-99m is the commonest radionuclide in nuclear medicine because it can be incorporated into a wide variety of molecules. It has a half-life of 6 h and is produced by elution from a bench-top generator consisting of the mother radionuclide (molybdenum-99) on an ion-exchange resin. Erythrocyte labelling allows imaging of the intra-cardiac blood pools and is usually performed in vivo with sequential intravenous injections of 5 mg stannous pyrophosphate and 740 MBq of sodium pertechnetate (Pavel et al. 1977).

Thallium-201 is a cyclotron-produced radio-nuclide with a physical half-life of 72 h. Following intravenous injection, clearance from the blood-stream is rapid with approximately 95% clearance after the first circulation, although only 5% of the injected dose is taken up by the myocardium (Okada et al. 1982). Myocardial distribution is proportional to myocardial blood flow over a wide range of values, hence its value (Neilson et al. 1980; Mueller et al. 1976).

Gamma camera

Different types of gamma camera are available, but they all use a crystal (or crystals) of sodium iodide in front of an array of photomultiplier tubes. Gamma photons absorbed by the crystal produce scintillations that are located upon the face of the camera according to the relative responses in each photomultiplier tube. A collimator, consisting of a honeycomb of holes in a disc of lead, sits in front of the crystal and ensures that only gamma photons travelling perpendicularly to the camera-face reach the crystal. The image represents a projection of the distribution of the radionuclide within the field of view. Specialised collimators are available, such as the slant-hole collimator which allows images to be acquired with cranio-caudal tilt without tilting the camera. The camera may be fixed or mobile, and it may rotate about the patient to allow emission tomography. The seven-pin-hole collimator or the rotating slant-hole collimator may also be used to produce tomograms.

Computers

A gamma camera alone produces static analogue images which may be adequate for planar thallium imaging, but for radionuclide ventriculography and for most other applications an on-line computer is necessary. The computer controls dynamic imaging, and is used for data processing and storage. If imaging is performed outside the nuclear medicine department, there must either be computer links to it, or the computer must be an integral part of the mobile camera.

Radionuclide Ventriculography

Radionuclide ventriculography involves imaging of the intracardiac blood pools following erythrocyte labelling with technetium-99m. Data can be obtained either during the first passage of a bolus of activity through the central circulation (a first-pass study) or after the activity is evenly dispersed throughout the blood pool (equilibrium study). Similar information is obtained from both types of study and it is possible to follow a first-pass study (in the right anterior oblique projection for instance) with an equilibrium study (left anterior oblique). Table 9.2 lists the information usually obtained by each study.

Table 9.2. Measurements commonly made during first-pass (FP) and equilibrium (Eq) radionuclide ventriculography.

Measurement	Study
Ventricular volume (absolute or relative)	FP or Eq
Left ventricular ejection fraction	FP or Eq
Right ventricular ejection fraction	FP or Eq
Regional ventricular wall motion	FP or Eq
Quantification of valvular regurgitation	FP or Eq
Quantification of systemic to pulmonary shunting	FP

Equilibrium Studies

Figure 9.1 shows an image of the intracardiac blood pools acquired in the left anterior oblique projection. Imaging is usually restricted to this projection so that there is no overlap between the left and right ventricular blood pools, and cranio-caudal tilt is also used to separate the left atrial and ventricular blood pools. The images are recorded on a 64×64 pixel matrix and the number of counts in each pixel is displayed using a colour scale. Data acquisition requires between 2 and 5 min, and electrocardiographic gating is used to produce a number of images (typically 16) representing an average cardiac cycle (Fig. 9.2).

Global Ventricular Function

Since the number of counts within any area of the image is proportional to the volume of blood represented by it, ventricular volume throughout the cardiac cycle can be plotted. Counts can be converted to absolute volumes if a sample of blood is imaged to measure its specific activity, and if a correction is made for attenuation of counts by tissue in front of the blood pool. In practice, this is not usually done since ejection fraction is a ratio of two volumes (stroke volume/end-diastolic volume) and does not require a knowledge of the specific

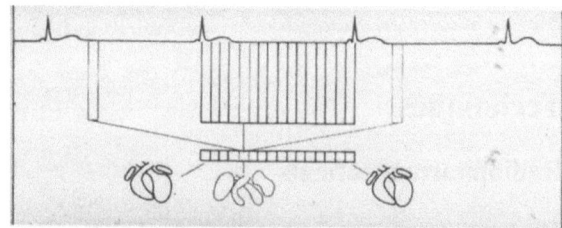

Fig. 9.2. Electrocardiographic gating: data acquired during each interval after the R wave is added into one of a number of frames (typically 16). The frames finally contain information from a number of cardiac cycles, but each represents part of an average cycle.

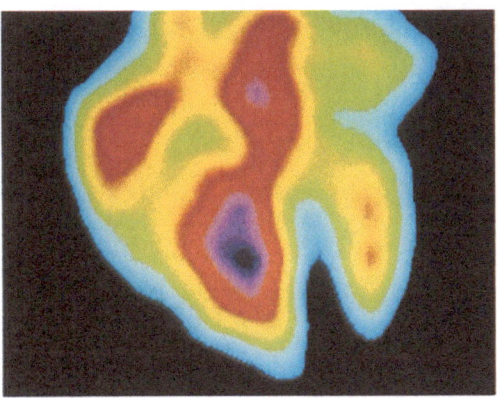

Fig. 9.1

Fig. 9.1. End-diastolic image of the intracardiac blood pools in the left anterior oblique projection with 30° of cranio-caudal tilt. The left and right ventricles are separated by the interventricular septum.

Fig. 9.4. Normal amplitude (*left*) and phase images (*right*). High values of amplitude (*red*) and uniform values of phase (*green*) are seen over both ventricles.

Fig. 9.5. Amplitude (*left*) and phase images (*right*) in a patient with anteroseptal infarction. The infarcted territory has low values of amplitude (hypokinesis) and high values of phase (tardykinesis).

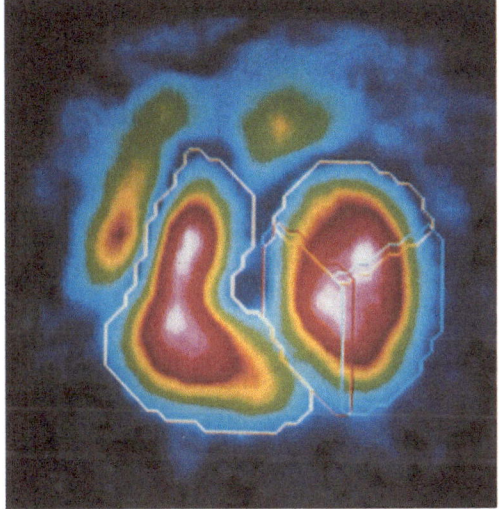

Fig. 9.4 Left

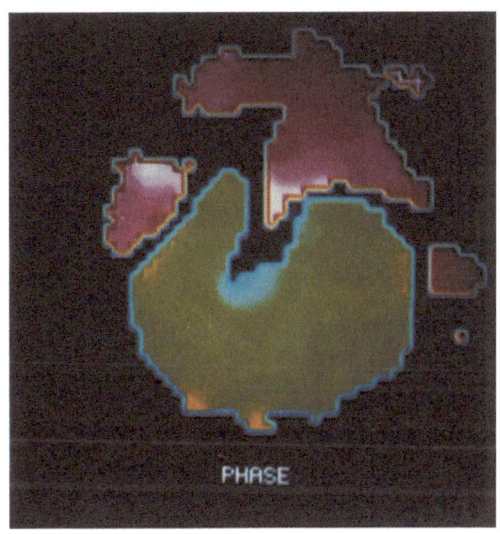

Fig. 9.4 Right

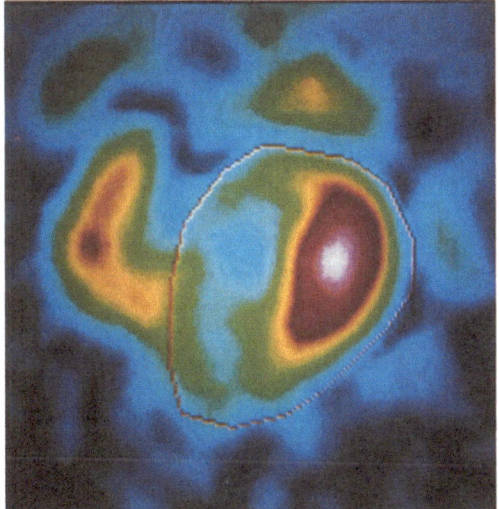

Fig. 9.5 Left

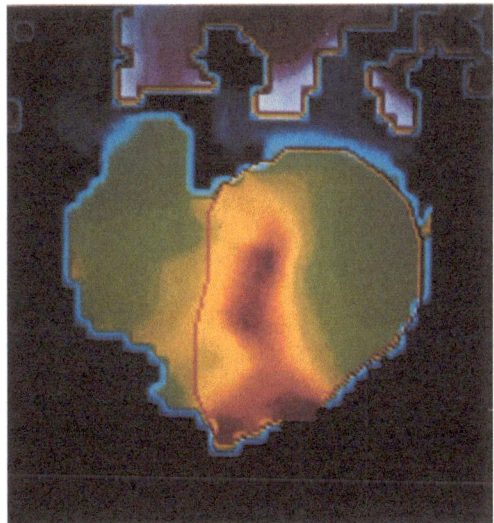

Fig. 9.5 Right

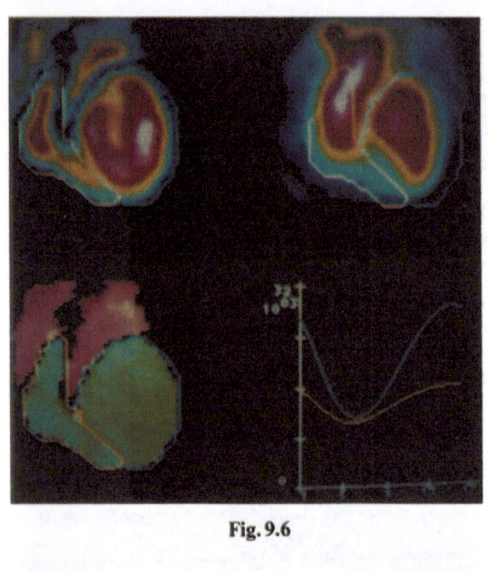

Fig. 9.6

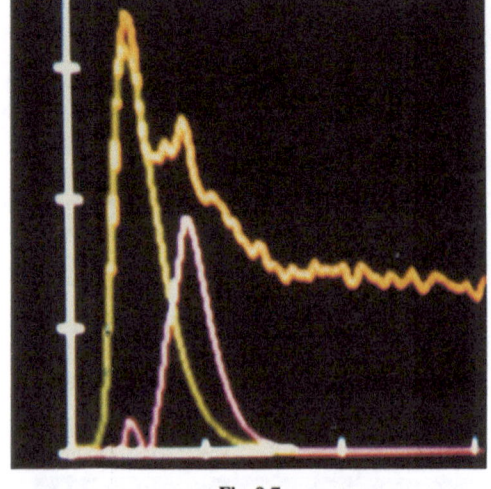

Fig. 9.7

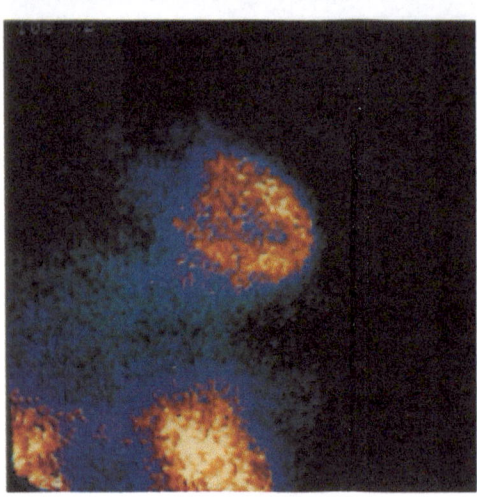

Fig. 9.9 AP

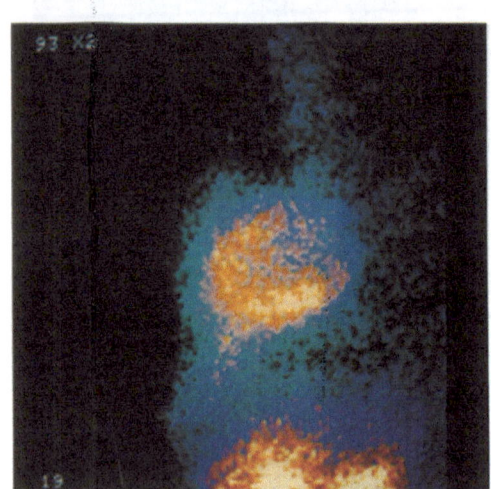

Fig. 9.9 LAT

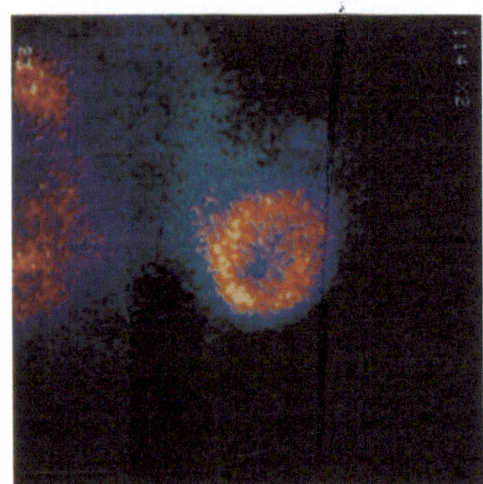

Fig. 9.9 LAO

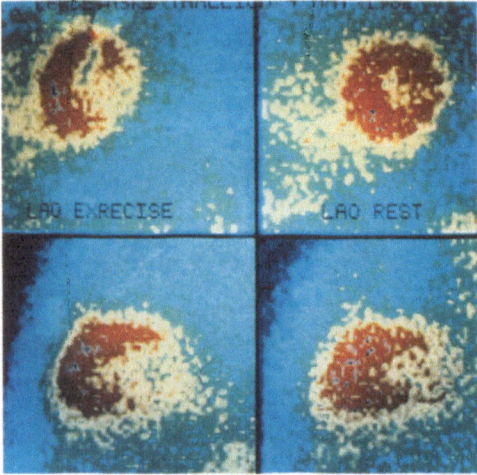

Fig. 9.10

Fig. 9.6. Aortic regurgitation. The end diastolic image shows a dilated left ventricle, and the left ventricular ejection fraction is 0.57 with a left to right ventricular stroke volume ratio of 2.9, indicating moderate left sided valvular regurgitation. The defect in the amplitude image is commonly seen in aortic regurgitation.

Fig. 9.7. Pulmonary activity–time curve (yellow) in a patient with a ventricular septal defect. The green and pink curves are computer fits to the main peak, and to the second peak of early recirculation through the defect respectively. The areas under these curves are proportional to pulmonary and shunt flow, and the pulmonary to systemic flow ratio is easily calculated.

◀────────────────────────

activity. Both left and right ventricular ejection fractions can be calculated, and since the measurements are independent of ventricular geometry they are more accurate than those made from echocardiograms and X-ray ventriculograms, particularly for irregularly shaped ventricles and for the right ventricle.

Before the ejection fraction is calculated, correction is made for counts arising from blood behind and in front of the ventricle. Background counts are usually estimated from a crescentic region beside the left ventricle, but other methods are available allowing background to be measured without assigning another region (Goris et al. 1979) and this improves the accuracy and reproducibility of the measurements. It is difficult to estimate background for the right ventricle because of overlap with the right atrium, and the right ventricular ejection fraction is usually underestimated.

Regional Ventricular Function

Regional ventricular wall motion can be assessed by displaying the 16 images as a cine loop, but it is more easily quantified using parametric images, such as the stroke volume image, the regional ejection fraction image, or the amplitude and phase images.

The amplitude and phase images display the extent and timing of motion of each point of the image respectively, and they are constructed from the volume–time curves of individual pixels. The curves for ventricular pixels are roughly sinusoidal

and the mathematical technique of Fourier transformation allows the curves to be reduced to a sine wave and defined by two only parameters – amplitude and phase (Fig. 9.3). The amplitude of a pixel is a measure of the extent of wall motion at that point and phase is a measure of the timing of its contraction. Amplitude and phase images can be constructed by colour-coding amplitude and phase values for each pixel, and normal images are shown in Fig. 9.4. High values of amplitude are seen over both ventricles and phase values are displayed in green, indicating uniform extent and timing of contraction. Figure 9.5 shows a patient with previous anteroseptal infarction. The anteroseptal wall has low values of amplitude (hypokinesis) and high values of phase (delayed contraction).

The phase image is of particular value in the detection of ventricular aneurysms, since dyskinetic areas (paradoxical contraction) appear with atrial phase. It also allows the contractile segment of the ventricle to be defined, and the ejection fraction of this can be used to predict function of the whole ventricle after aneurysmectomy (Yiannikas et al. 1985).

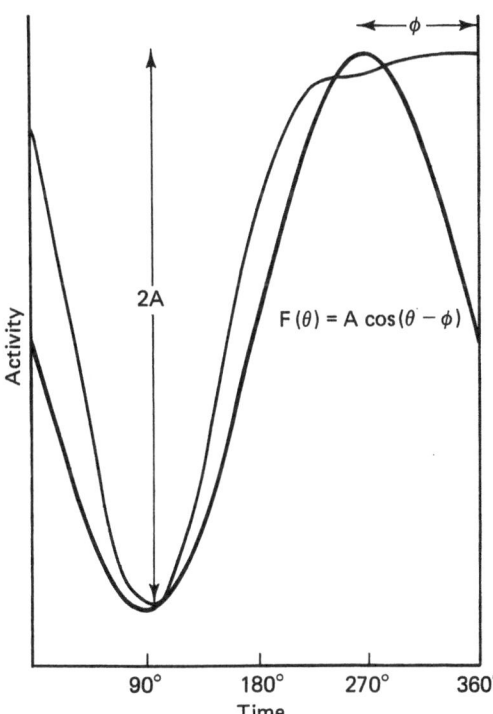

Fig. 9.3. A ventricular activity–time curve (thin line) with the corresponding fundamental frequency of its Fourier transform (thick line). The Fourier transform is a sinusoid and is completely described by two parameters, amplitude (A) and phase (φ), which represent the extent and timing of contraction respectively.

◀────────────────────────

Fig. 9.9. Normal planar thallium images in the antero-posterior, left anterior oblique, and left lateral projections.

Fig. 9.10. Left anterior oblique and left lateral thallium images at stress and following rest in a patient with disease of the left circumflex coronary artery. There is a reversible perfusion defect of the lateral and basal inferior walls.

Valvular Regurgitation

The ratio of the left and right ventricular stroke volumes is a measure of the severity of valvular regurgitation, since in the absence of regurgitation the output of both ventricles is the same (Rigo et al. 1979; Alderson 1982). Figure 9.6 shows a patient with aortic regurgitation. The left ventricle is dilated, but the ejection fraction is normal, and the stroke volume ratio of 2.9 indicates moderately severe regurgitation. In normal subjects the mean value of the stroke volume ratio is 1.4, since the equilibrium technique underestimates right ventricular stroke volume because of overlap between the atrium and ventricle. This does not limit its usefulness provided a normal range is established (Underwood et al. 1986).

The ratio provides a balance between left and right sided regurgitation, and it may be normal if regurgitation is equally severe on both sides of the heart. This is usually obvious clinically and does not often lead to confusion. The regurgitant fraction of individual valves can be measured from a first-pass study (Janowitz and Fester 1982; Walton et al. 1984).

First Pass Studies

If a bolus of technetium-99m (less than 0.5 ml) is rapidly flushed through a cannula in a medial antecubital vein, its passage through the central circulation can be recorded with high temporal resolution, and similar information can be obtained as from an equilibrium study. The main advantage of the first-pass study is that it can be recorded in any projection since the passage of the bolus through the left and right hearts is separated temporally and overlap of the blood pools is not a problem. A common practice is to perform a right anterior oblique first-pass study followed by a left anterior oblique equilibrium study (Underwood et al. 1983).

One disadvantage is that the study can only be performed once (or at most twice) because background blood pool activity complicates data analysis. In addition, not all cameras and computers are capable of handling the high count rates achieved whilst the bolus is within the field of view. Short-lived isotopes such as 195m-gold (half-life 30.5 s) allow multiple first-pass studies in rapid succession, and are ideal for monitoring changes in ventricular function induced by drugs or stress (Dymond et al. 1983).

Right Ventricular Ejection Fraction

A first-pass study avoids the problems of the equilibrium technique in determining right ventricular ejection fraction – overlap between the right atrium and ventricle can be avoided, and background estimation is less important (Xue et al. 1983). Incomplete mixing of the bolus within the ventricle can lead to an overestimation, however, and the best technique is the one that is in regular use in a centre and can be shown to be reproducible (Walton et al. 1980).

Intracardiac Shunting

The pulmonary activity–time curve generated from a first-pass study will show a single peak as the bolus passes through the lungs, and a later more diffuse one as the bolus recirculates. In the presence of left to right intracardiac shunting, there will be an early second peak which is usually superimposed upon the downslope of the first one, because of recirculation through the shunt (Fig. 9.7). The areas under the peaks allow the pulmonary and systemic flows to be calculated (Maltz and Treves 1973) and the measurements are more accurate than those made by oximetry at cardiac catheterisation (Underwood et al. 1986), particularly for atrial septal defects where true mixed venous saturation is unknown (Baker et al. 1985). Right to left shunting can also be detected from a left ventricular activity-time curve, but it is harder to quantify.

Stress Imaging

One of the great advantages of nuclear techniques is that functional information can be obtained during stress (Iskandrian and Hakki 1985b). Supine or upright bicycle exercise is usually performed with the upper body immobilised, and images are acquired for the last 2 min of 3-min stages, until significant symptoms are produced or an adequate rate–pressure product is reached. A normal response is for the left ventricular ejection fraction to increase by at least 0.05. Abnormality, or a new wall motion defect, implies stress-induced ischaemia which can be localised and its effect quantified (Borer et al. 1977). The value of these studies in the detection and management of coronary artery disease is discussed below.

Not all patients are able to perform dynamic exercise, and alternative forms of stress are isometric exercise (Bodenheimer et al. 1978) and cold pressor stress (Verani et al. 1982). In the former, the patient squeezes a bulb at 30% of maximal grip during acquisition, and in the latter, the forearm is immersed in iced water. They both produce a large pressor response and a slight tachycardia, and it is the increased afterload that constitutes the stress. These forms of stress are attractive for patients unable to exercise, but abnormalities are not so frequently produced. The development of a new wall motion abnormality is however a very specific indicator of the presence of disease (Underwood et al. 1984).

Non-Imaging Devices

Both first-pass and equilibrium studies may be performed with a non-imaging probe, which is relatively small and portable and consists of a scintillation crystal with a single photomultiplier tube and a focussing conical collimator. The count rate from the probe is displayed, and with suitable experience a real-time volume curve of the left ventricle can be obtained leading to beat-by-beat ejection fraction. Electrocardiographic gating can be used to sum beats over 30 or 60 s for greater statistical accuracy, and emptying and filling rates may be measured (Steele et al. 1974; Bacharach et al. 1977) (Fig. 9.8). The probe is particularly valuable on the intensive or coronary care units since a single

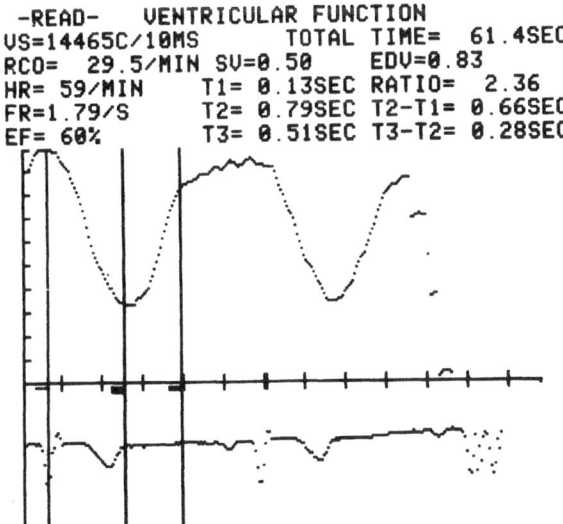

```
-READ-    VENTRICULAR FUNCTION
US=14465C/10MS        TOTAL TIME=   61.4SEC
RCO=  29.5/MIN SV=0.50      EDV=0.83
HR= 59/MIN    T1= 0.13SEC RATIO=    2.36
FR=1.79/S     T2= 0.79SEC T2-T1= 0.66SEC
EF= 60%       T3= 0.51SEC T3-T2= 0.28SEC
```

Fig. 9.8. Background corrected activity–time curve recorded over the left ventricle using a nonimaging scintillation probe. The recorded counts are electrocardiographically gated and averaged over 1 min, with a temporal resolution of 10 ms. Ejection fraction, emptying and filling rates may be measured, and absolute volumes are normalised to the end diastolic volume.

injection of technetium-99m allows monitoring of ventricular function for up to 24 h.

Portable detectors are being developed for ambulatory monitoring of ventricular volume. Current devices based on a cadmium telluride crystal are only just sufficiently sensitive for beat-by-beat monitoring, but sodium iodide detectors are feasible and ambulatory monitoring will soon be possible.

Thallium-201 Myocardial Perfusion Imaging

As described above, thallium-201 is taken up by the myocardium in proportion to blood flow, although at high values of flow, the rate of extraction becomes limiting and uptake does not increase proportionately. This is not clinically important because it is nearly always used to detect areas of decreased flow.

If thallium is injected intravenously at peak exercise, imaging within the first half hour reflects the distribution at the time of injection. Myocardial uptake should be homogeneous and, in patients with coronary artery disease, a defect represents either an old infarct, or an area of viable myocardium that is temporarily ischaemic because of the stress. Defects are visible when 5–7 g of myocardium have blood flow reduced to less than 60% of normal values (Pohost et al. 1977). After the first half hour, redistribution occurs and images acquired between 2 and 4 h distinguish between reversible and irreversible ischaemia. Both the site and the extent of ischaemia can be seen, and this is particularly important because the ability to do this is not shared by 12-lead exercise electrocardiography (Abouantoun et al. 1984).

For several reasons, thallium-201 is not an ideal radionuclide for imaging. Its principal emission is low energy leading to low resolution images, it has a long half-life so that small amounts must be used to limit radiation exposure, and only 5% of the injected dose is taken up by myocardium. Despite this it has found extensive use because its uptake by the myocardium is proportional to myocardial blood flow over a wide range of values, and myocardial perfusion may be imaged both at rest and during stress (Iskandrian and Hakki 1985a).

Figure 9.9 shows normal planar thallium images and Fig. 9.10 shows a defect of perfusion of the lateral wall during stress, with redistribution following rest in a patient with disease of the left circumflex coronary artery.

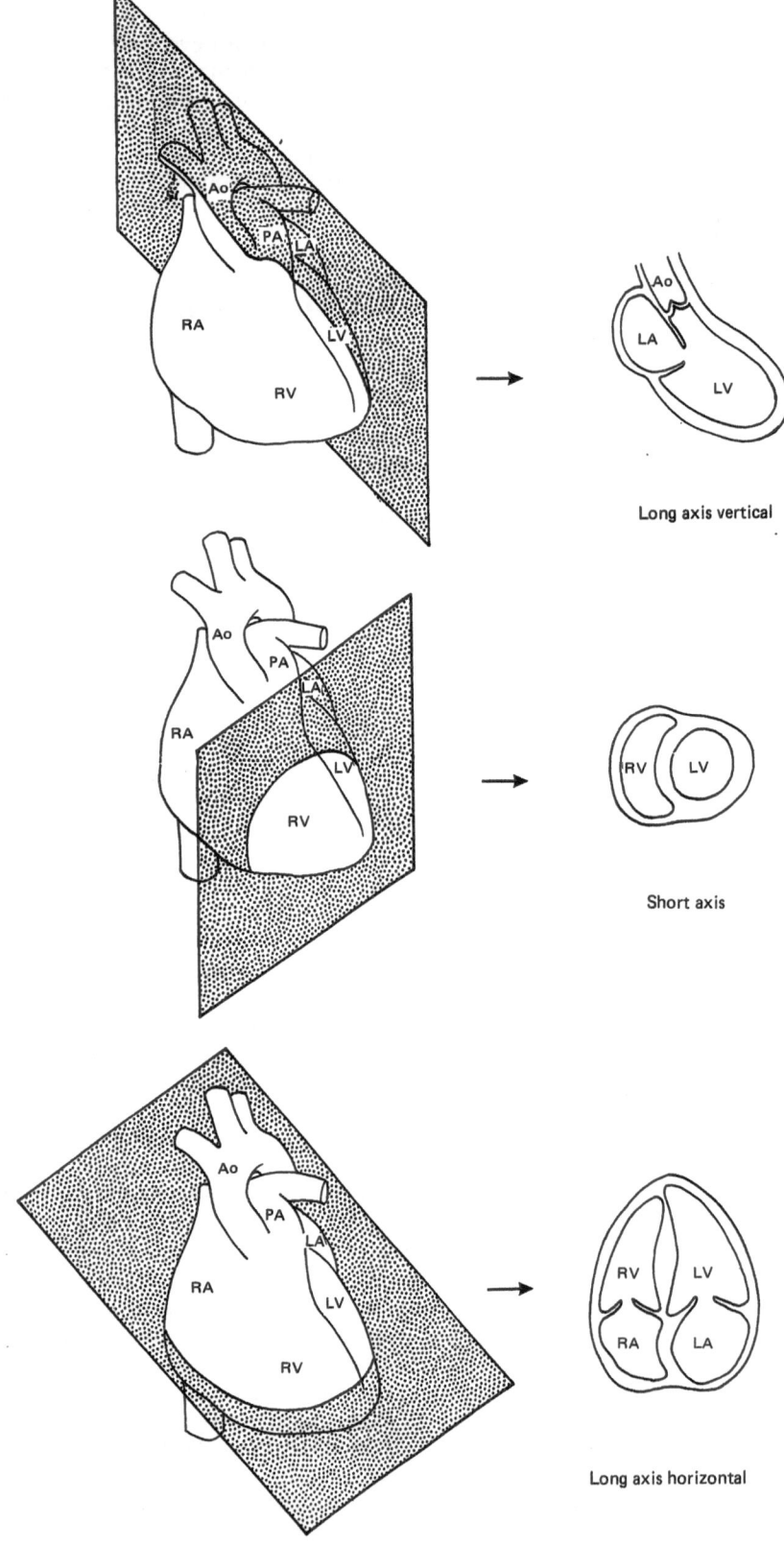

Long axis vertical

Short axis

Long axis horizontal

Fig. 9.11a

Fig. 9.11a,b. Planes perpendicular and parallel to the long axis of the left ventricle used in emission tomography (**a**) and normal thallium tomograms in the three planes (**b**).

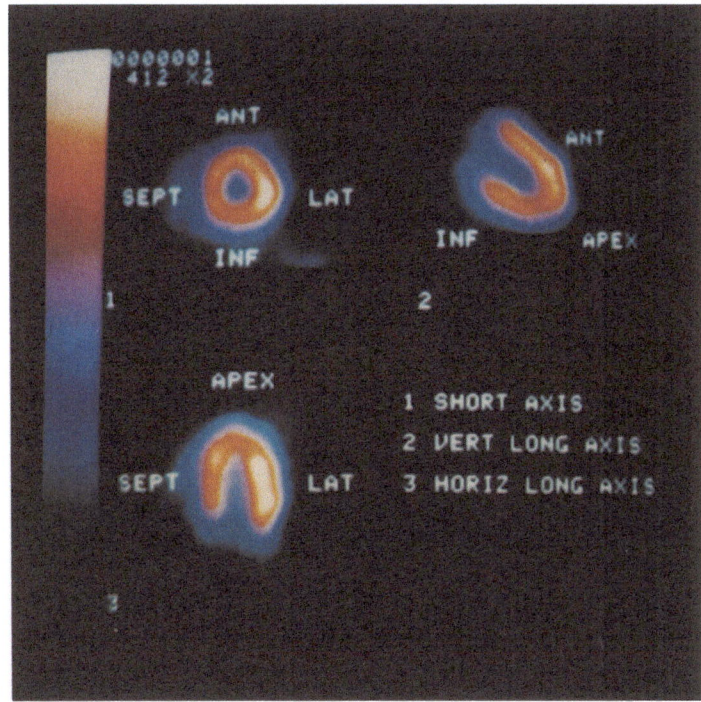

Fig. 9.11b

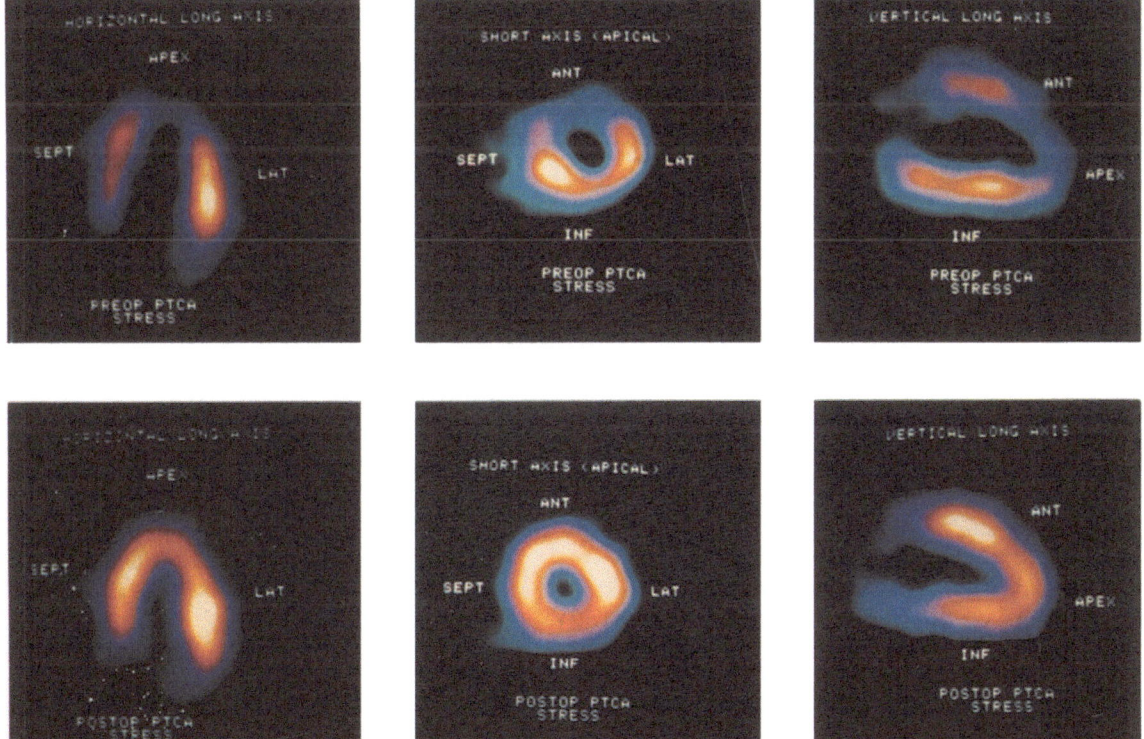

Fig. 9.12. Stress thallium tomograms before and after transluminal angioplasty in a patient with disease of the left anterior descending coronary artery. There is a perfusion defect of the distal anterior wall and apex which is not present following angioplasty.

Emission Tomography

Planar images such as the ones above can be difficult to interpret without considerable experience, but single photon emission tomography has helped greatly and makes the images more reliable as well as easier to interpret (Tamaki et al. 1981; Kirsch et al. 1983). The technique involves a rotating gamma camera to acquire multiple planar images, and from these, tomographic sections are reconstructed in the same way as in X-ray transmission tomography. The tomograms can be orientated in any plane, and sections perpendicular and parallel to the long axis of the left ventricle are usual (Fig. 9.11). Figure 9.12 shows tomograms demonstrating reversible septal ischaemia in a patient with disease of the left anterior descending coronary artery.

Although rotating camera tomography provides the best images, limited angle acquisition using either a rotating slant hole collimator or a seven-pin-hole collimator is also possible, with the advantage of being available on portable machines (Vogel et al. 1979; Bateman et al. 1983).

Quantification

Another technique that improves sensitivity in the detection of defects is quantification, both of planar images and tomograms (Berger et al. 1981; Maddahi et al. 1981). A narrow sector is swept around the image and the activity at each point plotted as a profile (Meade et al. 1978; Burow et al. 1979). The circumferential profiles can be compared with those from a bank of normal subjects, and any area where the activity is significantly less can be easily identified. Figure 9.13 shows circumferential profiles from vertical long axis tomograms. There is an anterior defect that is not present following rest, and the defect is not easily seen from the images alone.

Analysis of the rate of thallium wash-out from the myocardium also improves sensitivity (Watson et al. 1981; Garcia et al. 1981). Thallium washes out more slowly from areas served by a stenosed artery, and this allows the detection of ischaemia even when there is balanced three-vessel coronary artery disease and the whole heart is underperfused. When a lesion in one vessel is dominant, and a single defect is seen, there may be wash-out abnormalities in other areas reflecting disease in the other vessels. In practice, the interpretation of wash-out abnormalities in the absence of a defect must be made with care. Figure 9.13 shows slow wash-out from the anterior wall in the same region as the perfusion defect present during stress.

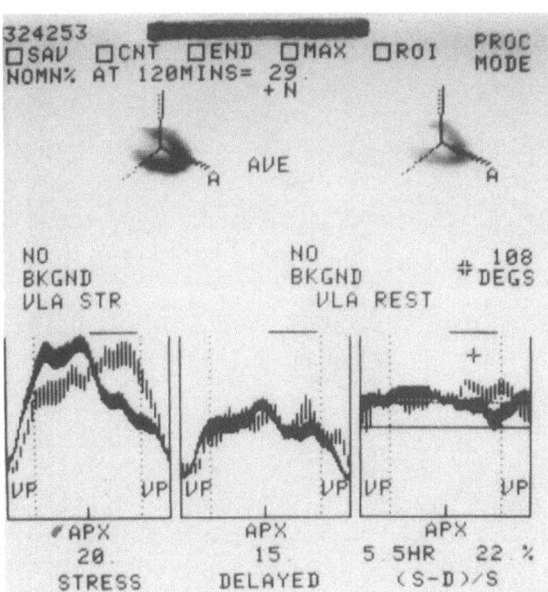

Fig. 9.13. Circumferential profiles from vertical long axis tomograms during stress (*top left*) and following redistribution (*top right*). The profiles sweep anticlockwise from the valve plane (*solid line*) and are compared with profiles from a bank of normal subjects. There is an anterior defect at stress (*bottom left*) which disappears with redistribution (*bottom centre*). The wash-out profile (*bottom right*) shows slow wash-out in the affected area.

Dipyridamole Stress

Intravenous dipyridamole is a powerful coronary dilator, and it has been used as an alternative to dynamic exercise as a form of stress in thallium imaging (Gould 1978; Gould et al. 1979; Albro et al. 1978). In a vessel with a fixed stenosis, vasodilatation will not lead to as large an increase in flow as in a normal vessel, and there will be a relative perfusion defect in the territory served by the vessel. In addition to this, normally perfused areas may steal blood from the abnormal territory, and it is possible to induce angina with intravenous dipyridamole in the presence of coronary artery disease. Although dipyridamole stress has been used successfully in some centres (Leppo et al. 1982; Francisco et al. 1982) it is usually reserved, along with cold pressor stress (Ahmad et al. 1982), for patients who are unable to perform dynamic exercise.

Acute Infarction Imaging

Imaging of acute infarction is not commonly performed because of the simplicity of conventional

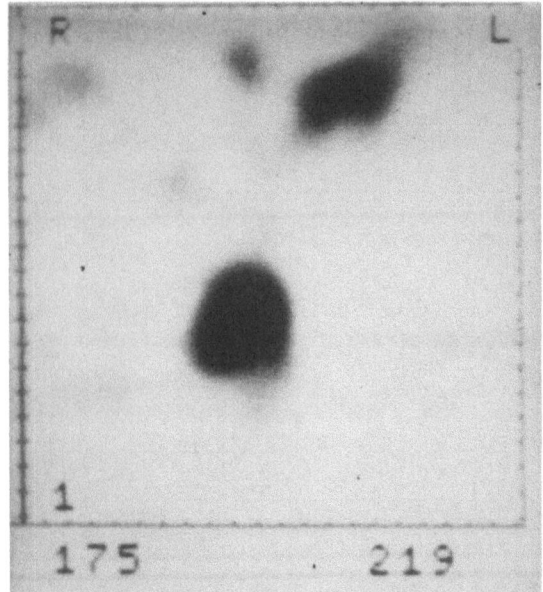

Fig. 9.14. Transaxial tomogram following injection of technetium-99m pyrophosphate in a patient with acute septal infarction. There is heavy uptake in the spine and some uptake by the sternum, but also a large area of abnormal uptake in the left ventricular septum.

methods for the detection of infarction. On the intensive care unit however, acute infarct imaging has a particular role, since cardiac enzymes may be elevated because of recent surgery, and the electrocardiogram may not be easy to interpret (Burdine et al. 1979; Righetti et al. 1977).

The infarct may be imaged either as a hot spot or as a cold spot. Thallium-201 will show an infarct as a cold spot, and it is particularly sensitive in the early hours after infarction. More commonly used is technetium-99m pyrophosphate which shows areas of acute infarction as a hot spot. If emission tomography is performed, the size of the infarct may be accurately measured, providing important prognostic information (Keyes et al. 1978) (Fig. 9.14).

Table 9.3. Sensitivity and specificity of exercise electrocardiography, thallium-201 scanning, and radionuclide ventriculography (RNV) in the diagnosis of coronary artery disease (Laird et al. 1984).

	Sensitivity (%)	Specificity (%)
Exercise electrocardiography	64	82
Exercise thallium	79	86
Exercise radionuclide ventriculography	86	82

One drawback of technetium pyrophosphate is that although uptake by infarcted myocardium is maximal on the second day, by 5–7 days there is very little uptake, so that there is only a narrow window in which to use the test.

The Role of Nuclear Cardiology in Coronary Artery Disease

Diagnosis

Because nuclear techniques are relatively non-invasive and are able to detect stress-induced myocardial ischaemia with high sensitivity, they are of value in the diagnosis of coronary artery disease. Although there is considerable variation in figures for sensitivity and specificity in the detection of coronary artery disease (Borer et al. 1979; Berger et al. 1979; Bodenheimer et al. 1979; Austin et al. 1982; O'Keefe et al. 1983) Table 9.3 shows representative figures for electrocardiography, radionuclide ventriculography, and thallium imaging. The nuclear techniques are more sensitive without a reduction in specificity, but electrocardiography is more widely available and will probably continue to be more widely performed. It should be noted that the figures given in Table 9.3 are for planar thallium imaging without quantification, and much higher values can be achieved with quantitative tomography (Tamaki et al. 1984; Laird et al. 1984).

The figures do not tell the whole truth, however, because a test can only be of value if it contributes towards the management of the patient. If there is a low probability of disease (for instance a young woman with atypical chest pain), then even if the test is abnormal it is likely to be considered a false-positive test and the patient will not be catheterised. Conversely, in a middle-aged male smoker with typical angina, a negative result is also unlikely to alter the diagnosis. It is only in patients with an intermediate pretest probability of disease that a positive result is likely to lead to the decision to perform coronary arteriography, or a negative result will allow reassurance without catheterisation (Becker 1980; Timmis 1985).

Management

If nuclear techniques have a limited but definite role in the diagnosis of coronary artery disease, they have a very large part to play in the management of established disease (Bonow et al. 1984a; Beller 1984).

Traditionally, coronary-artery disease is managed according to the anatomy of the coronary arteries and judgement is made on the significance of lesions from the coronary arteriogram. Setting aside the fact that the coronary arteriogram is not as exact a test as is usually assumed, the demonstration of the functional significance of a lesion allows a more logical approach to treatment. It is now well established that prognosis in patients with coronary artery disease depends upon ventricular function, and upon the amount of myocardium in jeopardy, and patients in whom it is not possible to demonstrate reversible ischaemia have a low probability of future cardiac events, whatever the anatomy of the coronary arteries (Fioretti et al. 1984; Iskandrian et al. 1985a,b; Bonow et al. 1984b; Pryor et al. 1984; Brown et al. 1983; Wahl et al. 1985). Ideally, all patients with coronary artery disease should be studied in order to pick out those at high risk for aggressive treatment.

Conclusion

Nuclear cardiology provides a wide range of information, and differs from other techniques in that the information is predominantly about function rather than structure. Portable cameras and the smaller non-imaging detectors allow information to be obtained on the intensive care unit, and measurements may be made during stress if appropriate. A logical approach to cardiovascular disease is possible with a knowledge of structure and function, and widespread use of nuclear techniques will benefit all those with disease of the cardiovascular system.

References

Abouantoun S, Ahnve S, Savvides M, Witztum K, Jensen D, Froelicher V (1984) Can areas of myocardial ischaemia be localised by the exercise electrocardiogram? A correlative study with thallium-201 scintigraphy. Am Heart J 108: 933–941

Ahmad M, Dubiel JP, Haiback H (1982) Cold pressor thallium-201 myocardial scintigraphy in the diagnosis of coronary artery disease. Am J Cardiol 50: 1253–1257

Albro PC, Gould KL, Westcott RJ, Hamilton GW, Ritchie JL, Williams DL (1978) Noninvasive assessment of coronary stenoses by myocardial perfusion imaging during pharmacologic coronary vasodilatation. III Clinical trial. Am J Cardiol 42: 751–760

Alderson PO (1982) Radionuclide quantification of valvular regurgitation. J Nucl Med 23: 851–855

Austin EH, Cobb FR, Coleman RE, Jones RH (1982) Prospective evaluation of radionuclide angiocardiography for the diagnosis of coronary artery disease. Am J Cardiol 50: 1212–1216

Bacharach SL et al. (1977) ECG-gated scintillation probe measurement of left ventricular function. J Nucl Med 18: 1176–1173

Baker EJ, Ellam SV, Lorber A, Jones ODH, Tynan MJ, Maisey MN (1985) Superiority of radionuclide over oximetric measurement of left to right shunts. Br Heart J 53: 535–540

Bateman T, Garcia E, Maddahi J et al. (1983) Clinical evaluation of seven-pinhole tomography for the detection and localization of coronary artery disease: comparison with planar imaging using quantitative analysis of myocardial thallium-201 distribution and washout after exercise. Am Heart J 106: 263–271

Becker LC (1980) Diagnosis of coronary artery disease with exercise radionuclide imaging: state of the art. Am J Cardiol 45: 1301–1304

Beller GA (1984) Quantitative thallium-201 scintigraphy. Internat J Cardiol 5: 234–239

Berger BC, Watson DD, Taylor GJ et al. (1981) Quantitative thallium-201 exercise scintigraphy for detection of coronary artery disease. J Nucl Med 22: 585–593

Berger HJ, Reduto LA, Johnstone DE et al. (1979) Global and regional left ventricular response to bicycle exercise in coronary artery disease. Assessment by quantitative radionuclide angiocardiography. Am J Med 66: 13–21

Bodenheimer MM, Banka VS, Fooshee CM, Gillespie JA, Helfant RH (1978) Detection of coronary heart disease using radionuclide determined regional ejection fraction at rest and during handgrip exercise: correlation with coronary arteriography. Circulation 58: 640–648

Bodenheimer MM, Banka VS, Fooshee CM, Helfant RH (1979) Comparative sensitivity of the exercise electrocardiogram, thallium imaging and stress radionuclide angiography to detect the presence and severity of coronary heart disease. Circulation 60: 1270–1278

Bonow RO, Green MV, Bacharach SL (1984a) Radionuclide angiography during exercise in patients with coronary artery disease: diagnostic, prognostic, and therapeutic implications. Internat J Cardiol 5: 229–233

Bonow RO, Kent KM, Rosing DR et al. (1984b) Exercise-induced ischaemia in mildly symptomatic patients with coronary artery disease, and preserved left ventricular function: identification of subgroups at high risk for death during medical therapy. New Engl J Med 311: 1339–1345

Borer JS, Bacharach SL, Green MV, Kent KM, Epstein SE, Johnston GS (1977) Real-time radionuclide cineangiography in the noninvasive evaluation of global and regional left ventricular function at rest and during exercise in patients with coronary artery disease. New Engl J Med 296: 839–844

Borer JS, Kent KM, Bacharach SL et al. (1979) Sensitivity, specificity and predictive accuracy of radionuclide cineangiography during exercise in patients with coronary artery disease. Comparison with exercise electrocardiography. Circulation 60: 572–580

Brown KA, Boucher CA, Okada RD et al. (1983) Prognostic value of exercise thallium-201 imaging in patients presenting for evaluation of chest pain. J Am Coll Cardiol 1: 994–1001

Burdine JA, DePuey EG, Orzan F, Mathur VS, Hall RJ (1979) Scintigraphic, electrocardiographic, and enzymatic diagnosis of perioperative myocardial infarction in patients undergoing myocardial revascularisation. J Nucl Med 20: 711–714

Burow RD, Pond M, Schafer AW, Becker L (1979) "Circumferential profiles:" a new method for computer analysis of thallium-201 myocardial perfusion images. J Nucl Med 20: 771–777

Dymond DS, Elliot AT, Flatman W et al. (1983) The clinical validation of gold-195m: a new short half life radiopharmaceutical for rapid, sequential, first pass angio-cardiography in patients. J Am Coll Cardiol 2: 85–92

Fioretti P, Brower RW, Simoons ML et al. (1984). Prediction of mortality in hospital survivors of myocardial infarction. Comparison of predischarge exercise testing and radionuclide ventriculography at rest. Br Heart J 52: 292–298

Francisco DA, Collins SM, Go RT, Ehrhardt JC, VanKirk OC, Marcus ML (1982) Tomographic thallium-201 myocardial perfusion scintigrams after maximal coronary artery vaso-dilation with intravenous dipyridamole: comparison of quali-tative and quantitative approaches. Circulation 66: 370–379

Garcia E, Maddahi J, Berman D, Waxman A (1981) Space/time quantitation of thallium-201 myocardial scintigraphy. J Nucl Med 22: 309–317

Goris ML, Briandet PA, Huffer E (1979) Automation and oper-ator independent data processing of cardiac and pulmonary functions: role, methods, and results. In: Di Paolo R, Kahn E (eds) Information processing in medical imaging. Pro-ceedings of the 6th international conference. Paris: INSERM 88: 427–448

Gould KL (1978) Noninvasive assessment of coronary stenoses by myocardial perfusion imaging during pharmacologic cor-onary vasodilatation. I Physiologic basis and experimental validation. Am J Cardiol 41: 267–278

Gould KL, Westcott RJ, Albro PC, Hamilton GW (1978) Non-invasive assessment of coronary stenoses by myocardial perfusion imaging during pharmacologic coronary vasodilatation. II Clinical methodology and feasibility. Am J Cardiol 41: 279–287

Iskandrian AS, Hakki A-H (1985a) Thallium-201 myocardial scintigraphy. Am Heart J 109: 113–129

Iskandrian AS, Hakki A-H (1985b) Radionuclide evaluation of exercise left ventricular performance in patients with coronary artery disease. Am Heart J 110: 851–856

Iskandrian AS, Hakki A-H, Kane-Marsch S (1985a) Prognostic implications of thallium-201 scintigraphy in patients with suspected or known coronary artery disease. Am Heart J 110: 135–143

Iskandrian AS, Hakki A-H, Goel IP, Mundth ED, Kane-Marsch SA, Schenk CL (1985b) The use of rest and exercise radionuclide ventriculography in risk stratification in patients with suspected coronary artery disease. Am Heart J 100: 864–872

Janowitz W, Fester A (1982) Quantification of left ventricular regurgitant fraction by first pass radionuclide angio-cardiography. Am J Cardiol 49: 85–92

Keyes JW, Leonard PF, Brody SL, Svetkoff DJ, Rogers WL, Luchessi BR (1978) Myocardial infarct quantification in the dog by single photon emission computed tomography. Cir-culation 58: 227–232

Kirsch C-M, Doliwa R, Buell U, Roedler D (1983) Detection of severe coronary heart disease with Tl-201: comparison of resting single photon emission tomography with invasive arteriography. J Nucl Med 24: 761–767

Laird EE, Rajathurai A, Williams ED, Mittra B, Rankin D (1984) Quantitative analysis of rotating gamma camera thal-lium-201 scintigrams of myocardium. Nucl Med Commun 5: 577–586

Leppo J, Boucher CA, Okada D, Newell JB, Strauss HW, Pohost GM (1982) Serial thallium-201 myocardial imaging after dipy-ridamole infusion: diagnostic utility in detecting coronary stenoses and relationship to regional wall motion. Circulation 66: 649–656

Maddahi J, Garcia EV, Berman DS, Waxman A, Swan HJC, Forrester J (1981) Improved noninvasive assessment of cor-onary artery disease by quantitative analysis of regional stress myocardial distribution and washout of thallium-201. Cir-culation 64: 924–935

Maltz DL, Treves S (1973) Quantitative radionuclide angio-cardiography: determination of Q_p/Q_s in children. Circulation 47: 1049–1056

Meade RC, Bamrah VS, Horgan JD, Ruetz PP, Kronenwetter C, Yeh E-L (1978) Quantitative methods in the evaluation of thallium-201 myocardial perfusion images. J Nucl Med 19: 1175–1178

Mueller TM, Marcus ML, Ehrhardt JC, Chandhuri T, Abboud FM (1976) Limitations of thallium-201 myocardial perfusion scintigrams. Circulation 54: 640–646

Neilson AP, Morris KG, Murdock R, Bruno FP, Cobb FR (1980) Linear relationship between the distribution of thal-lium-201 and blood flow in ischaemic and nonischaemic myo-cardium during exercise. Circulation 61: 797–801

Okada RD, Leppo JA, Strauss HW, Boucher CA, Pohost GM (1982) Mechanisms and time course for the disappearance of thallium-201 defects at rest in dogs. Relation of time to peak activity to myocardial blood flow. Am J Cardiol 49: 699–706

O'Keefe JC et al. (1983) Comparison of exercise elec-trocardiography, thallium-201 myocardial imaging and exer-cise gated blood pool scan in patients with suspected coronary artery disease. Aust NZ J Med 13: 45–50

Pavel DG, Zimmer AM, Patterson V (1977) In vivo labelling of red blood cells with 99m-Tc: a new approach to blood pool visúalisation. J Nucl Med 18: 305–308

Pohost GM, Zir LM, Moore RH, McKusik KA, Guiney TE, Beller GA (1977) Differentiation of transiently ischaemic from infarcted myocardium by serial imaging after a single dose of thallium-201. Circulation 55: 294–302

Pryor DB, Harrell FE Jr, Lee KL et al. (1984) Prognostic indicators from radionuclide angiography in medically treated patients with coronary artery disease. Am J Cardiol 53: 18–22

Righetti A, O'Rourke RA, Schelbert H et al. (1977) Usefulness of preoperative and postoperative Tc-99m (Sn) pyro-phosphate scans in patients with ischaemic and valvular heart disease. Am J Cardiol 39: 43–49

Rigo P, Alderson PO, Robertson RM, Becker LC, Wagner HN Jr (1979) Measurement of aortic and mitral regurgitation by gated cardiac blood pool scans. Circulation 60: 306–312

Steele PP, Van Dyke D, Trow RS, Anger HO, Davies H (1974) Simple and safe bedside method for serial measurement of left ventricular ejection fraction, cardiac output, and pulmonary blood volume. Br Heart J 36: 122–131

Tamaki N, Mukai T, Ishii Y et al. (1981) Clinical evaluation of thallium-201 emission myocardial tomography using a rotat-ing gamma camera: comparison with seven-pinhole tom-ography. J Nucl Med 22: 849–855

Tamaki N, Yonekura Y, Mukai T et al. (1984) Segmental analy-sis of stress thallium myocardial emission tomography for localisation of coronary artery disease. Eur J Nucl Med 9: 99–105

Timmis AD (1985) Probability analysis in the diagnosis of cor-onary artery disease. Br Med J 291: 1443–1444

Underwood SR, Walton S, Laming PJ, Ell PJ, Swanton RH, Emanuel RW (1983) Differential sensitivity of the Fourier phase and amplitude images in the detection of abnormal anterior and inferior left ventricular wall motion (Abstract). Nucl Med Commun 4: 135

Underwood SR, Walton S, Ell PJ, Emanuel RW, Swanton RH (1984) Isometric exercise in the detection of coronary artery disease – specific but not sensitive. In: Hoefer R, Bergman H (eds) Radioactive isotopes in clinical medicine and research. Verlag H Egermann, Vienna, 16: 443–450

Underwood SR, Klipstein RH, Firmin DN et al. (1986) Mag-netic resonance assessment of the accuracy of radionuclide methods for the quantification of valvular regurgitation and

113

atrial shunting. In: Hoefer R, Bergman H (eds) Radioactive isotopes in clinical medicine and research. Verlag H Egermann, Vienna, 17: 299–305

Verani MS, Zacca NM, DeBauche TL, Miller RR, Chahine RA (1982) Comparison of cold pressor and exercise radionuclide angiocardiography in coronary artery disease. J Nucl Med 23: 770–776

Vogel RA, Kirch DL, LeFree MT, Rainwater JO, Jenson DP, Steele PP (1979) Thallium-201 myocardial perfusion scintigraphy: results of standard and multi-pinhole tomographic techniques. Am J Cardiol 43: 787–793

Wahl JM, Hakki AH, Iskandrian AS (1985) Prognostic implications of normal exercise thallium 201 images. Arch Intern Med 145: 253–256

Walton S, Jarritt PH, Ell PJ (1980) Improved reproducibility of ejection fraction estimation using the phase image. Use of the technique to determine the heart's response to isometric exercise. In: Nuklearmedizin. Schattauer Verlag, Stuttgart, 1980; 220–224

Walton S, Underwood SR, Ell PJ, Swanton RH, Emanuel RW (1984) Measurement of valvular regurgitation by first pass radionuclide angiocardiography (Abstract). Br Heart J 54: 91P

Watson DD, Campbell NP, Read EK, Gibson RS, Teates CD, Beller GA (1981) Spatial and temporal quantitation of plane thallium myocardial images. J Nucl Med 22: 577–584

Xue QF, Macnee W, Flenley DC, Hannan WJ, Adie CJ, Muir AL (1983) Can right ventricular performance be assessed by equilibrium radionuclide ventriculography? Thorax 38: 486–493

Yiannikas J, MacIntyre WJ, Underwood DA et al. (1985) Prediction of improvement after ventricular aneurysmectomy using Fourier phase and amplitude analysis of radionuclide cardiac blood pool scans. Am J Cardiol 55: 1308–1312

Chapter 10

Magnetic Resonance

S. Rees, S. R. Underwood and D. Firmin

The phenomenon of magnetic resonance was first described in 1946 (Purcell et al. 1946) and for many years it has provided chemists with an invaluable analytical tool. More recently, it has also been applied in the fields of biology and medicine (Pykett et al. 1982) for such diverse applications as the provision of in vivo metabolic information (Hoult et al. 1974), and the non-invasive imaging of most organs of the body (Steiner 1983).

The brain and spinal cord provide particularly good images, and whilst magnetic resonance imaging (MRI) has not had quite the impact on the practice of neurology that computed tomography (CT) had, it is eventually likely to replace it in cerebral imaging. The special advantages of MRI are not only the excellent spatial resolution of the images in any of the three orthogonal planes, and their wide range of contrast between different soft tissues, but also the variation of the parameters displayed in the images according to the biochemical environment. Other organs are more difficult to image, mainly because of the problem of image degradation by motion artefact, and it is not yet clear whether magnetic resonance will compete successfully with CT in the abdomen. With respiratory gating, these images are much improved (Bailes et al. 1985), and although clinical experience is still relatively limited, metastatic disease of the liver is readily detected. Motion of the heart presents even greater problems, and cardiac gating is essential in order to demonstrate both anatomy and function. Nevertheless, it is already possible to show detailed cardiac anatomy (Steiner et al. 1983; Higgins et al. 1985a, b) (Fig. 10.1) and to measure ventricular function (Longmore et al. 1985) and

blood flow (Bryant et al. 1984), and the prospect of extending this to anatomy and blood flow in the coronary arteries is real. The potential applications of MRI are thus numerous, and will certainly assure it a place in the investigation of the heart.

The purpose of this brief survey is to describe the application of MRI to the study of the heart; to demonstrate the information that can already be obtained, and to speculate upon its future place in the management of cardiac disease.

Global Ventricular Function

It has been shown that ventricular volumes can be measured with an accuracy of approximately 2% (Longmore et al. 1985). This exceeds the accuracy of all other techniques, the reason being that volumes are calculated by summing the areas of the chamber shown in 1 cm-thick contiguous sections. The method is applicable to both left and right ventricles (or atria), so that both left and right ventricular stroke volumes, ejection fractions, and output can be calculated. Any plane may be used, although in the sagittal plane it is difficult to define the position of the tricuspid valve. Table 10.1 shows mean normal values for these measurements: the true value of the stroke volume ratio (LVSV/RVSV) is 1, since left and right ventricular outputs have to be the same over the period of imaging.

This multi-slice method of measuring ventricular volume is accurate but relatively lengthy. A simpler approximation to left ventricular volume may be obtained from a central oblique slice containing the long axis of the ventricle (Fig. 10.2). The area (A)

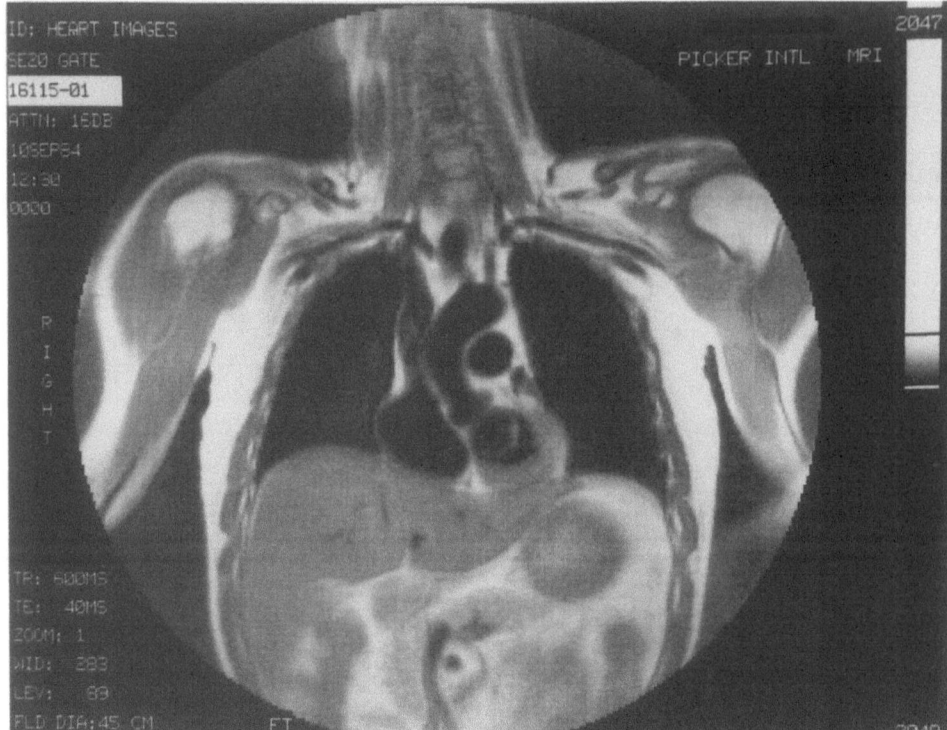

Left

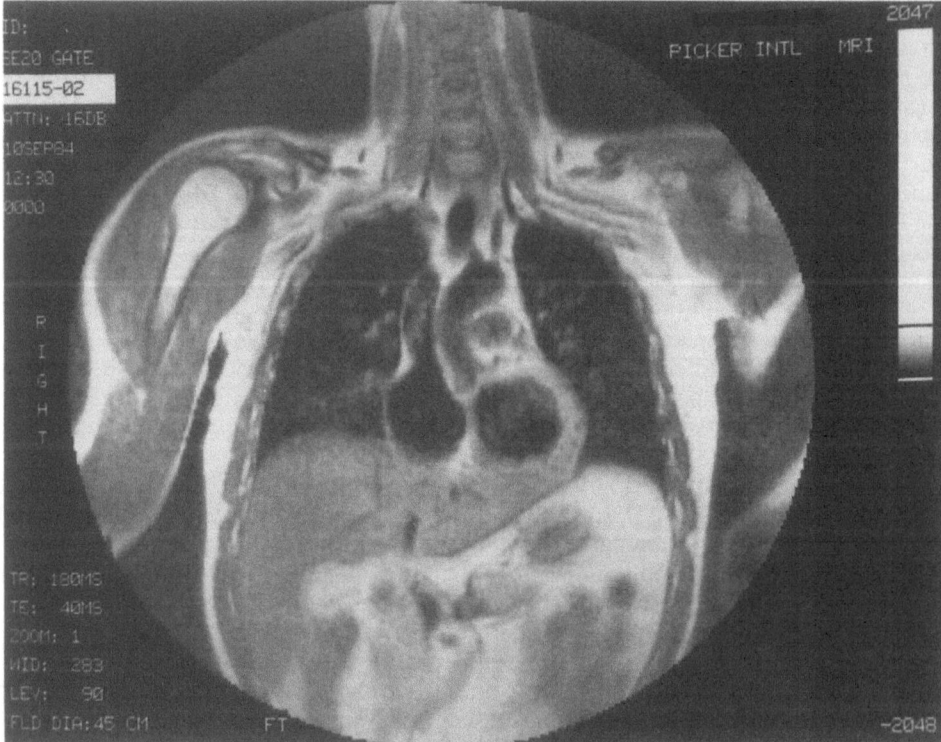

Right

Fig. 10.1. Coronal images through the aortic valve at end diastole (*left*) and end systole (*right*). Signal from static blood is seen at end diastole in the ascending aorta and pulmonary artery, and also in the superior vena cava. At end systole, there is no signal within the great vessels because of rapid flow, but there is a small area of signal within the left ventricular cavity.

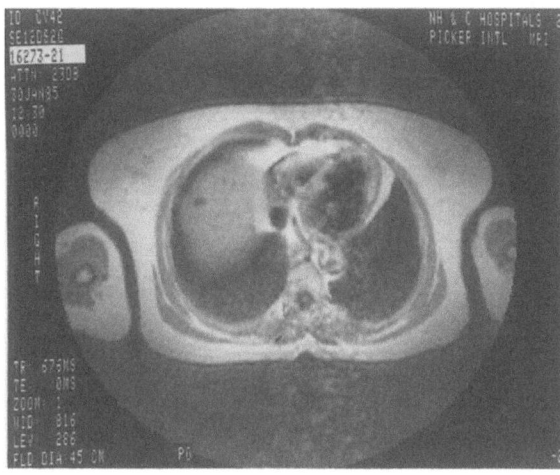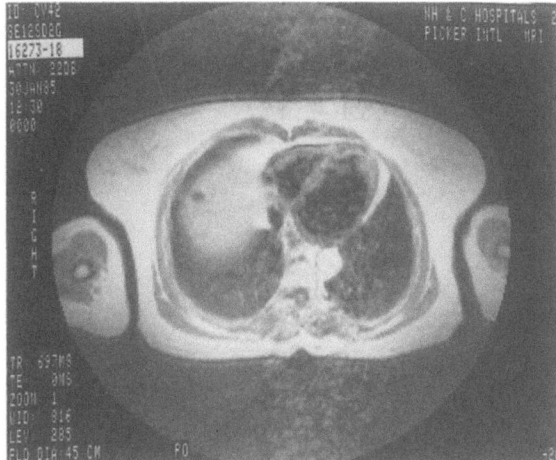

Fig. 10.2. A transverse plane tilted down by 30° towards coronal. The images are shown at end diastole (*left*) and end systole (*right*), and contain the long axis of the left ventricle.

Table 10.1. Mean values in 20 normal subjects, with standard deviations, for left and right ventricular end diastolic volume, stroke volume, and ejection fraction.

	Left ventricle			Right ventricle			
	End diastolic volume (LVEDV)	Stroke volume (LVSV)	Ejection fraction (LVEF)	End diastolic volume (RVEDV)	Stroke volume (RVSV)	Ejection fraction (RVEF)	Stroke volume ratio (LVSV/RVSV)
Mean	132 ml	81 ml	61%	152 ml	80 ml	53%	1.01
SD	14.7	16.2	7.2	20.9	16.4	7.4	0.067

and length (L) of the cavity are measured, and assuming the ventricle to be an ellipsoid of revolution, its volume is given by the formula:

$$V = 8 \times A^2/3\pi \times L$$

Figure 10.3 shows a subject with coronary artery disease and previous myocardial infarction. The left ventricle is dilated and the ejection fraction is low. The left ventricular myocardium is thin and hypokinetic at the site of infarction.

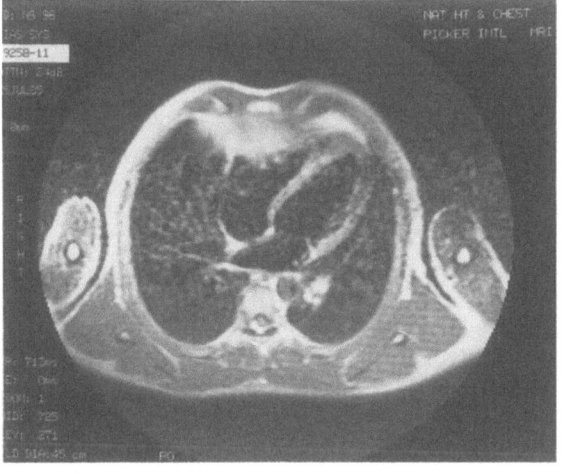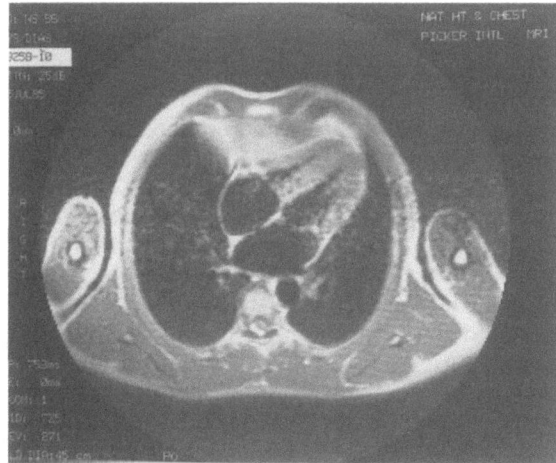

Fig. 10.3. Transverse sections at end diastole (*left*) and end systole (*right*) in a subject with coronary artery disease and previous myocardial infarction. The left ventricle is dilated (228 ml) with an ejection fraction of 25%. The distal septal and basal lateral walls are thinned, and at end systole they do not contract.

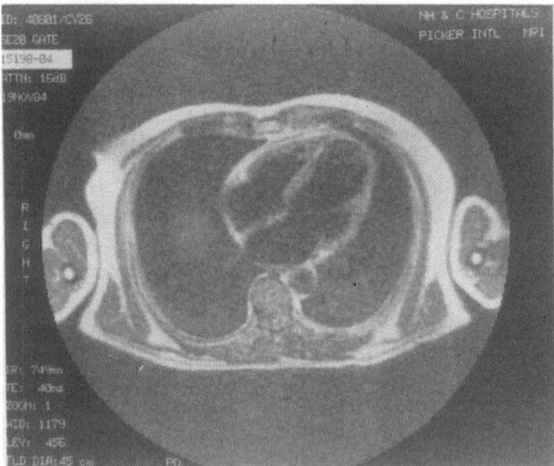 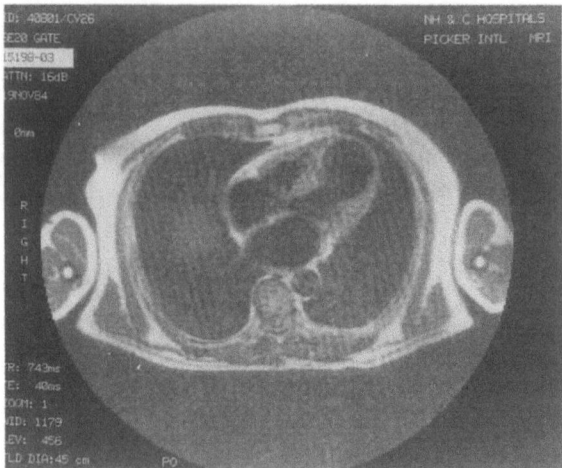

Fig. 10.4. Transverse section at end diastole (*left*) and end systole (*right*) in a patient with previous myocardial infarction and an apical left ventricular aneurysm. The basal myocardium contracts, but the whole of the apex is thin and dyskinetic.

Ventricular Wall Motion

Comparison of diastolic and systolic left ventricular contours allows the detection of areas of abnormal ventricular wall motion (Underwood et al. 1986). The myocardium at areas of previous infarction is also usually thin, although this may take up to 3 months to develop. Figure 10.4 shows a patient with an apical left ventricular aneurysm. A combination of cine imaging and functional images displaying different parameters of wall motion (such as regional ejection fraction, amplitude, or phase) will allow simple quantification of wall motion.

Myocardial Ischaemia

The effects of myocardial ischaemia are seen in a variety of ways. Myocardial infarction reduces ventricular ejection fraction and produces abnormalities of wall thickness and motion, as has been seen in the examples above. There has also been considerable interest in the changes in T_1 and T_2 produced by acute ischaemia (McNamara et al. 1985). Both T_1 and T_2 increase within a number of hours, in part due to an increased water content. An acute infarct can therefore be seen as an area of increased signal in a T_2-weighted spin-echo image, and over a period of 3 to 4 months T_2 values fall again to below those of normal myocardium. This provides a means for the detection and sizing of acute infarction.

It has been shown in animal experiments that the reduction in T_1 caused by gadolinium-DTPA is proportional to myocardial perfusion (at least at reduced levels of perfusion) (Goldman et al. 1982). Whether this will allow the detection of ischaemia induced by intravenous dipyridamole in areas served by diseased arteries remains to be seen.

Ventricular Hypertrophy

The ventricular myocardium is well demonstrated, and its volume can be measured with an accuracy similar to that of ventricular volume measurement. Measurements of ventricular thickness are however only significant if the plane of section is perpendicular to the wall. Figure 10.5 shows a subject with severe symmetrical left ventricular hypertrophy secondary to hypertension. Compare the myocardium with that of the normal subject in Fig. 10.1.

Hypertrophic cardiomyopathy is also readily seen and, in particular, it can be appreciated that the distribution of hypertrophy is very variable, and is not solely confined to the septum. T_2 values are different from those of normal myocardium.

Valvular Regurgitation

The left and right ventricular stroke volumes are identical over the period of imaging provided there is no valvular regurgitation or intracardiac shunting. If there is regurgitation on the left, the left to right stroke volume ratio will rise, and if there is regurgitation on the right, it will fall. From the stroke volume ratio, the regurgitant fraction can be calculated, although if there is both left- and right-sided regurgitation, the ratio may be either high or

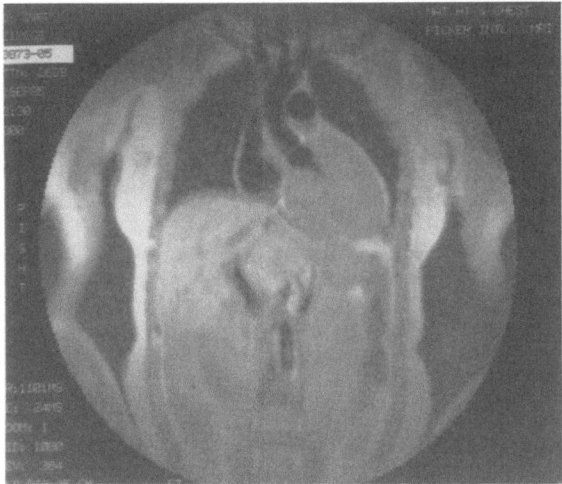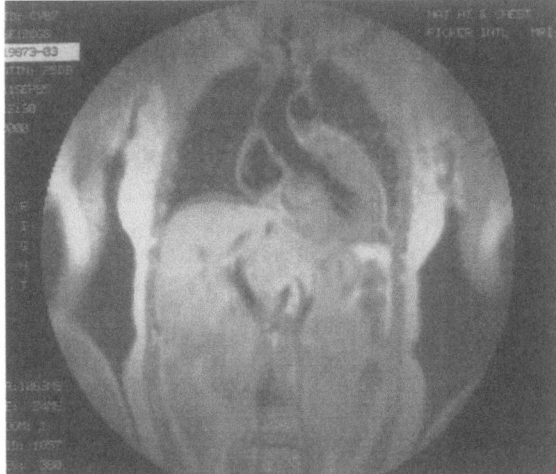

Fig. 10.5. Severe hypertensive heart disease. Transverse and coronal sections at end diastole (*left*) and end systole (*right*) in a patient with severe left ventricular hypertrophy. The volume of left ventricular myocardium is 752 ml. The ventricular cavity is almost totally obliterated at end systole.

low depending upon which is predominant. Figure 10.6 shows a patient with aortic regurgitation due to Marfan's syndrome. The ascending aorta is enormous compressing the pulmonary trunk (Fig. 10.6a). The left ventricle is dilated (Fig. 10.6b) with a diastolic volume of 542 ml and a stroke volume of 328 ml giving a stroke volume ratio of 3.5 and a regurgitant fraction of 71%.

Figure 10.7 shows a dilated left atrium in a subject with mitral regurgitation due to valve prolapse. The left ventricle was also dilated (403 ml), although the ejection fraction was normal (57%). The stroke volume ratio of 1.9 indicated a regur-

gitant fraction of 47% and valve replacement was performed.

Congenital Heart Disease

The ability to show cardiac anatomy so clearly means that MRI will be valuable in the investigation of congenital heart disease (Higgins et al. 1985b), although it is likely to complement rather than replace echocardiography. With conventional spin-echo sequences, children and neonates may need to be sedated for imaging, because of the long acqui-

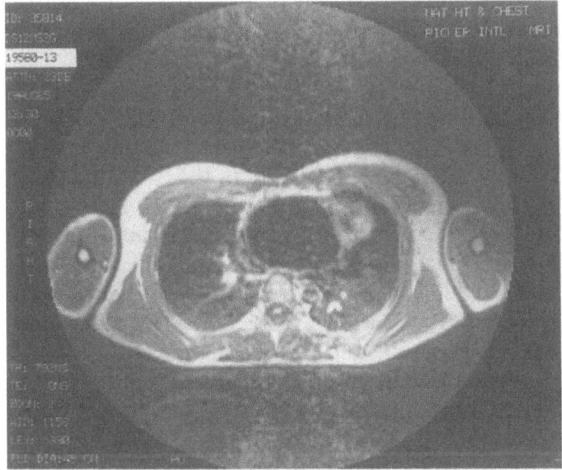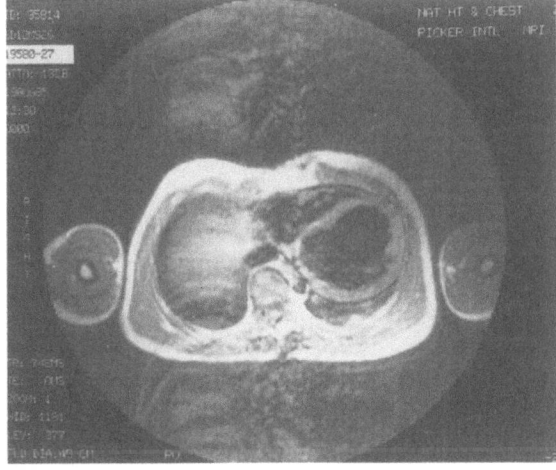

Fig. 10.6. Marfan's syndrome. Grossly dilated ascending aorta (*left*) in a patient with severe aortic regurgitation. The left ventricle is also grossly dilated (*right*) with a stroke volume of 328 ml and an ejection fraction of 61%.

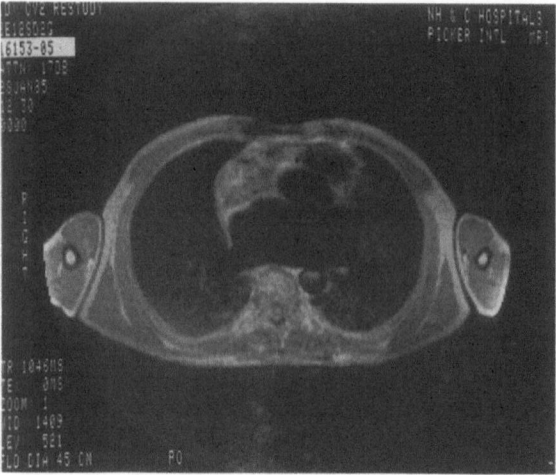

Fig. 10.7. Transverse section in a patient with severe mitral regurgitation due to mitral valve prolapse, showing a dilated left atrium. The left ventricle was also dilated (403 ml) but with reasonable function (ejection fraction 57%). The left to right ventricular stroke volume ratio was 1.9 and the regurgitant fraction 47%). The patient was in atrial fibrillation, but despite this image quality is good enough to see the left circumflex and anterior descending coronary arteries.

sition time for each slice, but real-time imaging using echo-planar techniques has already been successful at relatively low resolution (Ordidge et al. 1982).

Atrial and ventricular septal defects may be seen, and pulmonary to systemic flow ratio can be calculated from the left and right ventricular stroke

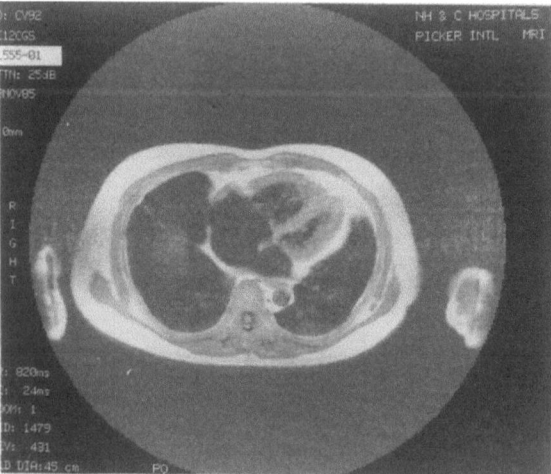

Fig. 10.8. Ostium secundum atrial septal defect: the atrial septum is present close to the mitral valve. The right heart is dilated (410 ml) due to the volume overload, but its function is preserved (ejection fraction 60%). A pulmonary to systemic flow ratio of 3.6 to 1 was calculated from the left and right ventricular stroke volumes. The moderator band is particularly well seen at the right ventricular apex.

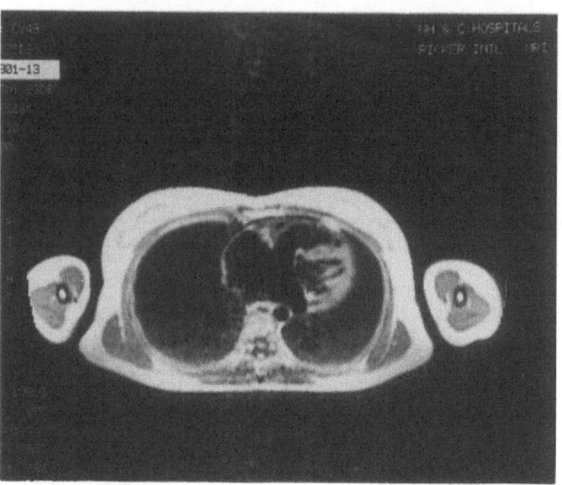

Fig. 10.9. Ostium primum atrial septal defect: no septum is present beside the mitral valve. The right heart is dilated (right ventricular end diastolic volume 329 ml, ejection fraction 67%), and the pulmonary to systemic flow ratio is 3.0 to 1.

volumes in atrial septal defect. Figure 10.8 shows an ostium secundum atrial septal defect with a dilated right heart due to the volume overload, and a pulmonary to systemic flow ratio of 2.3. If the defect is ostium primum, it can be seen to involve the septum right down to the atrio-ventricular valve plane (Fig. 10.9). Care is necessary however, since even in normal subjects, an apparent septal defect can sometimes be seen in the region of the foramen ovale. This is less common in oblique sections that are perpendicular to the septum, and a cine sequence should be acquired if there is any doubt.

More complex anomalies may also be unravelled. Fig. 10.10 shows a subject with atrio-ventricular canal which was associated with other complex lesions including right isomerism.

Diseases of the Great Vessels

CT has proved to be helpful in the investigation of aortic aneurysms and aortic dissection, although infusion of contrast medium is necessary. MRI can be equally valuable without contrast infusion (Geisinger et al. 1985; Amparo et al. 1985). Fig. 10.11 shows a type B aortic dissection. The entry point was in the arch, and the aneurysm was shown to extend to the diaphragm but not beyond. The true lumen was compressed by a large false lumen which was lined with clot.

Angiograms may be acquired without the use of contrast media by subtracting an image acquired with a sequence that does not give signal from

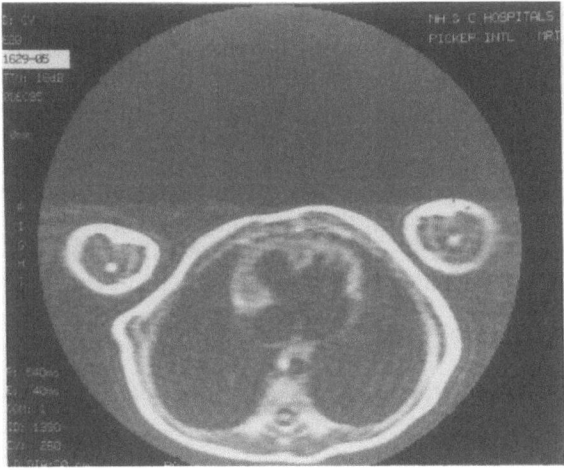

Fig. 10.10. Atrio-ventricular canal in a patient with right isomerism. Transverse section showing deficiency of atrial and ventricular septa extending through the atrio-ventricular orifices.

moving blood, from the same image acquired with a sequence that does. In this way vascular anatomy is demonstrated, and stenoses due to atheroma may be seen.

Coronary Vessels

Blood vessels are easily shown by MRI because of the absence of signal from flowing blood contrasting with the signal from surrounding tissue. The coronary vessels are no exception, and they can nearly always be seen provided that images are acquired in the right plane (Fig. 10.12). Coronary artery bypass grafts may be assumed to be patent if seen (Fig. 10.13). With a tomographic technique, however, it is difficult to follow a single vessel more than a few centimetres, and therefore to say whether an apparent narrowing is due to atheroma or to the vessel moving out of the plane of section.

Flow Imaging

Measurement of coronary flow or the use of contrast agents as flow markers are more likely to allow the detection of coronary artery disease and in fact soon after magnetic resonance was first described in 1946, its use in the measurement of flow was investigated both for industrial and biological applications. In the 1970s it was realised that a combination of MRI and flow measurements would allow flow to be measured in even the most inaccessible blood vessels (Singer 1978).

Phase mapping has become the most popular method for the measurement of flow because it has proved the easiest to quantify (Bryant et al. 1984). It uses the fact that any magnetic resonance signal has both amplitude and phase, and that phase can be encoded to give a measure of flow velocity. A conventional image is a display of the amplitude of signal at each point, but a display of phase quantifies velocity at each point. Stationary tissues have zero phase and are shown as mid-grey, but flowing blood has a phase shift that is displayed as either a

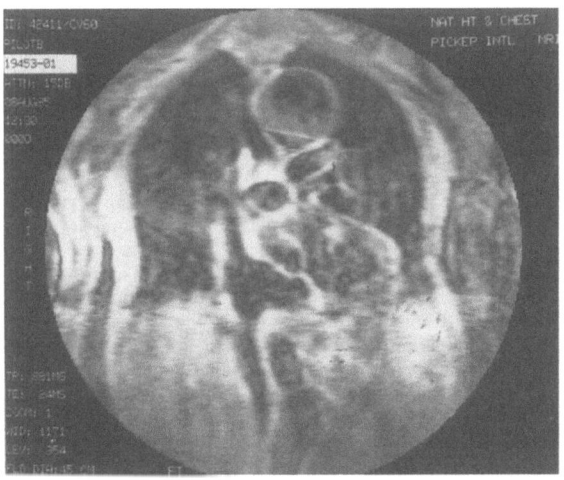

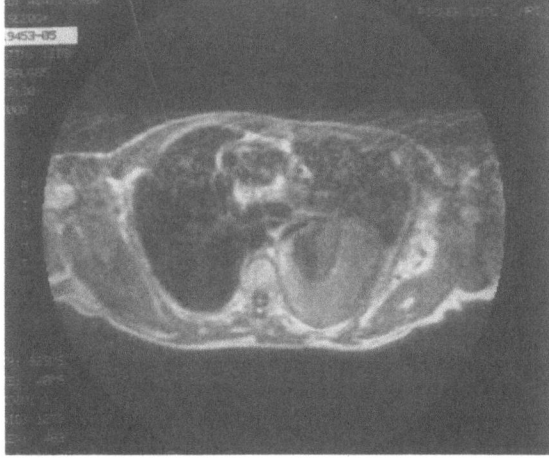

Fig. 10.11. Dissecting aortic aneurysm in coronal and transverse sections. In the coronal section (*left*) the intimal flap is seen in the aortic arch dividing the true (inferior) from the false (superior) lumen. The transverse section (*right*) was acquired without cardiac gating and so there is a lot of motion artefact. The true lumen is a small slit and the false lumen is lined with thrombus.

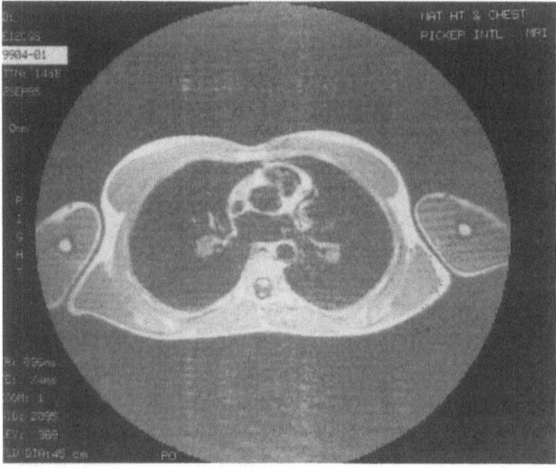

Fig. 10.12. Transverse section through the aortic root and roof of the left ventricle to show the coronary arteries. The left main stem divides to the left anterior descending and circumflex arteries, and the right coronary artery is also seen.

darker or a lighter shade depending upon its direction and velocity. The maps may also be colour-coded to aid interpretation.

An example of a phase map through the great vessels is shown in Fig. 10.14 with blood flowing towards the feet shown in white (descending aorta and superior vena cava), and blood flowing towards the head in black (ascending aorta and pulmonary artery). The gradients can be arranged to quantify velocity of flow within the plane as well as perpendicular to it, and in this way a complete description of flow is provided at any desired point of the

cardiac cycle. The accuracy of these measurements has been validated in the ascending aorta by comparison with left ventricular stroke volume. The techniques have already been of value in the investigation of the peripheral arterial system, and progress towards flow angiograms of the coronary arteries is advancing. When these can be produced reliably and accurately, the diagnosis and assessment of coronary artery disease will be greatly enhanced and simplified.

Future Prospects

At the present time magnetic resonance equipment is expensive and bulky. Image acquisition is relatively slow compared to other techniques, so that imaging during exercise is not yet possible. In addition the patient has to lie in the magnet during the study where he is virtually inaccessible. Nevertheless, there is a very real prospect of smaller machines operating at low magnetic field strengths being able to produce images rapidly, and even possibly in real time. Coupled with the ability to measure ventricular function and to demonstrate coronary anatomy and flow noninvasively, MRI is a potentially valuable technique in the management of the critically ill patient.

References

Amparo EG, Higgins CB, Hricak H, Sollitto R (1985). Aortic dissection: Magnetic Resonance Imaging. Radiology 155: 399–406

Bailes DR, Gilderdale DJ, Bydder GM, Collins AG, Firmin DN (1985) Respiratory ordered phase encoding (ROPE): a method for reducing respiratory motion artefacts in MR imaging. J. Comput Assist Tomogr 9: 835–838

Byrant DJ, Payne JA, Firmin DN, Longmore DB (1984) Measurement of flow with NMR imaging using a gradient pulse and phase difference technique. J Comput Assist Tomogr 8: 588–593

Geisinger MA, Risius B, O'Donnell JA, Zelch MG, Moodie DS, Graor RA, George CR (1985) Thoracic aortic dissections: Magnetic Resonance Imaging. Radiology 155: 407–412

Goldman MR, Brady TJ, Pykett IL et al. (1982) Quantification of experimental myocardial infarction using nuclear magnetic resonance imaging and paramagnetic ion contrast enhancement in excised canine hearts. Circulation 66: 1012

Higgins CB, Kaufman L, Crooks LE (1985) Magnetic resonance imaging of the cardiovascular system. Am Heart J 109: 136–152

Higgins CB, Byrd BF, McNamara MT, Lanzer P, Lipton MJ, Botvinik E, Schiller NB, Crooks LE, Kaufman L (1985) Magnetic Resonance Imaging of the heart: a review of the experi-

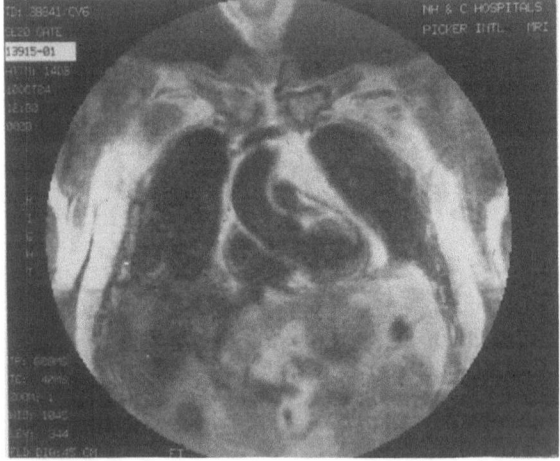

Fig. 10.13. Coronary artery bypass graft. The fact that the vessel is seen with no signal in the lumen means that it is patent with good flow.

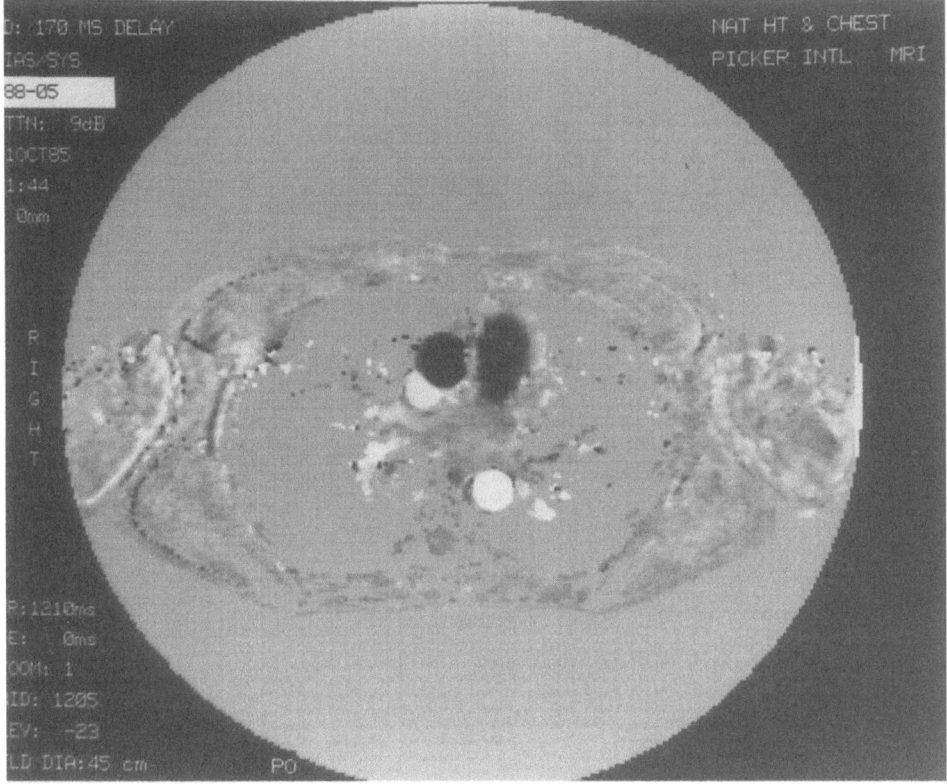

Fig. 10.14. Example of phase map obtained through the great vessels in a transverse slice, showing velocity in a direction perpendicular to the plane. Stationary material appears in mid-grey, flow towards the head in increasing shades of black (ascending aorta and pulmonary artery), and towards the feet in increasing shades of white (descending aorta and superior vena cava).

ence in 172 subjects. Radiology 155: 671–679

Hoult DI, Busby SJW, Gadian DG, Radda GK, Richards RE, Seeley PJ (1974) Observation of tissue metabolites using ^{31}P nuclear magnetic resonance. Nature 252: 285

Longmore DB, Klipstein RH, Underwood SR, et al. (1985) The dimensional accuracy of magnetic resonance in studies of the heart. Lancet I: 1360–1362

McNamara MT, Higgins CB, Schechtmann N, Botvinick E, Lipton MJ, Chatterjee K, Amparo EG (1985) Detection and characterisation of acute myocardial infarction in man with use of gated magnetic resonance. Circulation 71: 717–724

Ordidge RJ, Mansfield P, Doyle M, et al. (1982) "Real-time" moving images by NMR. In: Witcofski RL, Karstaedt N, Partain CL (eds). Proceedings of the international symposium in NMR imaging. Bowman Gray School of Medicine Press, Winston-Salem NC pp 89–92

Purcell EM, Torrey HC, Pound RV (1946) Resonance absorp-

tion by nuclear magnetic moments in a solid. Phys Rev 69: 37–38

Pykett IL, Newhouse JH, Buonanno FS, Brady TJ, Goldman MR, Kistler JP, Pohost GM (1982). Principles of nuclear magnetic resonance imaging. Radiology 143: 157–168

Singer JR (1978) NMR diffusion and flow measurements and an introduction to spin phase graphing. J Phys E Sci Instrum 11: 281–291

Steiner RE (1983) The Hammersmith clinical experience with nuclear magnetic resonance. Clin Radiol 34: 13–23

Steiner RE, Bydder GM, Selwyn A, et al. (1983) Nuclear magnetic resonance imaging of the heart. Current status and future prospects. Br Heart J 50: 202–208

Underwood SR, Rees RSO, Savage PE, Klipstein RH, Firmin DN, Fox KM, Poole-Wilson PA, Longmore DB (1986) The assessment of regional left ventricular function by magnetic resonance. Br Heart J 56: 334–340

Section IV

The Abdomen

Chapter 11

Abdominal Ultrasound in Intensive Care

J. Boultbee and W. Kox

Ultrasound has been used in diagnostic medicine for nearly 30 years and scanners have been commercially available since the mid 1960s. The first generation of bi-stable scanners displayed the two-dimensional scan information on a cathode ray tube as a series of bright dots where only echoes above a certain threshold were displayed. These corresponded to relatively large reflecting surfaces within the body, such as the capsule of the liver, the portal vein or the great vessels. In modern scanners a grey-scale display is now standard whereby each echo signal amplitude is related to a shade or level of grey, the stronger echoes delineated by the more reflective surfaces, thus giving information on the appearances of soft tissue parenchyma which was not available previously with bi-stable equipment. Real-time ultrasound units which we consider suitable for intensive care scanning are of two basic types; either mechanical sector or multiple transducer systems.

The one big advantage of mechanical transducer systems is their relatively low cost. Mechanical sector heads have been refined considerably over the last five years and many of the problems formerly associated with them have been overcome. The mechanical head rotates within a sealed fluid bath; the rotating type has a number of probes, usually three, which move past an acoustic window. Single probe mechanical sectors function on a fixed probe with either an oscillating acoustic reflector or an oscillating probe which moves from side to side in the fluid bath. The linear array which is the cheapest and most popular multiple transducer comprises a set of small elements arranged in a line and fired in sequential groups to produce a rectangular type of sectional image. Subtle control over the sequential firing of the elements provides focussing control within the image section. The disadvantage of the linear array probe has been its overall bulk, weight and size which make it difficult to use in the upper abdomen and chest wall. Their advantage of an extended field is often lost because of lack of contact between the straight linear probe and the curved surfaces of body contact. Recent improvements by the manufacturers have resulted in a very short linear array probe or curved (convex) linear array probes. The latter, although very often slightly more costly, are in our opinion quite useful and we have tried various forms in the intensive care environment. The ideal probe for our use should offer a good field of view, be light and easy to handle with high resolution throughout the whole field. Phased array promises most of these advantages but so far it is very expensive and may be at least twice the cost. The phased array transducer consists of a small curved group of elements. Delays applied to the elements not only enable the control to be focussed but also steer the beam through the section to be imaged.

The real-time or moving image is produced by these various systems whether they are a fan-shape image of the mechanical sector and phased array systems or a square or rectangular field as in the linear array. These real-time images are ideal for visualising movements within the body, whether it is peristalsis, vascular pulsation, heart valve or wall movement. On most scanners, 30 frames a second are possible but the moving images may be frozen and photographed on to any of the available image systems. Alternatively, a videotape recording may be made and a tape image frozen and recorded on to a hard copy. Although there are many options depending on individual requirements, the use of a polaroid camera has the advantage of instant review with the existing images such as the plain abdomen and chest radiographs.

Ultrasound equipment has become so mobile and in some instances portable in the last 5 years that good quality two-dimensional images with static hard copies are readily obtainable at the patient's bed side. Plain abdominal radiographs have an essential part to play and should always precede the ultrasound examination. Ultrasound should be seen as a method by which the findings on the radiography may be further interrogated, particularly with reference to the soft tissue organs and the presence of free or loculated fluid. It is worth remembering that visualisation of the abdominal soft tissue organs is very limited on the plain radiographs but with ultrasound imaging is relatively good. While ultrasound scanning has been mainly used for diagnostic purposes, a real-time probe is often used for directing needles or drainage tubes into the thoracic or abdominal cavities. Where ultrasound and plain-film radiography have failed to supply adequate information, a computed tomography (CT) examination becomes the method of choice.

Technique

Performing ultrasound in the intensive therapy unit (ITU) sometimes presents a challenge. The patient is immobile on life-support equipment, often including dialysis as well as the respiratory-cardiac life support. Our procedure is to scan patients in the position in which they are being nursed at the time, which is normally semi-erect. Patients can easily then be lowered into the supine position. Rolling the patient into the decubitus position is often necessary especially for coronal views. Sagittal, coronal and transverse cuts should be ideal. In some cases, it is necessary to get movement for contrast, for instance injecting water into the stomach via a nasogastric tube or injecting water into the rectum for differentiation of the large bowel from the contents of the pelvis. In the abdomen as a whole, an actively peristalsing small bowel is very useful as it enables the examiner to distinguish between the bowel itself and any static masses or collections of fluid which may surround or lie between the loops of bowel. In a postoperative situation, where there are large surgical incisions and open wounds, it is necessary to scan over these areas but to keep probe contact to the skin or the abdominal wall surface. Two methods of choice in this sort of situation are available. One is to place a sterile probe cover filled with contact gel over the scanning head. The patient is then scanned through this sterile cover with a sterile gel on the abdominal or wound surface. Sometimes, with small probes, a sterile surgical glove can be used instead of the commercially available scan-head covers. Another method which works very well is to use a sterile gel spread liberally over the wound and then covered with a sterile plastic membrane which can be scanned over without interference.

Indications

In the past, surgical procedures have been necessary to explore the abdominal cavity for purulent material or foreign bodies and to insert drains. Ultrasound investigations can localise collections of fluid, haemorrhage or ascites and give useful assistance when draining these collections. Patients in ITUs quite frequently develop jaundice. In order to distinguish between obstructive or haemolytic jaundice, an ultrasound should be performed routinely. Septicaemia or post-haemorrhagic shock is associated with low serum-albumin levels. This can lead to extravasation of fluid into the abdominal cavity and can cause not only hypotension but also an ileus. The most common clinical finding after blunt abdominal trauma is often the rupture of the spleen (Fig. 11.1). Hepatic lacerations also occur but are less frequent. If the capsule of the injured organ remains intact, clinical signs of haemorrhage may be delayed. Severe pain in the left or right upper quadrant which is normally a reliable indicator of a ruptured spleen may be masked by the administration of sedatives or pain killers when the patient requires these for mechanical ventilation or other invasive procedures in intensive care. Abdominal aortic aneurysms may be asymptomatic or may present as a life-threatening event (Fig. 11.2) if they are dissecting. Active leakage is best seen by CT as often ultrasound will not provide the dynamics of the situation.

Patients in ITUs often develop acute tubular necrosis (ATN) (Fig. 11.3) after haemorrhagic or septicaemic shock. The first sign of ATN is a drop in urine production to less than $50\,\mathrm{ml^{-1}h^{-1}}$ followed by complete anuria. It is indicated already in the oliguric state to examine these patients for pre- or post-renal obstruction by ultrasound. Patients with bleeding problems because of disseminated intravascular coagulation, low platelet counts or

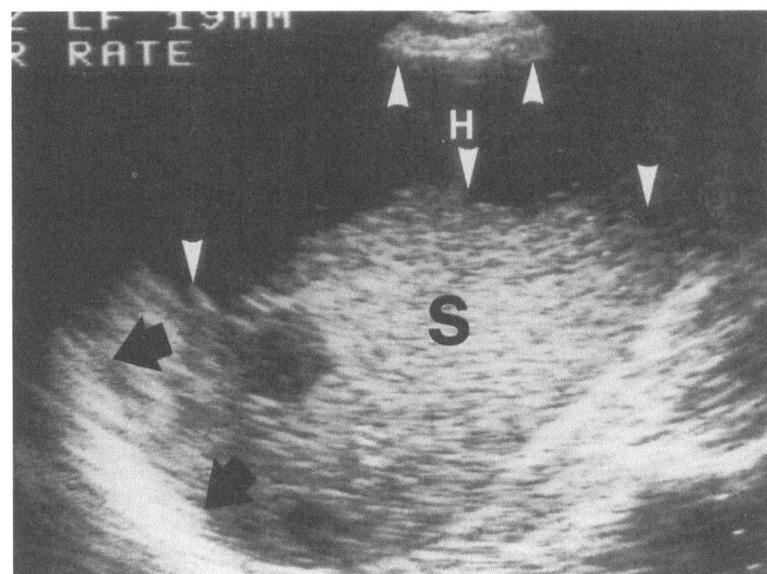

Fig. 11.1. Longitudinal scan through the spleen. The dark area denoted by white arrow heads is a subcapsular haematoma (*H*). The splenic parenchyma (*S*) is posterior. Black arrows demonstrate the left hemidiaphragm.

liver problems, and with indwelling urinary catheters, may be prone to bleeding into the bladder and thereby obstructing both ureters with clots (Fig. 11.4). When post-renal obstruction is diagnosed it can be relieved by percutaneous nephrostomy under ultrasound guidance at the bed side.

Ultrasound examination of the liver, spleen and biliary tree in the patient in intensive care should include the careful assessment of the inferior margins of these organs and of the hemidiaphragms

for free fluid. Size measurement is still relatively subjective. The shape of the organs is often a good indicator. Comparison can also be made with the size of the kidneys. The liver parenchyma produces a uniform grey echo-pattern throughout the organ only to be interrupted by the appearance of the portal vessels or the hepatic veins (Fig. 11.5). The portal tree appears much the brighter of the two with thick walls mainly because of the presence of the biliary and arterial vessels which run with them.

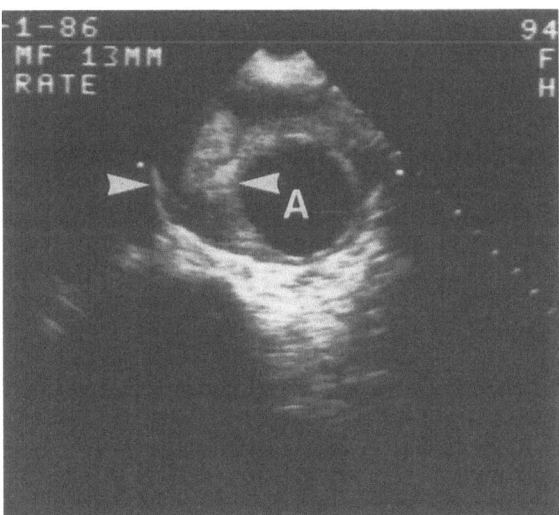

Fig. 11.2. Transverse scan through the abdominal aorta (*A*). The overall transverse diameter is 94 mm, although the diameter of the lumen is considerably less. Two white arrows demonstrate a thickened lateral wall, partly composed of blood clot.

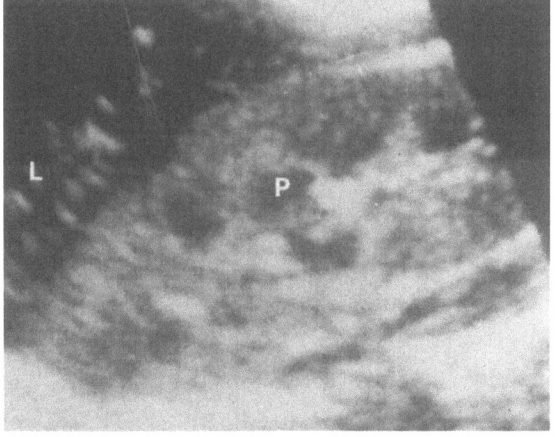

Fig. 11.3. Longitudinal scan through the right kidney (upper and middle thirds). This patient was in renal failure with acute tubular necrosis. The renal cortex is abnormally echogenic (white) and the normal liver (*L*) is darker than the renal cortex. *P*, portal vein.

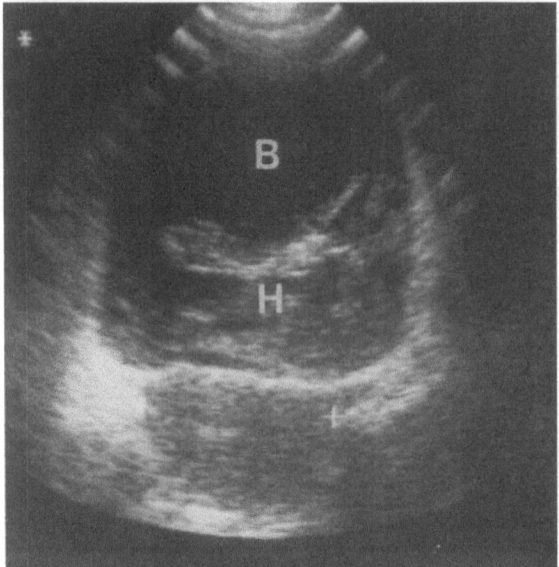

Fig. 11.4. Transverse scan through the bladder (B) which contains blood clot (H).

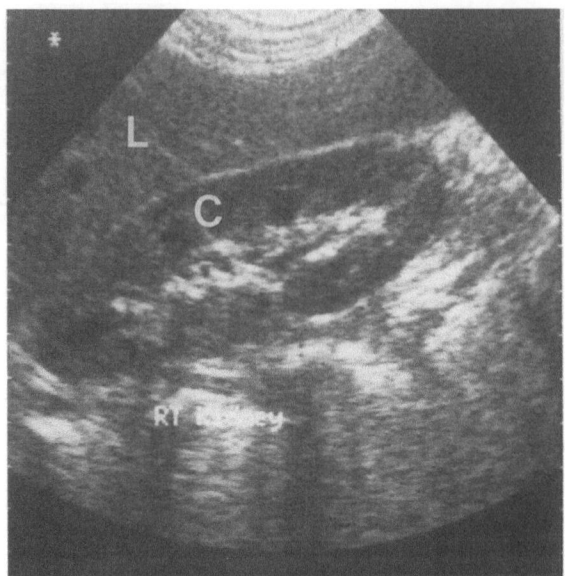

Fig. 11.6. Longitudinal section through the right lobe of the liver (L) and right kidney of a normal adult. Note the cortex (C) of the kidney is normally darker than surrounding liver (L).

There is no readily available method of assessing the intensity of the liver pattern but, in the right lobe of the liver, comparison can be made with the cortex of the right kidney and the immediate liver echo pattern (Fig. 11.6), the renal cortex being slightly darker in its appearance than that of the liver. Enlargement of the liver and spleen may be seen in patients on life-support equipment due

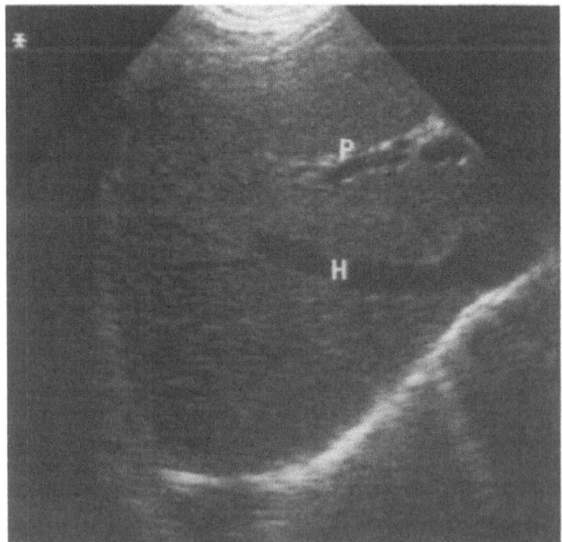

Fig. 11.5. Transverse cut through a normal liver, demonstrating hepatic vein (H) and portal vein (P) and associate vessels.

either to poor cardiac performance of the patient and/or to septicaemia. Focal abnormalities are much more easily detected than subtle diffuse changes. Liver abscesses for instance are usually relatively echo-poor and well circumscribed and have the effect of causing some distal enhancement of the echo pattern behind the lesion (Fig. 11.7). Serial examinations of a liver abscess should demonstrate progression of the lesion (Dewbury et al. 1980). Subphrenic collections are relatively echo-free but on occasions are complicated by the formation of gas in the collection which will thereby cause echoes. These collections are usually semilunar representing the abdominal surface of the diaphragm and the capsule of the liver and show well on ultrasound (Fig. 11.8). However, sometimes there is a transonic mass under the capsule of the liver in which case the lesion is made more ovoid and clearly circumscribed. Drainage of this area can often be achieved with the aid of ultrasound either for a complete evacuation with a drainage tube or procuration of small samples with a fine needle for bacteriology. Other echogenic or mixed lesions may present in the liver as a chance finding. A not-infrequent ¨finding is a capillary haemangioma which is often about 1–3 cm in diameter and usually appears as a highly echogenic area in the echo pattern in normal liver (Fig. 11.9). These lesions are a relatively common cause of an echogenic focus in the liver (Leopold 1984). Needle aspiration of these lesions is not recommended.

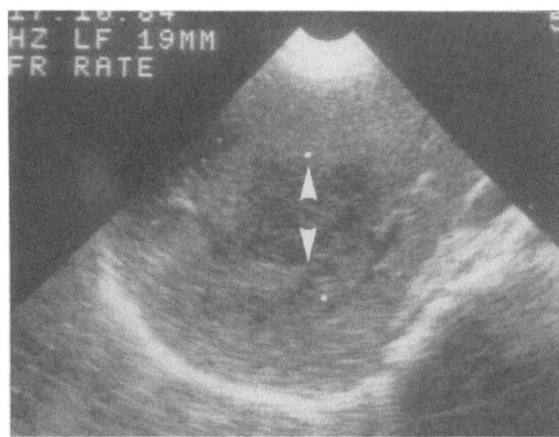

Fig. 11.7. A longitudinal scan through the right lobe of the liver. A large irregular mass with fewer echoes (darker) than the surrounding liver is present. This is a liver abscess.

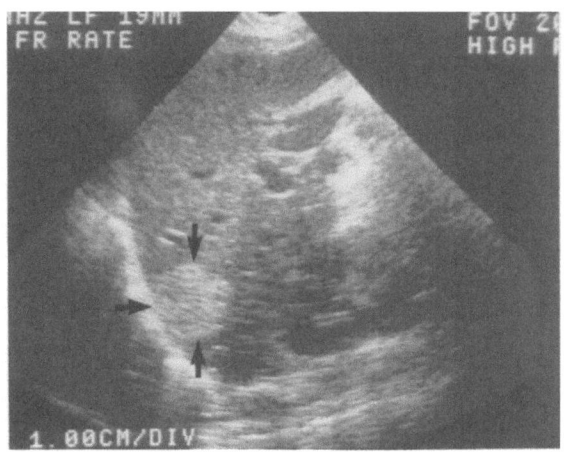

Fig. 11.9. Longitudinal section through the right lobe of the liver. A well circumscribed echogenic lesion (*arrowed*) lying next to the right hemidiaphragm is shown. This lies within normal liver. The patient was 23 years old and suffered from acute peritonitis following a ruptured appendix. This lesion has the appearance of an isolated haemangioma.

Metastatic carcinoma of the liver produces varied appearances. These can be relatively well-defined or mixed (Fig. 11.10) in their echo pattern and even in their shape, some being relatively echo-free while others are significantly echo-dense (Green et al. 1977). As this pattern is likely to change the prognosis and management of the patient, needle aspiration of one of these lesions is in fact very useful. Jaundice is a frequent clinical problem in the patient in intensive care and ultrasound is the method of

choice for exclusion of obstructive jaundice (Taylor and Rosenfield 1977). In a normal subject the common bile duct is visible and lies relatively superior in position to the portal vein as it leaves the hilum of the liver (Fig. 11.11). With modern scanners, it is possible to obtain accurate measurements of the diameter of the common bile duct and biliary tree. Often further information is obtainable giving the cause of the obstruction such as stones within the common bile duct or a mass at the head

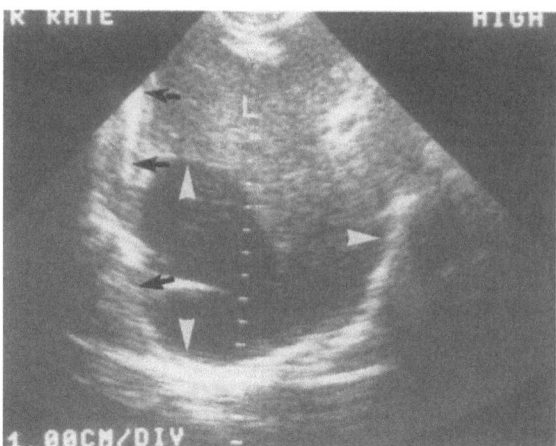

Fig. 11.8. Longitudinal section through the right lobe of the liver (*L*). Large echo-free (dark) area (*white arrows*) is a subphrenic collection. Black arrows define the right hemidiaphragm. This collection was aspirated under ultrasound control.

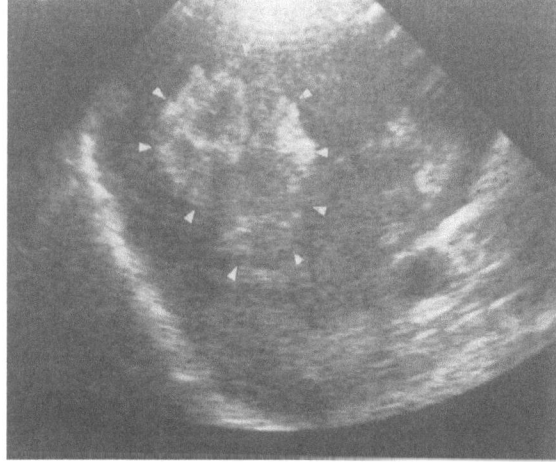

Fig. 11.10. Longitudinal section through the right lobe of the liver. There is a large irregular echogenic area within the right lobe of the liver. This is a large secondary from colon.

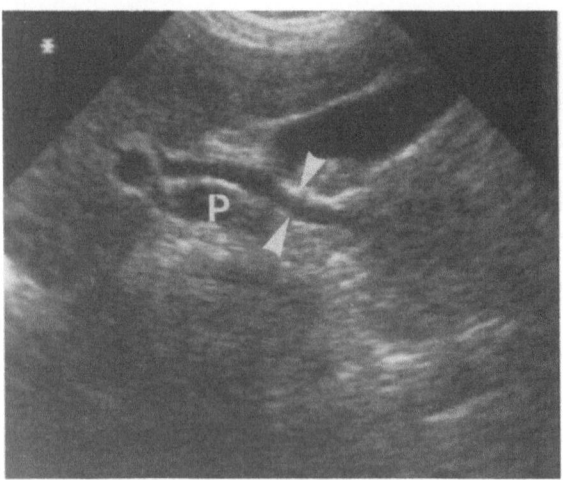

Fig. 11.11. The relationship of the portal vein (*P*) to the common bile duct (*arrow heads*) which lies in an anterior position.

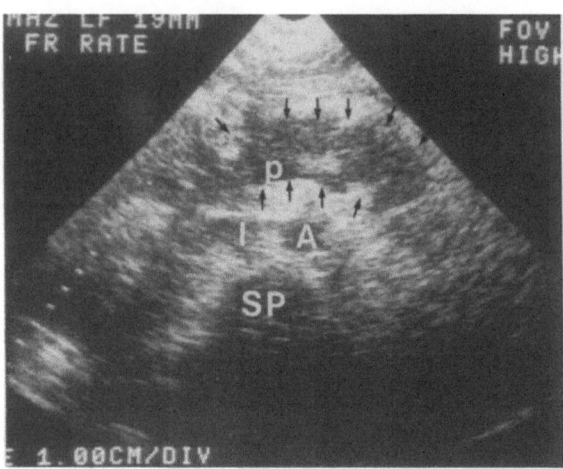

Fig. 11.13. Transverse scan of the pancreas. The patient has acute pancreatitis. The pancreas is enlarged and has fewer echoes than normal. *I*, IVC; *A*, aorta; *Sp*, spine; *P*, portal vein.

of the pancreas. The gall bladder can be relatively easily visualised with ultrasonography. However, the gall bladder in a patient who has been feeding parenterally for a number of days is often very prominent and quite large, there being no stimulus for it to contract. It has been suggested (Slasky, et al, 1983) that this may predispose to acalculous cholecystitis. Although ultrasound is very accurate in the detection of calculi in the gall bladder (Slasky et al, 1983) the presence of stones in the adult patient in the ITU is often coincidental and it is

perhaps more important to reveal the appearances of the gall bladder wall which in acute cholecystitis is often very significantly thickened (Fig. 11.12). Thickening of the gall bladder can occur with hepatitis and hypoalbuminaemia of any cause (Shlaer et al. 1981). When a patient is conscious, clinical history and examination with an ultrasound scan makes diagnosis much simpler. However, acute cholecystitis becomes a difficult diagnosis to make in the unconscious patient on life-support systems. In acute pancreatitis, ultrasound may be diagnostic: a large uniformly echo-free pancreas (Fig. 11.13) is characteristic in acute pancreatitis (Lawson 1983) although in some cases the pancreas can be ultra-

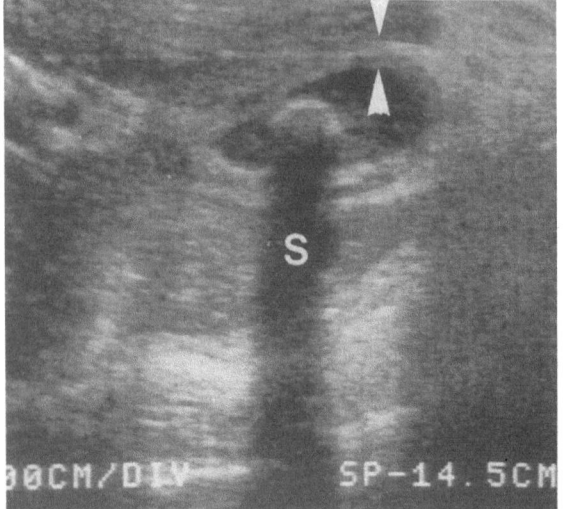

Fig. 11.12. Longitudinal scan through a small gall bladder with a gallstone which is casting a shadow (*S*). The gall bladder has a thickened wall (*white arrowhead*). These may be incidental findings.

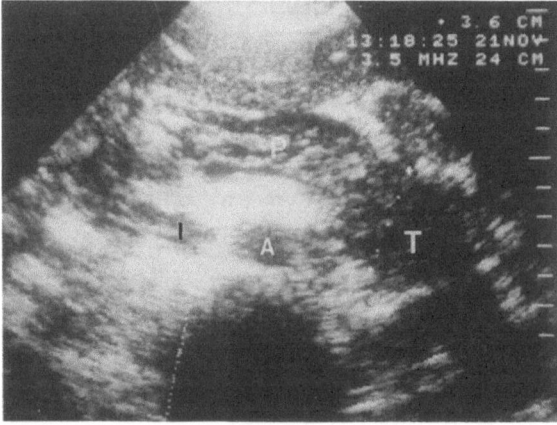

Fig. 11.14. Transverse scan through the pancreas. Pancreas (*P*) lies across the inferior vena cava (*I*) and the aorta (*A*). A mass at the tail of the pancreas is 4½ cm AP diameter. Acute on chronic pancreatitis.

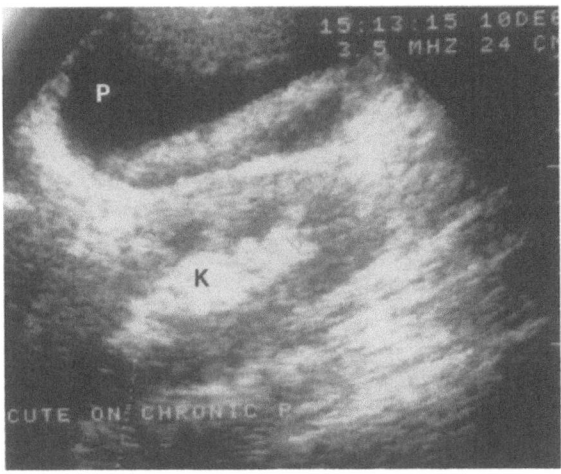

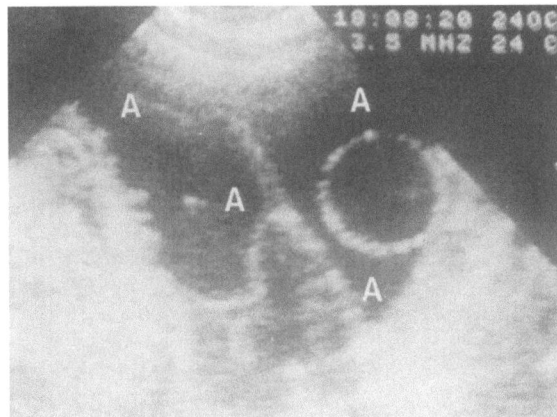

Fig. 11.17. Loops of bowel surrounded by free fluid ascites (*A*).

Fig. 11.15. Longitudinal section through the right kidney (*K*) with a collection anterior (*P*). This is a pseudo-cyst of the head of the pancreas, which, until it was aspirated under ultrasound control, caused acute obstruction at the level of the second part of the duodenum.

sonically normal. Localised abnormalities producing a mass effect may be demonstrated (Fig. 11.14). Pseudocysts or abscesses are usually accessible to drainage. Two of the patients we have treated in ITUs were obstructed at the second part of the duodenum by pseudocyst formation (Fig. 11.15) and this was rectified by insertion of a drainage tube in each case.

In many cases satisfactory images are obtained in the bowel. Sonographic patterns occurring in peristalsing bowel produce motion artefacts of the contents (Fig. 11.16) (Fleischer et al. 1980) which makes it much easier to demonstrate static collections outside the bowel: these may be sometimes enhanced by gas outside the bowel (Fig. 11.17) (Burt et al. 1983). Free abdominal fluid whether it

be from perforation, penetration injury or peritonitis presents normally as a relatively echo-free fluid area. Although ultrasound is very sensitive to the demonstration of free fluid (Ferrucci et al. 1981), fluid containing necrotic material is more echogenic and some gas-containing lesions are frankly confusing because of their extreme echogenicity. Percutaneous needle aspiration of these fluid collections (Fig. 11.18) is easily performed and well-justified, even when only small amounts are obtained for examination and culture (Ferrucci et al. 1981). Our approach is to use a small 7 or 8 French gauge catheter for continuous drainage and if needed increase the size of the catheter 12 h or more later if drainage is not satisfactory.

Demonstration of the great vessels is an important anatomical reference if a dissection is suspected. It is particularly worthwhile reviewing the aorta for the presence of an aneurysm or an intimal flap (Fig. 11.2) as these two conditions would contra-indicate

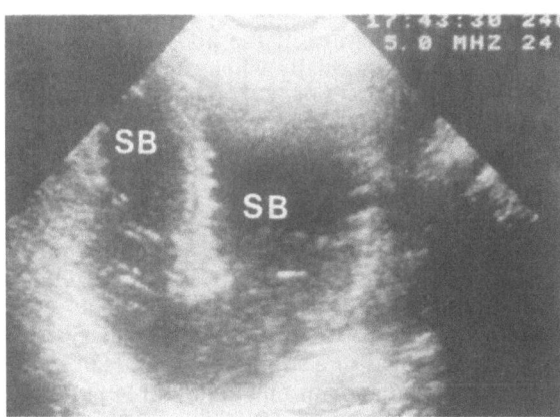

Fig. 11.16. Dilated loops of small bowel (*SB*).

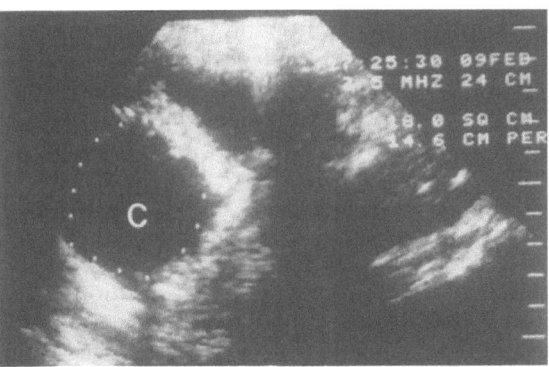

Fig. 11.18. Longitudinal scan through the splenic bed, post-splenectomy. *C* is a collection of pus which was aspirated under ultrasound control.

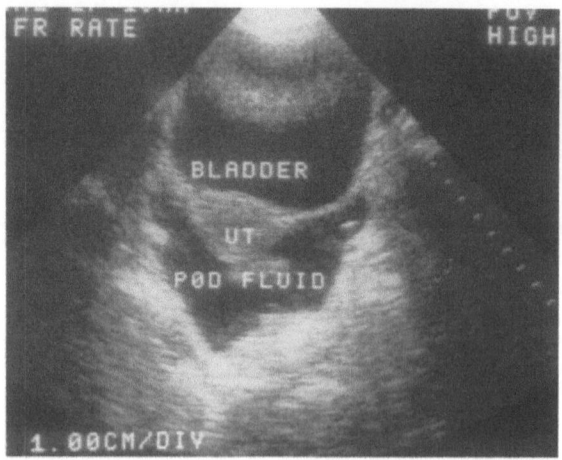

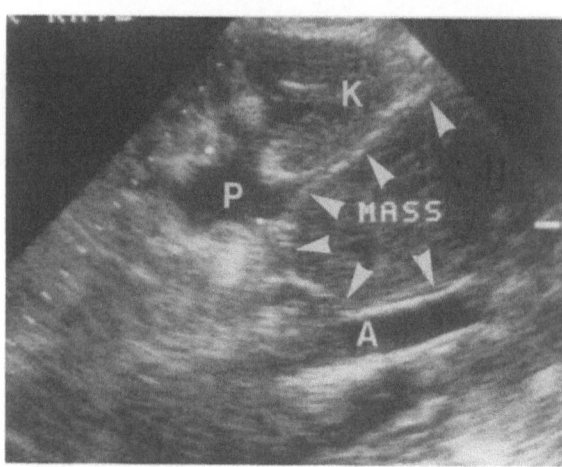

Fig. 11.19. A transverse scan through the female pelvis, demonstrating fluid (blood) in the pouch of Douglas (*POD*) behind the uterus (*UT*). This patient was bleeding from an ectopic pregnancy.

Fig. 11.20. Longitudinal (coronal scan) through the left kidney and aorta (*A*). There is a mass (glands from testicular teratoma) which is compressing the ureter (not shown) causing some dilatation of the renal pelvis (*P*). K, lower Pole of the kidney.

the use of aortic balloon pumps. Leaking aneurysms in the acute situation are ideally screened by CT scan using contrast and a rapid technique.

In the pelvis ultrasound is an ideal screening method for visualising the female organs (Fig. 11.19). The acute emergencies such as ectopic pregnancy may produce unexpected findings.

Septicaemia is often a cause of renal failure, usually in the form of acute tubular necrosis. Ultrasound is normally requested to exclude an obstructive uropathy although there are ultrasound changes seen in the kidneys in ATN which are non-specific (Rosenfield et al. 1978). The cortex of the kidney becomes relatively echo-dense when compared to the pattern of the right lobe of the liver (Fig. 11.3). Of 17 patients we have examined in acute renal failure in ITU only two were found to have an obstruction: these patients had malignancies involving the para-aortic region and the pelvis. An obstructive uropathy causes dilatation of the collecting systems which ultrasonically have the appearance of transonic fluid-filled areas representing the dilated calices and renal pelvis (Fig. 11.20). Examination of the bladder ultrasonically is useful because it is often very difficult to palpate the over-filled bladder when there is already distension of the abdomen. The bladder can be assessed for its volume and where there is a catheter in situ, it can be checked for its position quite easily. Visualisation of blood clot in the bladder has proved particularly useful in our experience (Fig. 11.4).

In patients with blunt trauma a CT examination of the whole abdomen is preferable as a first-time

investigation (see Chapter 12). Ultrasonically, trauma of the soft tissue organs is shown by visualisation of a sub-capsular haematoma initially echo-free, or by contusion of the parenchyma itself (echogenic). In the liver, spleen and kidney a large sub-capsular collection is usually echo-free and may cause considerable shift in position of the organ (Fig. 11.1). The pancreas may be considerably enlarged or swollen represented by decreased echoes. Sometimes a collection similar to a pseudo-cyst (Weill 1982), which is an echo-free fluid-filled space, will be present. When there is demonstrable intraperitoneal fluid following trauma, the presence of free intraperitoneal blood is most likely. It is important to make sure that ultrasound is performed before peritoneal lavage.

We have generally found that the small or average-sized patient is usually successfully examined by ultrasound, although in larger patients a negative ultrasound examination in the abdomen may be very misleading, expecially when there is a retro-peritoneal lesion present. CT then becomes the method of choice in spite of the logistic problem of moving the patient and all the life-support systems to the scanner.

The abdominal radiograph has an important place in the examination of patients with upper abdominal sepsis. Connell et al. (1980) reviewed the abdominal radiographs of 82 such patients and found that 71% abscess formation was suggested by extraluminal gas or a soft tissue mass. Halber et al. (1979) stated that plain-film radiography showed the diagnosis in over half of their proven cases of abdominal abscesses (Fig. 11.21). Ultrasound has

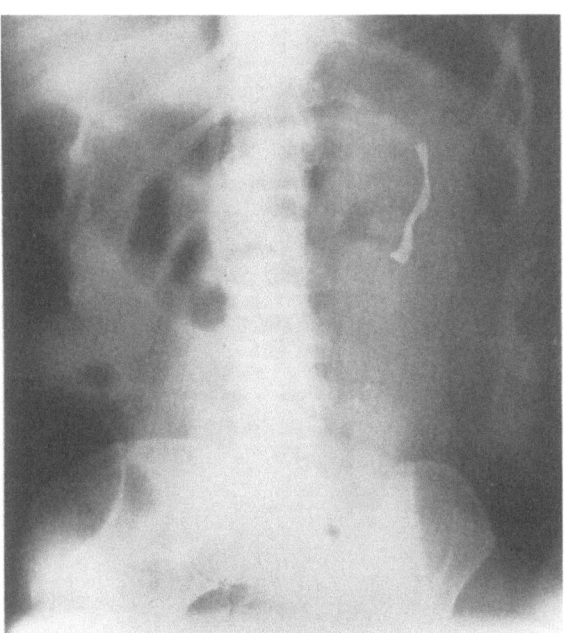

Fig. 11.21. Abdominal radiograph in a patient with stab wounds. A left nephrectomy and a splenectomy were performed. The patient developed persistent pyrexia. Ultrasound demonstrated a collection of fluid. The abdominal film taken afterwards has shown the cause of the pyrexia (a retained swab).

variable accuracy within the abdomen when searching for a cause for abdominal sepsis. Sinanan et al. (1984) found their diagnostic accuracy was 57%. Recently Dobrin et al. (1986) have found that CT was significantly more accurate than ultrasound in the diagnosis of intra-abdominal abscess except within the pelvis where ultrasound was more accurate. Ultrasound is still very operator-dependent and even more demanding in the ITU because of the physical difficulties involved when scanning patients surrounded by life-support machines.

Ideally, continuous presence of ultrasound in the ITU is justified. This, however, requires an experienced operator who is familiar with the operating problems. Ultrasound in conjunction with portable radiography will give a high diagnostic yield. When these two methods fail to give convincing information a CT scan should be performed without delay. In blunt abdominal injury an initial CT scan is recommended with follow-up by ultrasound where necessary.

References

Burt TB, Knockel JQ, Lee TG (1983) Gas as a contrast agent and diagnostic aid in abdominal sonography. J Ultrasound Med 1: 179–184

Connell TR, Stephens DH, Carlson HC, Brown ML (1980) Upper abdominal abscess: a continuing deadly problem. Am J Roentgenol 134: 759–765

Cooperberg PC (1982) Real-time ultrasonography of the gallbladder. Clin Diagn Ultrasound 10: 49–69

Dewbury KC, Joseph AEA, Millward Sadler GH, Birch SJ (1980) Ultrasound in the diagnosis of early liver abscess. Br. J Radiol. 53: 1160–1165

Dobrin PB, Gully PH, Greenlee HB (1986) Radiologic diagnosis of an intra-abdominal abscess. Arch Surg 121: 41–46

Ferrucci JT, Vansonnenberg E (1981) Intra-abdominal abscess. Radiological diagnosis and treatment. JAMA 246: 2728–2733

Fleischer AC, Mahletaler CA, James AE (1980) Sonographic patterns arising from normal and abnormal bowel. Radiol Clin North Am 18: 145–159

Green B, Bree RL, Goldstein HM, Stanley C (1977) Gray scale ultrasound evaluation of hepatic neoplasms. Patterns and correlations. Radiol. 124: 203–208

Halber MD, Daffner RH, Morgan CL, Trought WS, Thompson WM, Rice RP (1979) Intra-abdominal abscess. Current concepts in Radiologic evaluation. Am J Roentgenol 133: 9–13

Lawson TC (1983) Acute pancreatitis and its complications. Computed tomography and sonography. Radiol Clin North Am 21: 495–513

Leopold GR (1984) Liver. In: BB Goldberg (Ed) Abdominal ultrasonography Second edn. John Wiley & Sons, Chichester

Rosenfield AT, Taylor KJW, Crade M, De Graff CS (1978) Anatomy and pathology of the kidney by gray scale ultrasound. Radiology 128: 737–744

Shlaer WJ, Leopold GR, Scheible FW (1981) Sonography of the thickened gall bladder wall: a non-specific finding. Am J Roentgenol 136: 337–339

Sinanan M, Maier RV, Carrico CJ (1984) Laparotomy for intra-abdominal sepsis in patients in an intensive care unit. Arch Surg 119: 652–658

Slasky BS, Auerbach D, Skjolnick ML (1983) Value of portable real-time ultrasound in I.C.U. Crit Care Med 11: 160–164

Taylor KSW, Rosenfield AT (1977) Gray-scale ultrasonography in the differential diagnosis of jaundice. Arch Surg 112: 820–825

Weill F. (1982) Real-time ultrasonography in emergencies Clin Diagn ultrasound. 10: 95–116

Chapter 12

Computed Tomography of the Abdomen of the Critically Ill

A. Dixon

Introduction

Because of wider availability of modern computed tomography (CT) machines, much of the original work illustrating the use of abdominal CT in the critically ill patient has emanated from North America (Federle et al. 1981; Toombs et al. 1981). However, in those centres in Europe with on-site CT, the role of abdominal CT has long been appreciated in those patients with severe trauma or possible intraabdominal sepsis. These two clinical entities constitute the bulk of referrals for abdominal CT from the intensive care unit.

Technique

The preparation of the patient for abdominal CT is an integral part of the examination (Dixon 1983). Ideally the patient should be given an oral preparation of 300 ml of dilute sodium and meglumine diatrozoate (Gastrografin) about 40 min before the study begins. The object is to render the whole of the small bowel opaque by the time the patient is brought to the CT unit. A further similar drink, given immediately before the examination begins, will opacify the stomach and duodenum. However, many of the patients being referred for CT examinations from the intensive care unit are being fed parenterally and there may be serious contra indications to oral fluids (e.g. renal failure). So there must be discussion between the radiologist and the clinician in charge of the patient as to the desir-

ability of oral medium preparation, accepting that omission of oral contrast medium may lead to errors in diagnosis. If the patient's clinical condition necessitates general anaesthesia for the duration of the CT examination, there will again be a contra-indication to oral contrast-medium preparation. If need be, the anaesthetist can give the oral preparation via a nasogastric tube when the patient is fully anaesthetised although this technique will usually only opacify the proximal small bowel.

Discussion will also be needed as to whether the patient will be able to cooperate with the radiographer in terms of suspending respiration to command with enough reliability to ensure satisfactory images. Most modern scanners have a scan time of around 3 s or less and the patient must not move and should ideally not breathe at all during this data-acquisition period. The patient should be able to comply with the request to suspend respiration at a fixed point in the respiratory cycle so that supposedly sequential slices are indeed sequential. Ideally, the radiologist should examine a critically ill patient on the ward together with the clinician to assess the need for a full anaesthetic. As a general rule, the severely injured unconscious patient who is breathing very gently in a regular fashion can often be managed satisfactorily without a general anaesthetic. Furthermore, respiratory control is a much greater problem in the upper abdomen than in the lower abdomen/pelvis where adequate images can be obtained even in dyspnoeic patients. Body habitus is a further factor here; respiratory movement usually causes more problems of image degradation in the thin patient than in the fat patient. With these generalisations in mind the decision as to whether or not to give a full general anaesthetic can be rationally considered. There may be other factors involved, such as the need for CT examination of the chest as well where anaesthesia is often even more essential. If anaesthesia is required some system is needed to ensure that each CT image is obtained at the same phase of the respiratory cycle. If the chest is also being examined, this will usually be on inspiration. For abdominal work alone the precise phase of inspiration/expiration is less critical.

Most radiologists will want to give intravenous contrast medium immediately before starting the CT study. This will allow better assessment of the homogeneity of the major organs (e.g. liver/spleen) and will give better demonstration of abscesses by virtue of increased differentiation in contrast medium between the fluid density central pus and the enhancing rim of inflammatory material. Some radiologists may prefer a system of a routine series of images at outset and using a more rapid post-contrast medium run zoned in to a particular organ of interest (e.g. splenic rupture).

Trauma

General Considerations

The overall clinical condition of the patient may necessitate urgent resuscitation before investigations can be carried out. However, when the patient's condition has been stabilised it is often worthwhile proceeding with investigations forthwith so that a base-line assessment can be established. In our hospital there are geographic advantages in obtaining radiological tests at the outset as the main X-ray department is situated almost adjacent to the admissions unit. The admitting officer rings the department to check when a space on the CT machine might be available and the whole investigation can be timed accordingly. Frequently, when a cranial CT is requested, it seems likely that an abdominal CT might be helpful. As it is much more economical to perform this at the same session, we sometimes contact the clinicians and suggest this course of action. Abdominal CT is much easier to interpret *before* peritoneal lavage – any free fluid can then be fairly safely assumed to be blood. Furthermore, it is easier to perform CT before the patient is put into complicated traction devices.

The ability of CT to demonstrate all the major organs in virtually every patient means that it is the technique of choice in evaluating abdominal trauma. However, it is not freely available in every hospital and it is probably not worthwhile moving a critically-ill patient a long way in order to obtain abdominal CT. Many of the specific questions can be answered by more widely available tests (ultrasound and scintigraphy for hepatic and splenic trauma; ultrasound and intravenous urography for renal trauma).

The Liver

Conservative treatment is the mainstay of management of hepatic trauma in this country. Accordingly some might argue that high-technology investigation is unnecessary. However, the circumstances leading to surgical intervention may develop quickly and may preclude emergency investigation. Hence the need for a base-line study. Furthermore, the characteristics of the hepatic injury, as shown by CT, may influence the decision as to appropriate management.

CT has been shown to be reliable in identifying hepatic trauma (Toombs et al. 1984). Intrahepatic haematomas may appear as high-density lesions (often wedge-shaped) within the hepatic parenchyma before the administration of intravenous contrast medium. After contrast medium they will appear lucent in relation to the rest of the hepatic parenchyma which should enhance avidly. As some lacerations may only be visible following such enhancement, most centres only perform a post-contrast series of images under these circumstances. Subcapsular haematomas, which will appear as low-density crescentic collections, should be carefully searched for at narrow window widths – particularly close to the site of injury. The anatomical site of any injury should be assessed, especially the relationship with major veins (inferior vena cava, portal veins and branches).

After a base-line CT, the lesion may be assessed by ultrasound (US) which is useful for follow-up evaluation. As time progresses the haematoma may develop a near-fluid attenuation at CT and an echo-free appearance at US. This is commonly due to liquefaction of the haematoma, but a biliary collection or the development of an abscess should also be considered. Fine needle aspiration may be needed to elucidate further depending on the clinical condition.

Spleen

The diagnosis of splenic rupture is often made on clinical grounds; the chest X-ray film may reveal the classical signs of a high left hemidiaphragm,

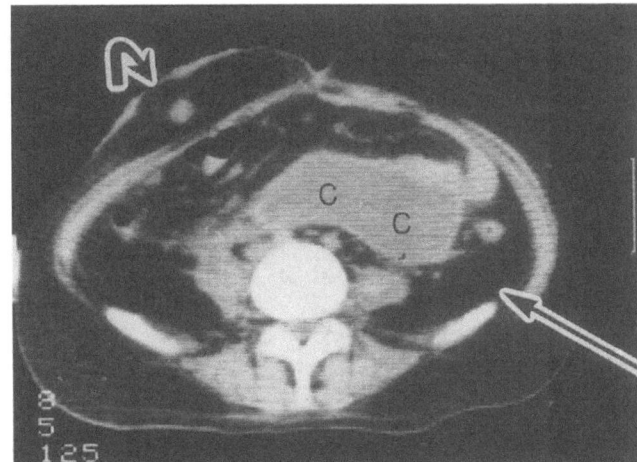

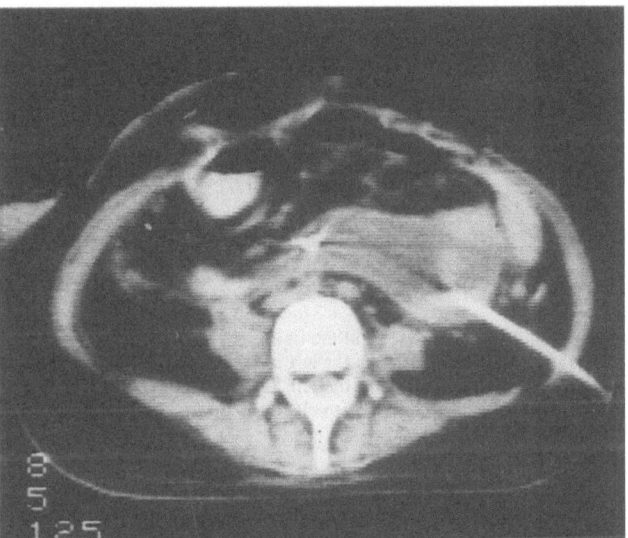

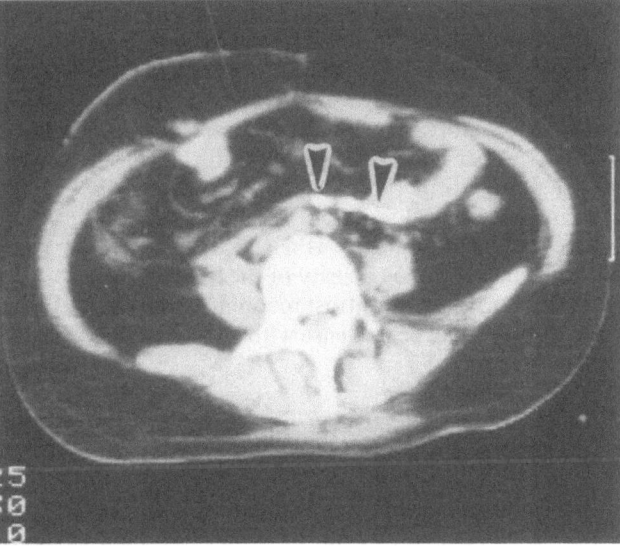

Fig. 12.1a–c. Pedestrian hit by a passing car. Multiple injuries leading to renal failure. Small bowel injury necessitating ileostomy. **a** CT image showing a fluid density collection (*c*) anterior to aortic bifurcation. More cranial cuts showed this to track to the tail of the pancreas. A suitable route for aspiration was chosen (*long arrow*). Note ileostomy (*curved arrow*).
b Percutaneous pigtail catheter in place following CT-guided insertion. This drained material consistent with infected pancreatic secretions. **c** Complete resolution of the collection four weeks later. Catheter no longer draining. No abnormality anterior to the bifurcation, just the loops of the pigtail still in situ (*arrowheads*).

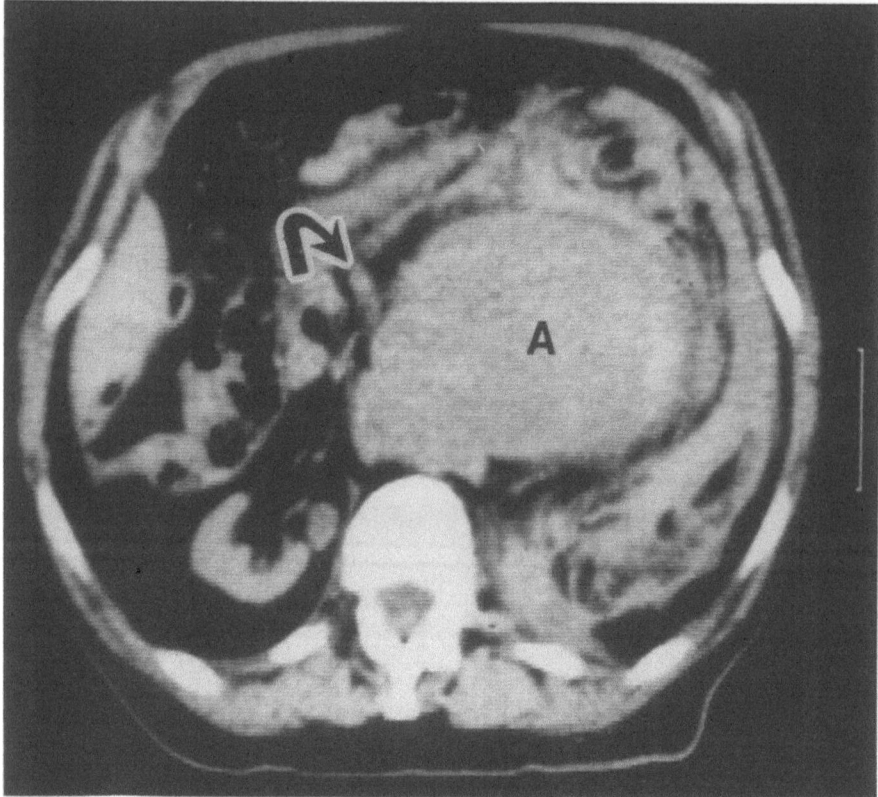

Fig. 12.2. Elderly gentleman admitted in a dire clinical state with low blood pressure and signs of internal haemorrhage. The abdomen was tense with fullness on the left. Abdominal CT shows a huge aortic aneurysm (*A*) and extensive haemorrhage in the left retroperitoneal tissues obscuring the left kidney. The aneurysm extends cranially to the origin of the superior mesenteric artery (distorted, curved arrow) and has involved the origin of the left renal artery. Features confirmed at emergency surgery which was sadly unsuccessful.

small left pleural effusion and some loss of volume in the lower lobe; sudden shock may necessitate an urgent laparotomy with no imaging.

In those patients in whom the diagnosis is in doubt, computed tomography is the optimal test with an overall accuracy of around 95% (Jeffrey et al. 1981). CT has the advantage of demonstrating all the adjacent organs which may be responsible for the left upper quadrant symptoms if the spleen is intact. Like US, it can identify small quantities of free intraperitoneal fluid.

The common appearance is a subcapsular crescentic haematoma. The density of the lesion varies with time; intravenous contrast medium is essential as some lesions may be isodense with splenic parenchyma.

Kidneys

CT is not essential for the evaluation of renal trauma. If this is the only question posed, a combination of urography and US will provide more than adequate information. However when a traumatised patient is being examined by CT, the kidneys should be carefully evaluated; this will usually prevent the need for further renal imaging (Federle 1981). CT will elegantly demonstrate haematomas and urine collections as well as the precise tissue planes involved. It is more sensitive than urography in identifying extravasation of contrast medium (Sclafani and Becker 1985).

Other Organs

The region of the duodenum and pancreas should be carefully inspected in patients undergoing CT following trauma (especially seat-belt injuries). Specks of air, usually loculated around the duodenum in an extraperitoneal fashion, may provide the first clue of traumatic duodenal perforation (Karnaze et al. 1981). Indistinctness of the outline of

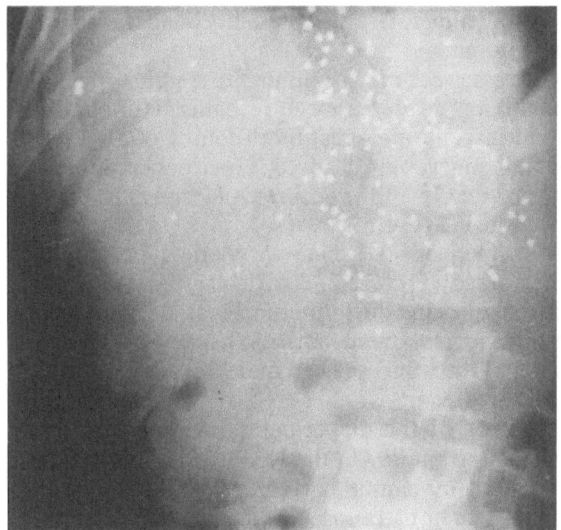

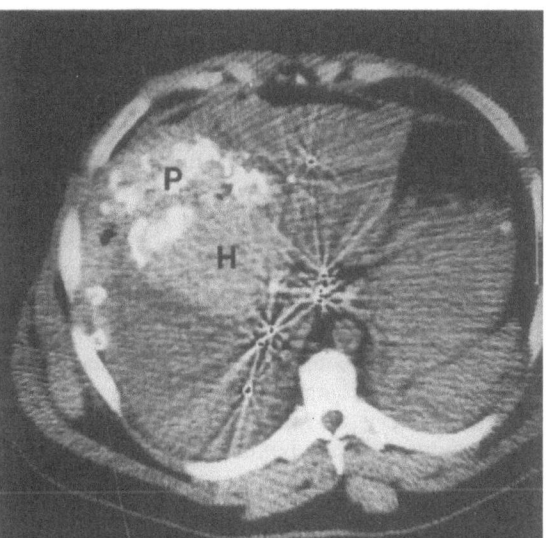

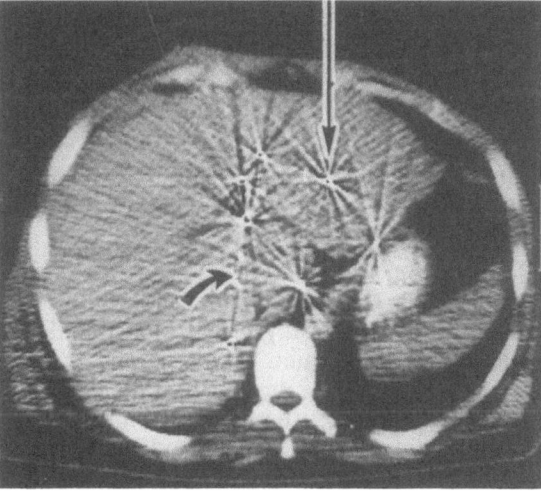

12.3a–c. Shotgun injury to right chest wall. Most of the pellets went through the right hemidiaphragm and entered the liver. At emergency surgery a pack was inserted into the hepatic laceration. **a** Plain abdominal X-ray showing the distribution of pellets. **b** CT of abdomen. The Pack (*P*) and haematoma (*H*) are well seen. So too is the distribution of bullets within the hepatic parenchyma. Considerable and inevitable artefacts from the high attenuation metallic density bullets. **c** A more caudal CT image shows pellets both within the left lobe (*straight arrow*) and caudate lobe (*curved arrow*). The pack was removed at subsequent surgery and the patient did well on lengthy conservative treatment.

the duodenum raises the possibility of an intramural haematoma.

The pancreas may be injured in a similar fashion and this may lead to the well-recognised CT changes found in acute pancreatitis (Toombs et al. 1981). Ductal injury may lead to a peripancreatic collection and CT allows accurate placement of drainage catheters (Fig. 12.1).

Retroperitoneal haemorrhage may be seen in other areas (Fig. 12.2), particularly around vertebral bodies in which fractures may be seen at CT despite normal plan films. A haematoma in the region of the vena cava can indicate a serious lesion to the great vein.

Rupture of the diaphragm is often overlooked following trauma. On the left such lesions may be diagnosed by simple barium studies. But CT, by virtue of demonstrating such a wide range of structures, can show defects close to the crura before major herniation develops. CT can also elegantly demonstrate the abdominal contents with the thoracic cavity, even omental fat which may not be well shown by other techniques (Gurney et al. 1985).

CT is now the optimal method of demonstrating the site of foreign bodies (eg, bullets, Fig. 12.3), even when these are not very radioopaque (wood, clothing etc. following blast injury).

Pitfalls

Uneven uptake of contrast medium in the spleen may occur due to coincidental infarcts or possibly even splenic artery spasm; such wedge-shaped areas of low attenuation may be mistaken for traumatic lesions.

Artefacts, especially caused by the movement of ribs during data acquisition, may simulate hepatic injuries: hence the need to control respiratory motion. Such artefacts are less of a problem with very modern CT machines with data-acquisition times of around 1–2 s.

Infection

General considerations

The use of CT in the evaluation of possible intraabdominal sepsis in critically ill patients should be considered in conjunction with US and scintigraphy. US can readily demonstrate many intraabdominal collections, especially those in the right upper quadrant, those in and around the kidneys and those situated in the pelvis. US also has the

advantage of being able to be performed at the bed side with minimal inconvenience to the patient. Scintigraphy (see Chapter 11), using some system of labelled white cells, carries the advantage of being able to identify an inflammatory process at *any* site within the abdomen and it can, in some hospitals, be performed using mobile equipment. However it is rather non-specific which has drawbacks in the immediate postoperative period. So CT is needed when US proves difficult (particularly left upper quadrant, beneath scars or drain sites, in the obese patient or in those in whom bowel gas obscures the region of interest) or in order to give anatomical delineation of a scintigraphic finding. Because many clinicians find CT relatively easy to interpret, there is an increasing tendency for CT to be used as the initial and definitive imaging test for possible sepsis. Some workers consider that CT provides the optimal images for planning the best route for percutaneous catheter drainage (see Figs. 12.1, 12.4 and 12.5).

The need for full bowel preparation has already been discussed. So too has the need for intravenous contrast medium. Indeed a collection of fluid which does *not* show an intense area of enhancement at its margin may well *not* be an abscess (simple cyst, pseudocyst, urinoma, etc).

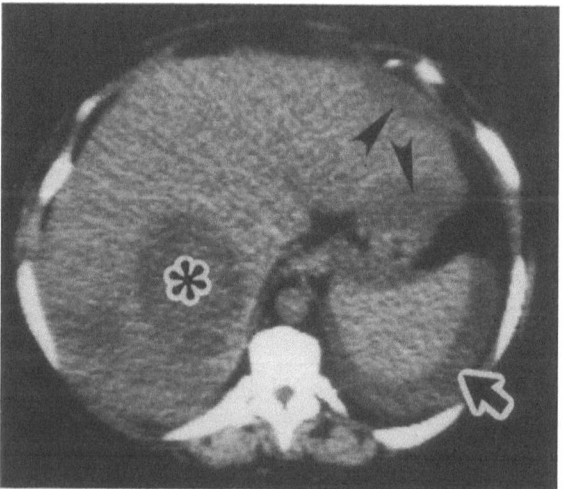

Fig. 12.4. Extremely obese (100 + kg) female with pyrexia of unknown origin. CT shows intra-hepatic abscess (*star*), perihepatic abscess (*arrowheads*) and left subphrenic abscess (*arrow*). These lesions could not be adequately demonstrated by ultrasound. All these sites were drained percutaneously using CT guidance. *Streptococcus milleri* identified in aspirate. Complete resolution with long-term antibiotics. The patient had underlying gall-bladder disease but surgery deemed too risky. Patient well four years later. Figure reproduced from Dixon: *Body CT* (1983) with kind permission of Churchill Livingstone.

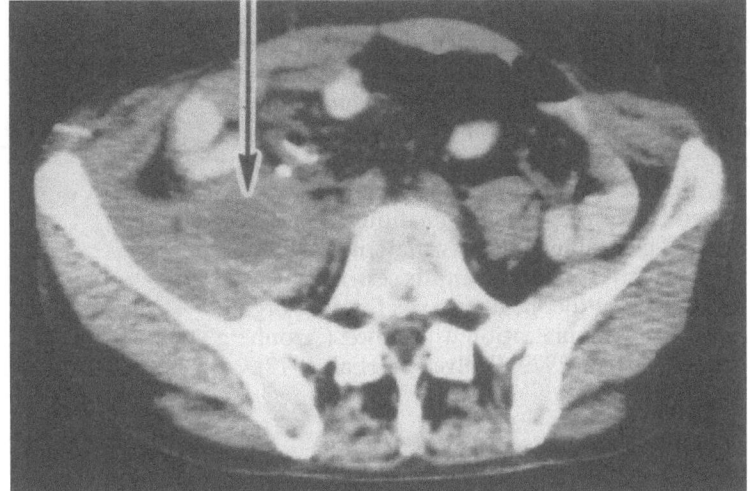

a

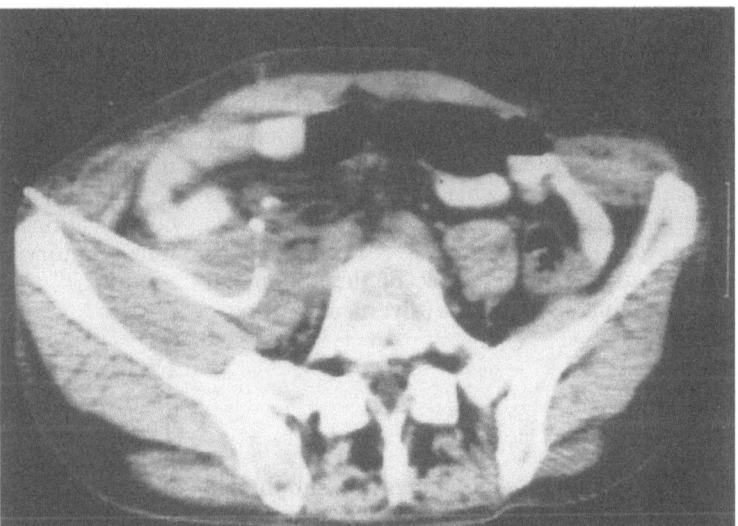

b

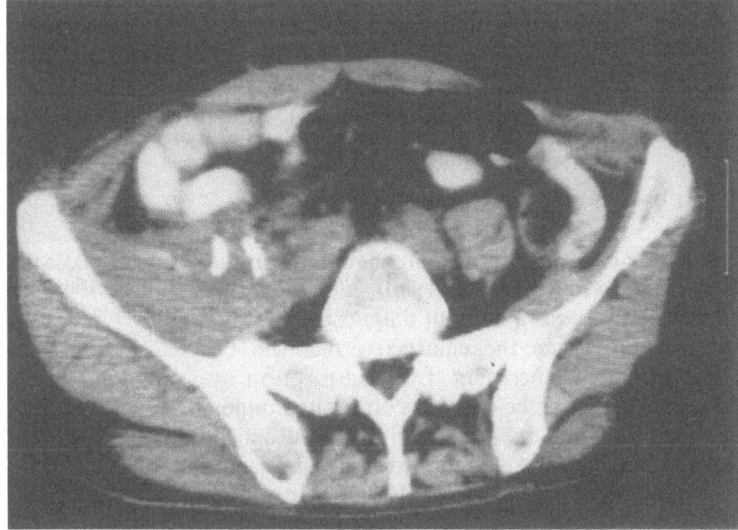

Fig. 12.5a–c. Patient with right hip/back pain and fever some months after colonic resection for carcinoma. **a** Lucent centre of pus (*arrow*) within inflammatory mass in right psoas merging with right iliacus. The tip of a needle used for local anaesthetic seen just anterior to anterior superior iliac spine. **b** Course of pigtail catheter leading to the psoas abscess. **c** Coils of pigtail within the abscess cavity.

c

A low-attenuation lesion with an enhancing rim is not necessarily diagnostic of an abscess. A necrotic neoplasm and even, as has been discussed, a resolving haematoma with surrounding inflammation can give similar appearances. There is therefore a need for fine needle aspiration in cases of doubt – either pus will be aspirated for culture or cells will be obtained for cytological examination. Air pockets within the central fluid density material, which are well shown by CT, make an abscess much more likely; this will either be due to gas forming organisms or to a communication with bowel (Aronberg et al. 1978; Callen 1979; Wolverson et al. 1979).

Hepatic/perihepatic abscess

These lesions will often be well seen at US. However, the whole liver may be difficult to demonstrate in the very obese patient (Fig. 12.4) and lesions in the very periphery of the liver may be hard to demonstrate. Furthermore, some multiloculated abscesses can be quite echogenic which causes further difficulty. Perihepatic abscesses should be well seen at US except when the overlying skin is inaccessible due to recent surgery.

Whenever an hepatic abscess is identified it is important to search the whole of the abdominal cavity for an underlying cause (diverticular abscess, gallstones, etc).

Subphrenic abscess

Ultrasound should reliably identify subphrenic abscesses on the right (Chapter 13). Gastric air and other bowel gas may hinder US on the left, although plain film and barium studies may be diagnostic. However CT will readily demonstrate the presence or absence of a subphrenic collection (on left or right) and allow guidance of draining catheters where this proves difficult on US (Fig. 12.4).

Psoas abscess

CT is the optimal technique for demonstrating a psoas abscess (Jeffrey et al. 1980), which in the past has often proved a difficult diagnosis. The low density lesion within the enlarged psoas will be well seen after enhancement. Either aspiration or catheter drainage can be easily accomplished under CT control (Fig. 12.5). The CT study should also include suitable cuts of vertebral discs to check for a possible tuberculous focus of infection. However, in this country nontuberculous causes (and indeed

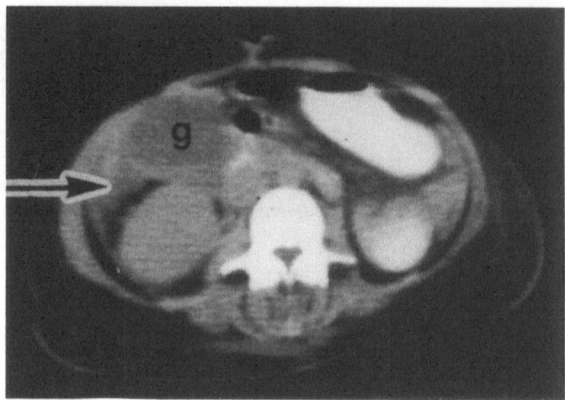

Fig. 12.6. A patient who had received severe skeletal and thoracic trauma, and was receiving artificial ventilation. CT performed because of pyrexia. Large distended gall bladder (*g*) together with small quantity of adjacent fluid (*arrow*) cited as a possible cause. Gall bladder normal at subsequent surgery, although large due to prolonged fasting. Figure reproduced from Dixon: *Body CT* (1983) with kind permission of Churchill Livingstone.

nonspinal causes) for a psoas abscess are more common (Williams 1986) and include postoperative complications and adjacent bowel disease, either inflammatory (eg. Crohn's disease) or malignant in nature.

Pitfalls

The potential problem of unopacified small bowel loops simulating a fluid collection has already been mentioned. Not all fluid density lesions are due to an abscess; small serous collections are quite common around surgical sites and fine-needle aspiration may be needed to distinguish them from abscesses. The gall bladder, so often responsible for intraabdominal sepsis, may become very distended when a critically-ill patient is being fed parenterally; this can be mistaken for an empyema (Fig. 12.6).

References

Aronberg DJ, Stanley RJ, Levitt RG, Sagel SS (1978). Evaluation of abdominal abscess with computed tomography. J Comput Assist Tomogr 2: 184–187

Callen, PW (1979) Computed tomographic evaluation of abdominal and pelvic abscesses. Radiology 131: 171–175

Dixon AK (1983) Body CT: a handbook. Churchill Livingstone, Edinburgh. pp 20–27

Federle MP (1981) Abdominal trauma: the role and impact of computed tomography. Invest Radiol 16: 260–268

Federle MP, Kaiser JA, McAninch JW et al. (1981) The role of computed tomography in renal trauma. Radiology 141: 455–460

Gurney J, Harrison WL, Anderson JC (1985) Omental fat simulating pleural fluid in traumatic diaphragmatic hernia: CT characteristics. J Comput Assist Tomogr 9: 1112–1114

Jeffrey RB, Callen PW, Federle MP (1980) Computed tomography of psoas abscesses. J Comput Assist Tomogr 4: 639–641

Jeffrey RB, Laing FC, Federle MP, Goodman PC (1981) Computed tomography of splenic trauma. Radiology 141: 729–732

Karnaze GC, Sheedy PF, Stephens DH, McLeod RA (1981) Computed tomography in duodenal rupture due to blunt abdominal trauma. J Comput Assist Tomogr 5: 267–269

Sclafani SJA, Becker JA (1985) Radiological diagnosis of renal trauma. Urol Radiol 7: 192–200

Toombs BD, Lester RG, Ben-Menachem Y, Sandler CM (1981) Computed tomography in blunt trauma. Radiol Clin North Am 19: 17–35

Toombs BD, Sandler CM, Rausch-Kolb EN et al. (1982) Assessment of hepatic injuries with computed tomography. J Comput Assist Tomogr 6: 750–756

Williams MP (1986) Non-tuberculous psoas abscess. Clin Radiol 37: 253–256

Wolverson MK, Jaganna IB, Sundaram M et al. (1979) CT as a primary diagnostic method in evaluating abdominal abscess. Am J Roentgenol 133: 1089–1095

Chapter 13

Radioisotopes in the Diagnosis of Abdominal Embarrassment in the Critically Ill

J. P. Lavender

Radioisotopes play relatively little part in the investigation of the acutely ill patient with abdominal disease. There are, however, two areas where, in my view, radioisotope tracers can play a significant role. The first is in the identification of the site of gastrointestinal bleeding where, together with angiography, tracers can make an important contribution to patient care. The second area is in the investigation of sepsis by the use of autologous labelled white blood cells. The object of this chapter is to review the generally available imaging techniques.

Liver

Colloid Liver Scan

The standard radioisotopic image of the liver is obtained by the intravenous injection of a colloid. This shows the liver parenchyma, by virtue of the removal of particles by the reticulo-endothelial cells lining the liver sinusoids. In the acutely ill patient, images may be useful in liver trauma but, if available, ultrasound (US) or computed tomography (CT) are more revealing investigations.

Biliary Scanning

Derivatives of immido-diacetic acid (HIDA) labelled with ^{99}Tc^m can be used to study both hepatic function and the biliary tracer. Following an intravenous injection of HIDA a rapid clearance of tracer into the liver is seen, with radioactivity appearing in the hepatic and common bile ducts (Fig. 13.1). The gall bladder should normally be seen in about 20 min, but may be seen in some patients at a later stage; however, it is usually seen within 60 min. The initial activity in the liver clears and later images demonstrate tracer in the small intestine. Acute liver failure and obstructive jaundice produce characteristic appearances on HIDA scans, but these problems are best explored by US.

Acute Cholecystitis

The appearance of a HIDA scan in a patient with an acute cholecystitis is characterised by no tracer entering the gall bladder even on delayed images. In the patient with an appropriate clinical picture, therefore, this finding is confirmatory of the disease. In patients with chronic cholecystitis, non-visualisation of the gall bladder frequently occurs.

Biliary leakage may be demonstrated reliably and simply by HIDA scanning. Rarely, such leaks may be spontaneous, due to a perforated gall bladder. More frequently, they are due to trauma, which may be accidental or surgical. One advantage of the technique is that of showing the proportion of tracer reaching the gut by normal anatomy compared with the extent of bile loss elsewhere. The combination of biliary scanning and US is a powerful diagnostic approach.

Spleen

Imaging of the spleen can be achieved, like that of the liver, through two functions. The first is its

a

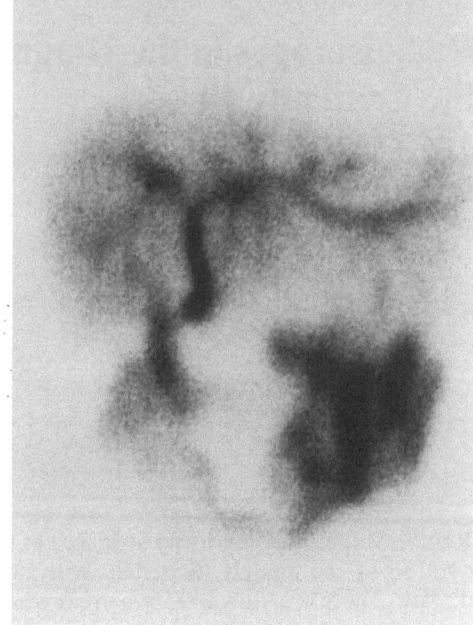

c

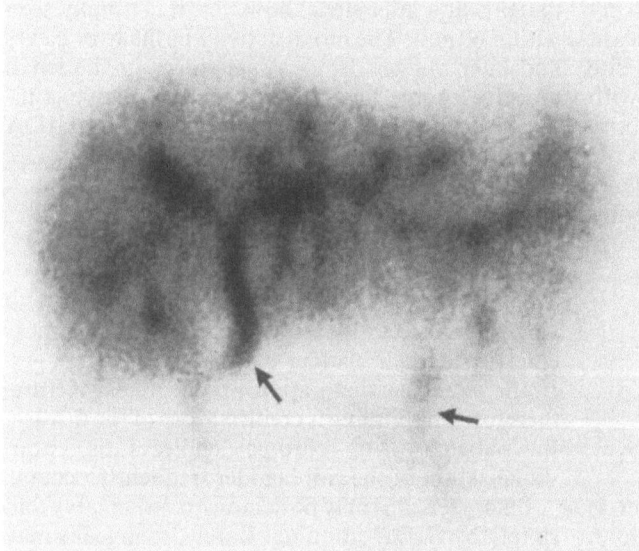

b

Fig. 13.1a–c. 20-yr-old patient with previous trauma to the liver. Images have been taken at 10a, 15b and 25c min after the intravenous injection of technetium-labelled HIDA and show the common bile duct (*left arrow*) and rather dilated hepatic ducts. A fistulous tract is seen between the bile ducts in the left lobe and loops of ileum (*right arrow*).

uptake of radioactive colloid and the second, more specialised function, is its ability to remove damaged cells. Applications in the acute abdomen are limited to trauma.

Gastrointestinal Tract

Gastrointestinal Bleeding

The majority of bleeds from the gut are identified by endoscopy. A proportion, however, present considerable difficulties and then isotopic studies and angiography may be used to demonstrate the site of bleeding. Angiography requires the patient to be actively bleeding and is less sensitive than isotopic tracers. Angiography is, however, anatomically more accurate and therefore the tracer study should logically precede the angiogram. If it is negative, it is unlikely that angiography will show bleeding, but it may show abnormal anatomy as, for example, in angiodysplasia. The tracer study may therefore aid angiography by indicating a region for selective study or may be abnormal when angiography is normal (Fig. 13.2) (Alavi et al. 1977; Winzelberg et al. 1982).

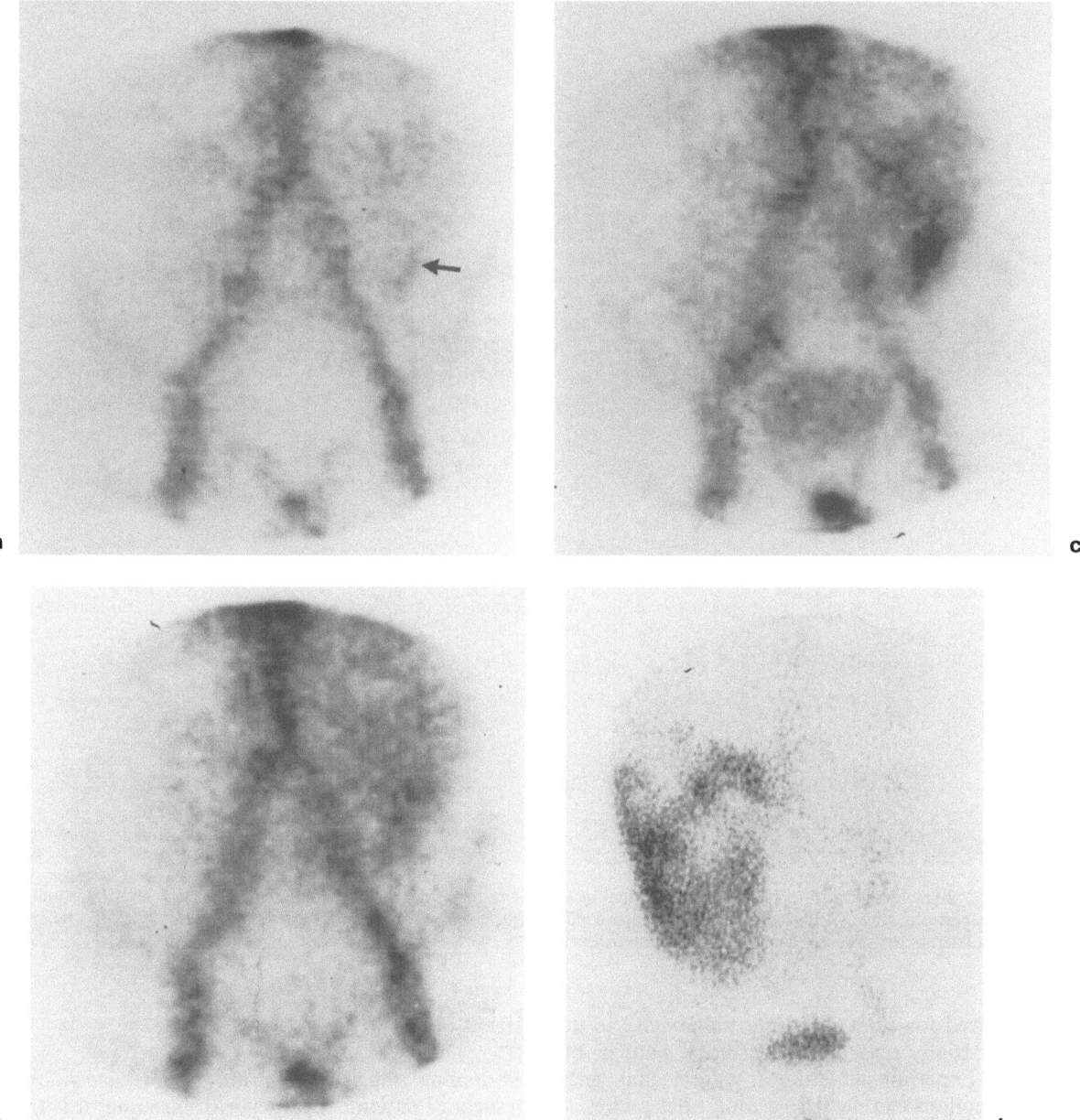

Fig. 13.2a–d. Technetium-labelled red-cell study in a patient with gastroentestinal bleeding. Angiography was negative. **a** View at 30 min after labelling red cells showing blood pool and early accumulation of activity in the left mid abdomen (*arrow*). **b, c** Increasing activity demonstrated in the ileum at 40 and 60 min. **d** View at 3 h showing activity in distal small bowel and ascending colon.

There are two techniques for identifying gastrointestinal bleeding by the use of radioactive tracers – radioactive colloid and the use of technetium-99m-labelled red cells – which each have advantages and disadvantages. Radioactive colloid is rapidly removed by the liver and the spleen: if a patient is actively bleeding, therefore, the intravenous injection of colloid will show the site of bleeding since the background activity is very low. However, patient may bleed intermittently and the alternative tracer in common use is technetium-99m-labelled red cells. Here, the leak of tracer can

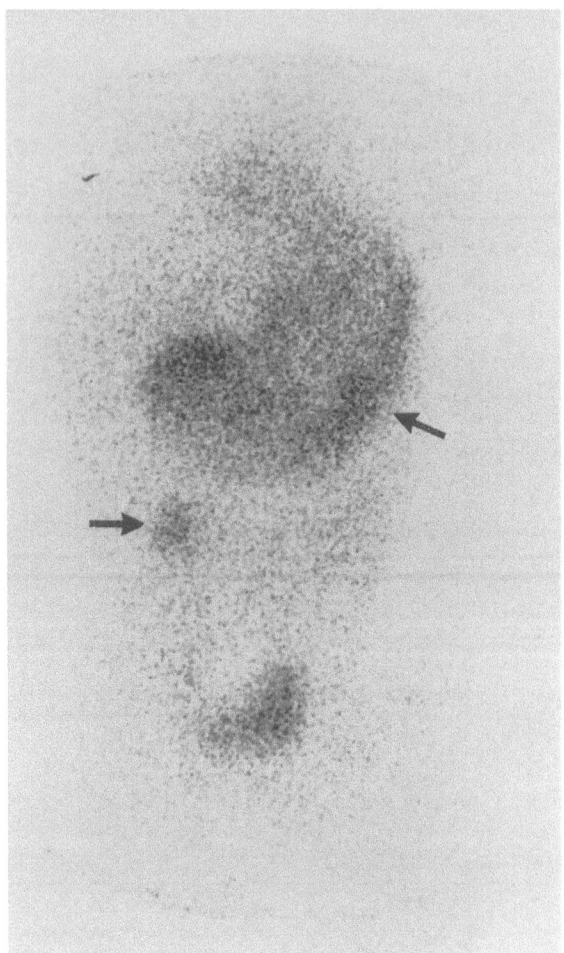
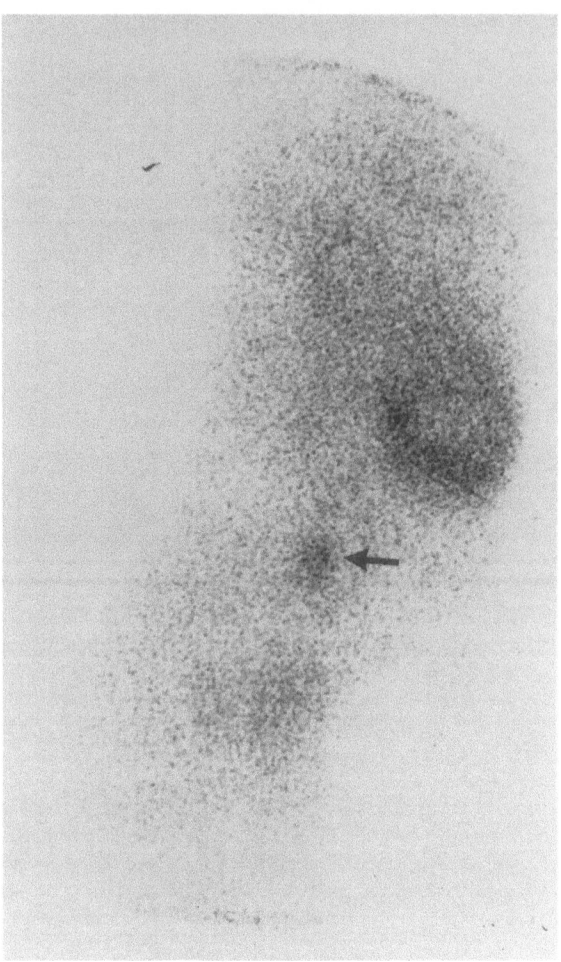

a   b

Fig. 13.3a,b. 2-yr-old child with episodic gastrointestinal bleeding. Images of the abdomen following an intravenous injection of technetium pertechnetate. **a** Anterior view showing gastric mucosa (*upper arrow*) and Meckel's diverticulum (*lower arrow*). **b** Same child, right lateral view to show Meckel's diverticulum (*arrow*).

be followed for up to 24 h, but the activity in the gut is partially masked by the blood pool in the vessels. Experimental studies suggest that technetium colloid can detect bleeding rates as low as $0.1 \, \text{ml}^{-1} \, \text{min}^{-1}$, but red-cell labelling requires 40–60 ml blood in the gut for successful imaging (Bunker et al. 1984).

Meckel's Diverticulum

Meckel's diverticulum is a relatively rare cause of gastrointestinal bleeding, more common in the infant than in the adult. Since the diverticulum contains gastric mocosa, sodium pertechnetate (technetium-99m), which shows uptake in gastric mucosa and salivary glands, will also show localisation in the diverticulum (Fig. 13.3).

Infection

Abdominal sepsis is of prime importance in the acutely ill patient; together with bleeding, it is the cause of shock.

Techniques for Detecting Infection

Gallium-67 Citrate

Gallium-67 citrate, when injected intravenously, shows protein binding and a slow clearance with localisation in liver, spleen and bone marrow and some 15% of activity excreted into the gastrointestinal tract. It was observed in 1969 that this tracer localised in neoplastic cells. Shortly there-

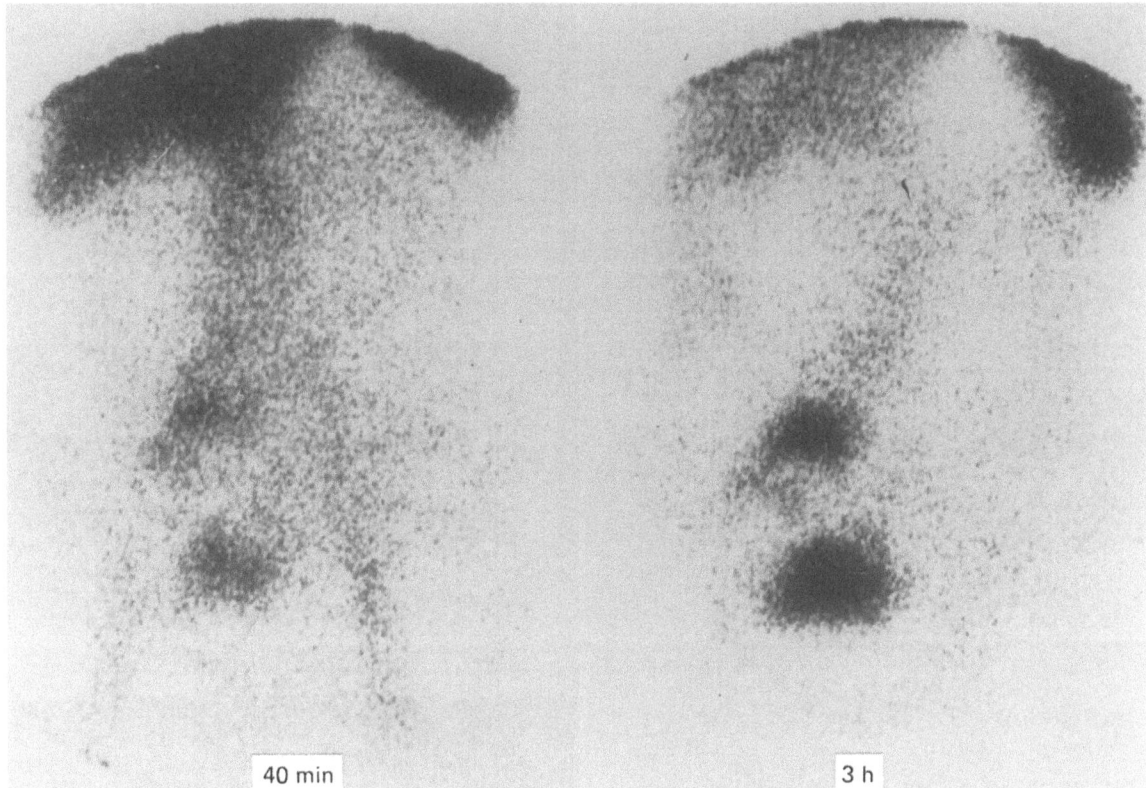

Fig. 13.4. Autologous white blood cells in patient with pelvic sepsis. Image on the left taken at 40 min after the infusion of Indium-111 labelled autologous granulocytes. This shows aorta and iliac vessels and early migration of cells to abscesses. Image on the right shows increasing accumulation of cells visible at 3 h.

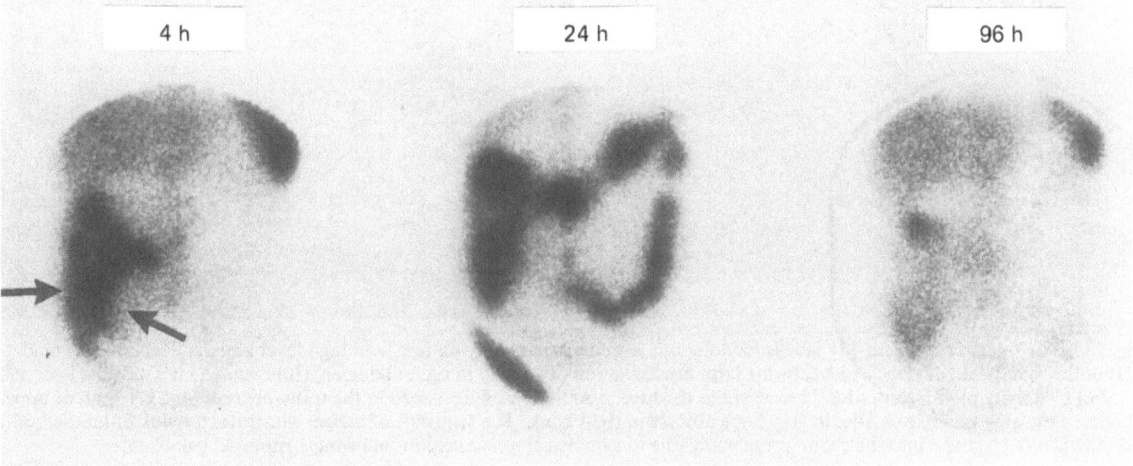

Fig. 13.5. Autologous white blood cells in patient with postoperative abdominal sepsis communicating with colon. Image at 4 h shows large accumulation of activity in right abdomen (*arrow*). At 24 h there is outlining of the transverse and descending colon and by 96 h activity is largely cleared.

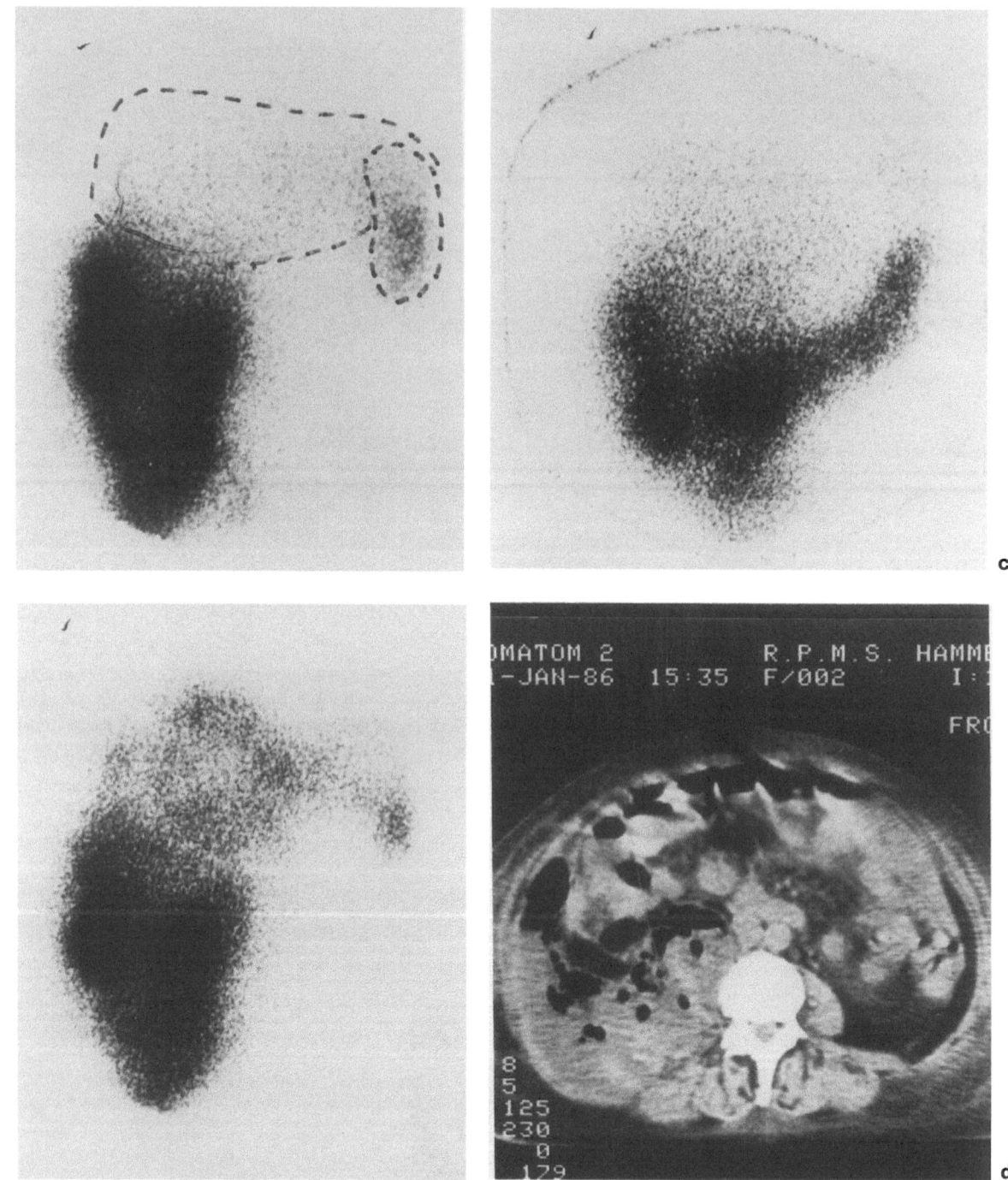

Fig. 13.6a–d. Images of Indium-111-labelled autologous leucocytes in elderly patient with high fever and acute abdominal tenderness in the right flank. **a** Image at 3 h showing large accumulation of activity in right abdomen. (Interrupted lines indicate liver and spleen.) **b** Activity at 48 h shows focal areas within the liver. **c** Activity at 4 days seen in the transverse colon. **d** CT scan of upper abdomen showing multiple cavities in very large abscess in right flank. The sequence of images illustrates a reflux of labelled cells into the biliary tract and into the colon, presumably due to fistulous communication following a ruptured gall bladder.

after, it was also shown that gallium will localise in inflammatory tissue (Staab and McCartney 1978). The difficulty with its use in the acute abdomen lies firstly in the delay of 12–24 h before imaging and secondly from the presence of activity in the gut. The interpretation of images is difficult. Subphrenic and perirenal regions, however, can be well-imaged by this method.

Indium-111 Labelled White Blood Cells

A method of labelling circulating cells with Indium-111 was developed some years ago (Thakur et al. 1977). This method utilises the lipophilic agent hydroxyquinoline (oxine) chelated to the radio-isotope Indium-111. The cells are separated from autologous blood and suspended in saline for labelling and then re-injected intravenously. This is a simple procedure but has certain drawbacks. Firstly, it is evident that non-migrating mononuclear cells are also labelled. There is also evidence that the granulocytes are not normal in behaviour after this procedure since they lodge in the lung following their re-injection, clearing slowly and only then becoming available for migration.

An alternative chelate of indium, tropolone, can be used in the presence of plasma and results in more rapid transit through the pulmonary vascular bed and earlier migration. A further refinement of the method uses a density gradient in order to obtain a pure population of granulocytes (Peters et al. 1983). Both methods can utilise donor white blood cells in children where volumes of blood may present a problem, and also in patients with aplasia.

Appearances after the re-injection of indium-labelled white blood cells maintained in plasma show a rapid transit through the lungs and activity distributed in spleen, liver and blood pool. The cells are cleared with a median survival of 6–7 h, activity then appearing in bone marrow. Cell migration to inflammatory sites can be seen from 10 min after re-injection; imaging is normally performed at 3 h and at 18–24 h.

Abdominal Sepsis

The common site of abdominal sepsis is the peritoneal cavity where pools of activity are frequently seen in the paracolic gutter and pelvis (Fig. 13.4). It is important to take the posterior view where possible to look at the pouch of Douglas. An abscess may be visualised within the first few minutes of the re-injection of the cells with activity increasing with time and most clearly seen at 18–24 h. It is important to take early and late views in order to differentiate white cells in an abscess from those which may be present in the bowel due either to inflammatory bowel disease or to swallowed sputum. Sepsis adjacent to or within the liver or spleen may require separate visualisation with technetium-labelled colloid.

Abscess cavities within the abdomen may communicate with gut. In such cases, a movement of activity can be seen ending up in outlining of the colon by Indium-111 (Figs. 13.5, 13.6).

Inflammatory Bowel Disease

This results in a characteristic series of images. Migration of cells to bowel wall is seen to occur very early. Such cells then migrate into the bowel lumen and can be followed through the gastrointestinal tract, the original site clearing of activity (Saverymuttu et al. 1983).

Comparisons of sensitivity and specificity between autologous white blood cell imaging and CT or US show high levels of accuracy for white blood cell imaging (Peters et al. 1983). This reflects the fact that although abscesses may appear as fluid collections, this is not always so and conversely they may be multiple collections of fluid, only some of which represent pus.

References

Alavi A, Dann RW, Baum S et al. (1977) Scintigraphic detection of acute gastroentestinal bleeding. Radiol 124:753–756

Bunker SE, Lull RJ, Tanascescu DE et al. (1984) Scintigraphy of gastrointestinal haemorrhage: superiority of technetium-99m red blood cells over technetium-99m sulphur colloid. Am J Roentol 143:543–548

Peters AM, Saverymuttu SH, Reavy H, Danpure H, Osman S, Lavender JP (1983) Imaging inflammation with 111-In-tropolonate labelled leucocytes. J Nucl Med 24:39–44

Saverymuttu SH, Peters AM, Lavender JP, Hodgson HJ, Chadwick VS (1983) Indium-111 autologous leucocytes in inflammatory bowel disease. Gut 24:293–299

Staab EV, McCartney WH (1978) Role of gallium-67 in inflammatory disease. Semin Nucl Med 8:219–234

Thakur ML, Coleman RE, Welch MJ (1977) Indium-111 labelled leucocytes for the localisation of abscesses. J Lab Clin Med 89:217–228

Winzelberg GG, McKusik KA, Froelich JW et al. (1982) Detection of gastrointestinal bleeding with technetium-99m labelled red blood cells. Semin Nucl Med 12:139–146

Section V

Special Techniques and Recent Advances

Chapter 14

Interventional Radiology and Digital Subtraction Angiography

J. McIvor and P. S. Treweeke

Interventional radiology is a term which covers a range of invasive procedures used by diagnostic radiologists to diagnose and treat disease. Most are extensions of long-established diagnostic techniques, such as arteriography and guided biopsy, but the scope has widened considerably during the last few years and now includes drainage procedures, therapeutic embolisation, angioplasty and catheter recovery. In general, these procedures replace open surgery and, although time-consuming and technically difficult, they can usually be carried out under local anaesthesia and have a low morbidity compared with surgery. However, most procedures require access to expensive and complicated X-ray equipment which is a disadvantage when managing patients in an intensive care unit as the patients have to be moved.

Digital subtraction angiography is a technique which increases the visibility of radio-opaque contrast medium by a process of electronic subtraction. The concept is simple, a positive image with contrast medium is superimposed on a negative image of the same area without contrast medium and the background structures, such as bones, soft tissues and gas "subtract" out leaving only the contrast medium visible. Photographic subtraction with conventional radiographic film has been in use for decades but recent advances in computer technology make it possible to subtract digital images in a way which demonstrates very low concentrations of radio-opaque contrast medium.

In practice, this means that the arterial tree can be demonstrated with an intravenous injection of normal strength contrast medium or with an intra-arterial injection of dilute contrast medium (25% normal).

Control of Haemorrhage by Therapeutic Embolisation

Arterial embolisation is an alternative to surgical ligation and has been used to control severe haemorrhage from the gastrointestinal, urinary, respiratory and female genital tracts. It is almost invariably carried out under local anaesthesia. Trans-hepatic venous embolisation will usually control haemorrhage from oesophageal or gastric varices, but requires general anaesthesia.

Splenic embolisation is an alternative to splenectomy and has been successfully used to treat severe haemorrhage caused by hypersplenism and idiopathic thrombocytopenic purpura in patients who are poor surgical risks.

A wide variety of materials has been used (Table 14.1) and the length of the list indicates that none

Table 14.1. Embolisation materials.

Physical
  Absorbable
    Blood clot
    Gel foam
  Non-absorbable
    Fat and muscle tissue
    Polyvinyl alcohol fragments (Ivalon)
    Plastic spheres
    Metallic spheres
    Steel coils
    Balloons
    Cyanoacrylate cement
    Silicone rubber

Chemical
    Ethanol (ethyl alcohol)
    Ethanolamine

is entirely satisfactory. Even if non-absorbable materials are used, much of the block is usually due to thrombus which propagates through the vascular tree when blood flow stops or is severely reduced. Thrombus can, of course, be rapidly resorbed by normal physiological processes and this may account for the short-lived therapeutic benefit of some embolisation procedures. Despite this limitation, therapeutic embolisation is usually effective, at least in the short term, and has a valuable role in the management of life-threatening haemorrhage in seriously ill patients.

Gastrointestinal Tract

Arterial embolisation has been successfully used to control upper gastrointestinal haemorrhage caused by peptic ulceration of the stomach and duodenum, haemorrhagic gastritis, Mallory–Weiss syndrome, haemorrhage pancreatitis, gastric and hepatic artery aneurysms, ulcerating tumours and vascular malformations (Irving and Northfield 1976; Allison 1980; Helliwell and Irving 1981; Rahn et al. 1982).

Selective arteriography of the coeliac axis, left gastric and superior mesenteric arteries are the initial arteriographic investigations and should demonstrate haemorrhage if blood loss exceeds $0.5\,\mathrm{ml\,s^{-1}}$ (Nusbaum and Baum 1963). Although gastrointestinal haemorrhage is usually intermittent, a bleeding point was demonstrated in 77% of 35 patients in one series (Irving and Northfield 1976) and in 63% of 52 patients in another (Rahn et al. 1982), but these figures are higher than usual. Embolisation of the bleeding artery is usually carried out with fragments of gel foam and requires selective catheterisation of the left gastric, gastroduodenal or inferior pancreatico-duodenal arteries. A vascular abnormality is sometimes demonstrated in the absence of haemorrhage and embolisation may be justified if there is reliable endoscopic evidence of bleeding from the site (Fig. 14.1). Stainless-steel coils are occasionally required for torrential haemorrhage and to occlude aneurysms.

Arterial embolisation has a much smaller role in controlling haemorrhage from the lower intestinal tract owing to the risks of necrosis, perforation and late stricture formation. The procedure is occasionally justified in massive haemorrhage from the small or large intestine when the patient's life is at immediate risk and a few successes have been reported (Rahn et al. 1982). Arteriography of the superior and inferior mesenteric arteries will sometimes demonstrate a bleeding point and diagnostic success in 39% of 33 patients has been reported (Rahn et al. 1982). The inferior mesenteric artery

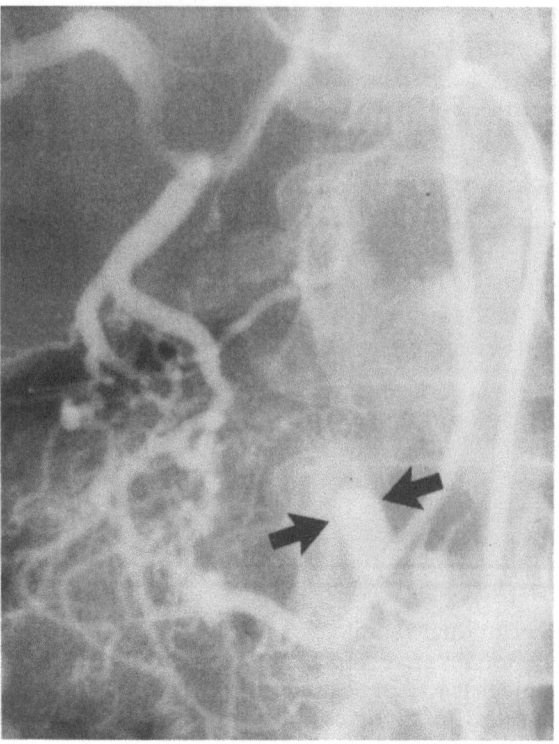

a

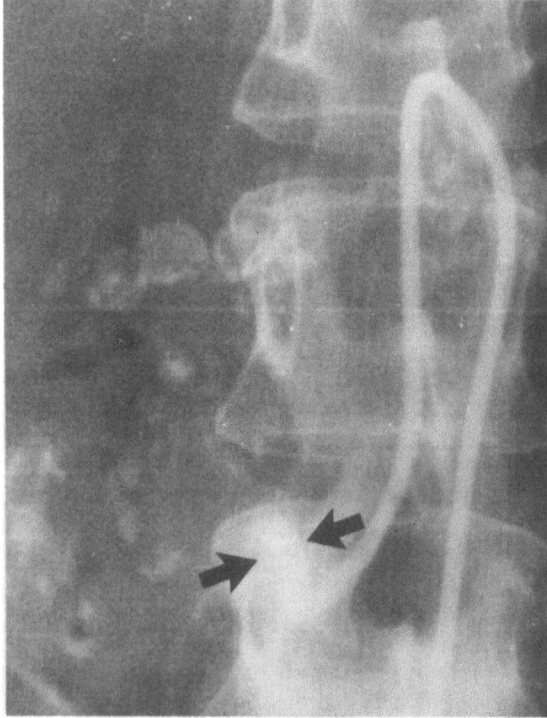

b

Fig. 14.1a,b. Before (**a**) and after (**b**) embolisation of the inferior pancreatico-duodenal artery in a 54-year-old woman with severe duodenal bleeding from chronic relapsing pancreatitis. The haemorrhage had been seen endoscopically and was controlled for several months.

should, if possible, be catheterised and injected before the superior mesenteric, as contrast medium rapidly accumulates in the bladder and obscures bleeding into the rectum and lower sigmoid colon. Arteriographic abnormalities in the absence of haemorrhage are more common and were demonstrated in 51% of 37 patients with intermittent haemorrhage arising in the lower gastrointestinal tract (Thompson et al. 1984). The most common abnormality in this series was angiodysplasia of the caecum, but Meckel's diverticula and smooth-muscle tumours were also seen. Vasopressin infusion is preferred to arterial embolisation in such cases and will control haemorrhage temporarily in the majority (Athanasoulis and Baum 1975).

Percutaneous transhepatic embolisation can be used to control severe haemorrhage from gastric or oesophageal varices. The procedure is usually carried out under general anaesthesia and is of value in patients who are unsuitable for endoscopic injection of varices due to oesophageal ulceration, or gastric varices. The technique is to pass a needle through one of the lower rib spaces into the right lobe of the liver and then into the right branch of the portal vein. This can usually be achieved under fluoroscopic control after a few passes of the needle. Using a modified Seldinger technique, a guide wire, followed by an arterial catheter, is passed into the splenic vein and into the veins feeding the varices. These can be occluded with various combinations of gel foam, ethanol and steel coils (Fig. 14.2). There are often technical difficulties as the veins feeding the varices may be small and difficult to catheterise, but if the feeding veins are successfully occluded then bleeding should be controlled and reports of therapeutic success in 80% of 116 patients have been recorded (Smith-Laing et al. 1981). Smaller series using ethanol reported slightly lower rates of therapeutic success (Keller et al. 1983, Uflacker 1983).

Therapeutic embolisation in the presence of severe haemorrhage is commonly associated with a mortality, which is more often due to the underlying disease than to the procedure itself. Vasopressin infusion also has complications as it reduces coronary blood flow and cardiac output and can result in severe hypotension.

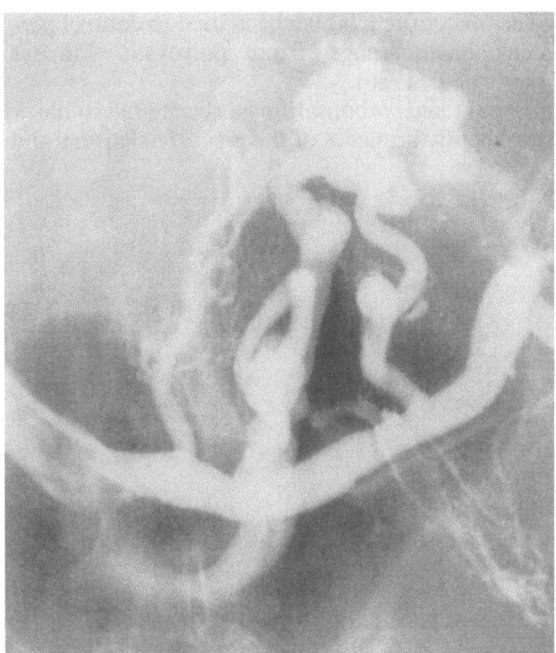

a

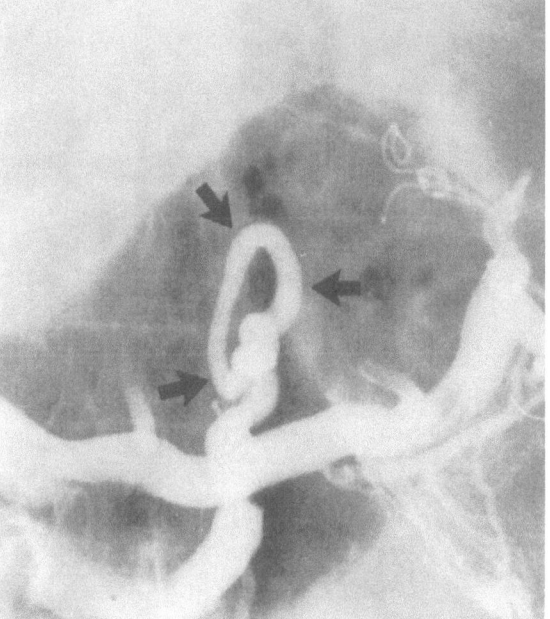

b

Fig. 14.2a,b. Before (**a**) and after (**b**) transhepatic embolisation of gastric and oesophageal varices in a patient with alcoholic cirrhosis and portal hypertension. A collateral vein draining into the left renal vein (*arrowed*) and not supplying the varices was not embolised. Bleeding stopped at once.

Urinary and Genital Tracts

Renal artery embolisation usually controls persistent severe haemorrhage from renal carcinoma (Ekelund et al. 1979; Macerlean et al. 1980). The procedure is carried out under local anaesthesia and has a negligible morbidity. It does, of course, destroy renal function, but is an alternative to surgical nephrectomy in these patients. The main indication is intractable haemorrhage in patients where nephrectomy is contra-indicated due to metastatic disease.

The procedure has also been used to control persistent haemorrhage from polycystic kidneys (Harley et al. 1980).

Partial renal embolisation has been used to block intra-hepatic branches of the main renal artery and

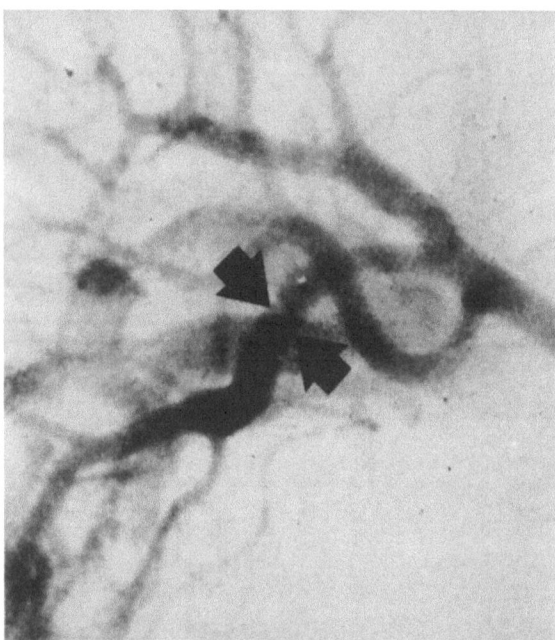

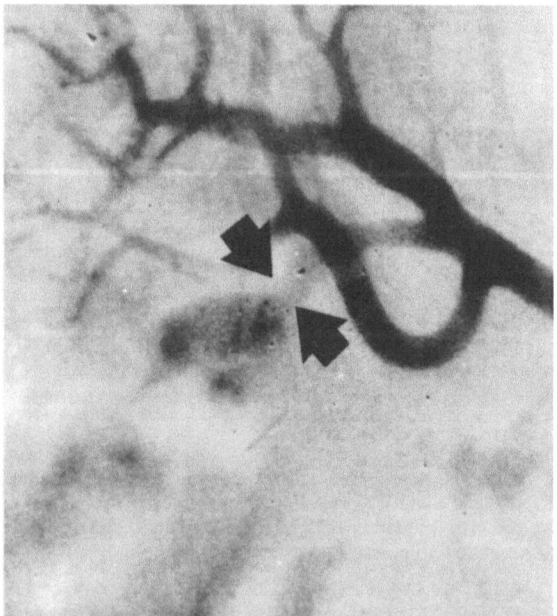

Fig. 14.3a,b. Subtraction arteriogram films before (**a**) and after (**b**) embolisation of an intra-renal branch (*arrowed*) of the right renal artery to control massive haematuria following renal biopsy. The haematuria cleared within a few hours.

to control haemorrhage resulting from biopsy and arterio-venous fistulae (Chuang et al. 1975; Richman et al. 1977; Wallace et al. 1978) (Fig. 14.3). Although the procedure is technically difficult and requires highly selective catheterisation, it does preserve a substantial proportion of renal perfusion and renal function. The procedure is particularly valuable in cases of severe haemorrhage following renal biopsy and is often an alternative to nephrectomy in these cases. Short-acting materials such as gelatin sponge are usually adequate if the procedure is carried out within a few days of injury, but more permanent materials, such as coils, or detachable balloons may be necessary if haematuria has been present for some weeks.

Embolisation of the internal iliac arteries will usually control haemorrhage from a carcinoma which has arisen in the bladder itself or invaded it from an adjacent organ, such as the rectum, colon or uterus. A review of the literature (McIvor et al. 1982) found a success rate of over 90%. Although haematuria from a tumour localised to one side of the bladder can be controlled by unilateral embolisation (Kobayashi et al. 1980), it is necessary to occlude the anterior divisions of both internal iliac arteries if the tumour is extensive (Carmignani et al. 1980), or if the patient had received radiotherapy, as haemorrhage in these cases may be due to post-irradiation telangiectasis. Short-acting materials, such as gelatin sponge, seem to be as effective as longer acting materials. The procedure is less traumatic than surgical ligation of the internal iliac arteries and seems to be more effective, probably because it occludes the small arteries within the tumour and not just the main feeding vessels (Fig. 14.4). Serious haemorrhage from arterio-venous malformations has been treated in the same way, but, even if the procedure is initially satisfactory, recurrence is common (Lang et al. 1979).

Gluteal pain, lasting a few days, is common if the posterior divisions of the internal iliac arteries are embolised, but the most serious complication is a neurological defect of one or both lower limbs (Carmignani et al. 1980; Hare and Holland 1983), which is probably due to ischaemic damage to the sciatic nerve. Although necrosis and gangrene of the bladder is frequently mentioned as a complication, it must be extremely rare as there is only one case in the literature, a patient with severe pelvic injuries and pelvic vein thrombosis in whom the pelvic circulation was already compromised at the time of arterial embolisation. The same case seems to have been reported twice (Braf and Koontz 1977; Hietala 1978).

Embolisation of the internal iliac arteries has also been used to control intractable post-partum

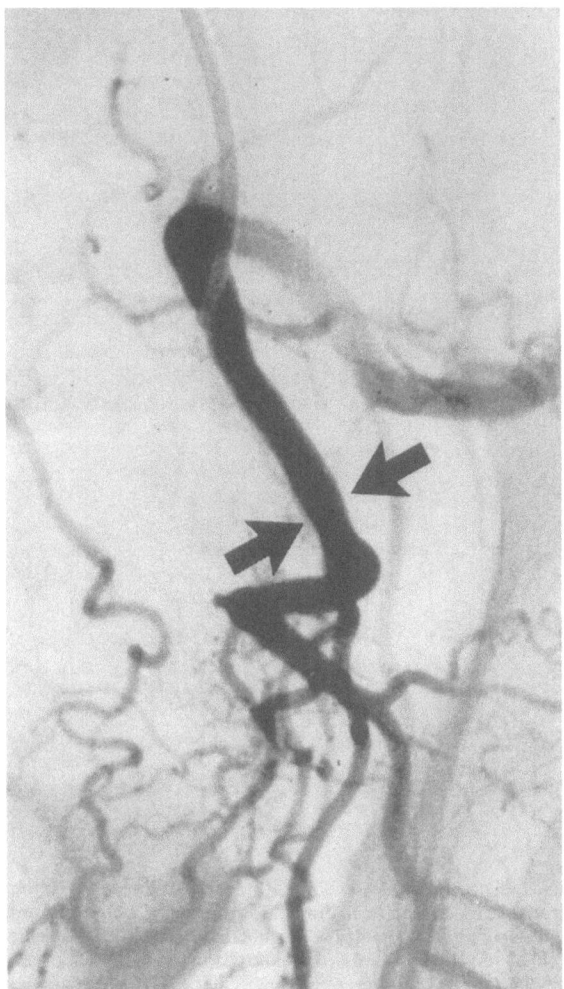 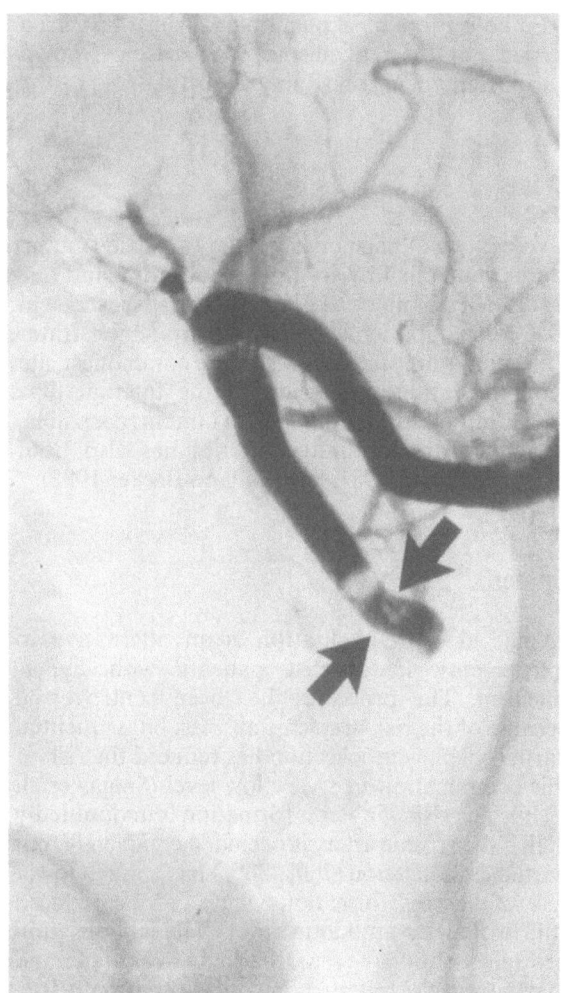

a   b

Fig. 14.4a,b. Subtraction arteriogram before (**a**) and after (**b**) embolisation of the anterior division (*arrowed*) of the left internal iliac artery in a 62-year-old man with uncontrollable haematuria from a colonic carcinoma invading the bladder. The anterior division of the right internal iliac artery was occluded at the same time and the haematuria cleared within a few hours.

haemorrhage (Pais et al. 1980) and severe haemorrhage from malignant uterine tumours (Lang 1981).

Respiratory Tract

Embolisation of the bronchial arteries has been used to control massive haemoptysis in patients unsuitable for surgery, often because of poor respiratory function. The underlying pathology is commonly bronchiectasis, pulmonary fibrosis with aspergilloma, or cystic fibrosis, but haemorrhage from carcinoma has also been successfully controlled (Remy et al. 1977; Vujic et al. 1982; O'halpin et al. 1984).

There are several reports of permanent damage to the spinal cord with resultant paraplegia and the risk of this complication should restrict the procedure to patients with life-threatening haemorrhage. It has been suggested that particulate materials, such as fragments of gel foam or polyvinyl alcohol sponge should be used in preference to liquid embolisation materials (White and Lundell 1984), as the particles impact in moderate sized arteries and do not pass into the very small arteries which supply the spinal cord.

In patients with bilateral lung disease bronchoscopy should be carried out prior to embolisation to identify the site of bleeding. Selective catheterisation of the bronchial arteries can be difficult, as the arteries are small and the anatomy is variable.

Embolisation of a pulmonary artery has been carried out to treat haemoptysis arising from a Rasmussen aneurysm (Remy et al. 1980).

Pelvis

Severe internal haemorrhage due to pelvic trauma can be controlled by arterial embolisation and one report (Matalon et al. 1979) claimed success in 70%–80% of patients. Arteriography demonstrates a bleeding point in most cases, the commonest site being the anterior division of the internal iliac artery, but bleeding from the 5th lumbar, deep iliac, circumflex and obturator arteries has also been described (Lang 1981; Sclafani and Becker 1982).

Spleen

Splenic artery embolisation is an alternative to splenectomy in selected patients with hypersplenism. The procedure has been controversial because of the risk of splenic abscess, but sequential partial splenic embolisation has reduced the risk of this complication to a very low level (Spigas et al. 1979). The risk of abscess formation is undoubtedly high if the splenic artery is occluded completely, but partial embolisation (70%–80%) has a much lower risk of abscess formation which can be reduced still further by antibiotic cover. The embolisation procedure should be repeated some weeks later and may have to be repeated on a third occasion before the splenic arterial tree is completely and permanently occluded.

There is no doubt that this procedure reduces the size of the spleen and results in an increase in the platelet count (Yoshioka et al. 1985). Short-acting materials, such as gel foam, seem to be effective, but it is more logical to use permanent materials, such as fragments of polyvinyl alcohol sponge or steel coils. Splenic embolisation can result in gas collections appearing within the spleen due to gas coming out of solution and this radiological abnormality does not necessarily indicate abscess formation. Gas has also been reported in the peritoneal cavity following splenic embolisation (Allison et al. 1981).

Therapeutic embolisation is particularly valuable in patients where surgery is contra-indicated due to a low platelet count and in patients where a grossly enlarged spleen would make the operation hazardous (Fig. 14.5). Splenic artery embolisation has also been used successfully to control haemorrhage from an injured spleen (Sclafani 1981).

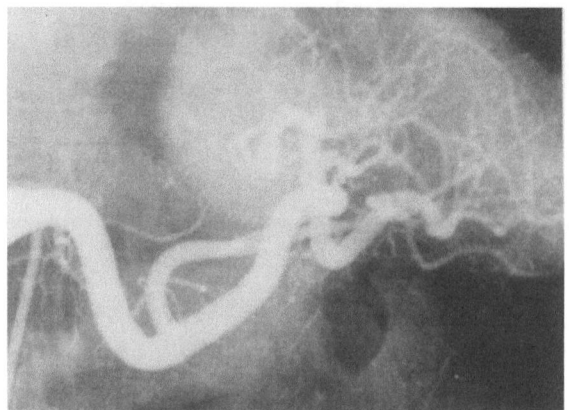

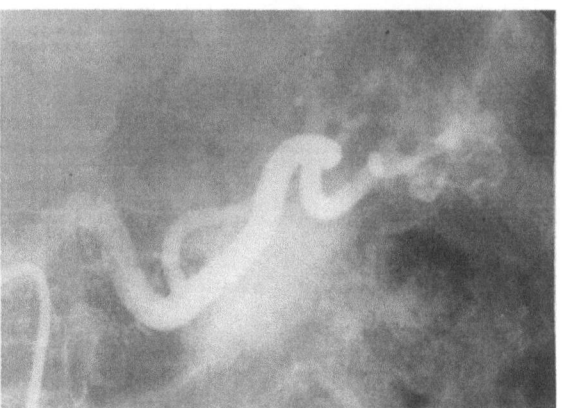

Fig. 14.5a,b. Before (**a**) and after (**b**) embolisation of the spleen in a 74-year-old man with idiopathic thrombocytopenic purpura and uncontrollable intestinal haemorrhage. There is no splenic "blush" on the post-embolisation arteriogram and most of the small arteries within the spleen are occluded. The platelet count rose from 30 000 to 120 000 after the procedure and bleeding stopped within 24 h.

Percutaneous Catheter Retrieval

Fragments of intravenous catheter and guide wire can be removed from the pulmonary artery, heart and large veins using percutaneous transluminal techniques. Loop catheters with a loop of wire passed through a 12FG catheter have been used in most reported cases. The earlier reports described a cut-down procedure on the jugular or femoral veins, but it is now more usual to use the Seldinger technique (Dotter et al. 1971). Loop catheters have the disadvantage that one end of the detached fragment has to be ensnared by the wire loop and this is impossible if both ends of the fragment are embedded in the endothelium, as is likely if it has been in situ for some weeks. Modified Dormia baskets have also been used but have the same limitation as loop catheters as it is necessary to engage a free end of the fragment within the basket (Dotter et al. 1971).

A more modern technique is to use a steerable catheter (Meditech) in which the tip of the catheter is wound tightly round the fragment and pulled back against the outer sheath. The sheath, catheter and fragment are then withdrawn. The earlier retrievals were carried out through a femoral cutdown (Davies et al. 1981; Mehta et al. 1983), but later retrievals have been carried out using the Seldinger technique.

One practical problem is that catheter fragments are often difficult to visualise fluoroscopically as their radio-opacity is similar to that of soft tissues and it has been suggested that catheters intended for long-term use should be more radio-opaque (Mehta et al. 1983).

Detached fragments in the heart and pulmonary artery are a serious threat to life and one survey reported that 17 out of 28 patients with a catheter fragment in the pulmonary artery died from related complications, such as sepsis, perforation, thrombosis and cardiac arrhythmias (Bernhardt et al. 1970). Catheter removal should be attempted early rather than late, as the fragment tends to migrate and removal is much more difficult once it has passed beyond the pulmonary valve into the pulmonary artery.

Although time-consuming and technically difficult, the procedure can be carried out under local anaesthesia and is an alternative to major surgery which is a substantial advantage when managing the complication in an intensive care unit.

Angioplasty

Transluminal angioplasty is of proven value in the treatment of atheromatous narrowing or occlusion of the iliac, femoral and popliteal arteries (Zeitler et al. 1983; Cumberland 1983) and in atheromatous narrowing of the coronary arteries (Cumberland 1983; Gruntzig 1981). The immediate patency rates and the patency rates 2 and 5 years later are roughly similar to the results of surgery, but no controlled trials have been carried out.

The technique is also valuable in treating renal artery stenosis, particularly if it is due to fibromuscular hyperplasia (Tegtmeyer et al. 1984) and has been successfully used to dilate arterial narrowing in transplanted kidneys. Successful dilatation of atheromatous lesions in other sites, including the aorta and its larger branches such as the axillary, subclavian, coeliac and mesenteric arteries, has been reported. Angioplasty has also been used to treat arterial narrowing caused by therapeutic radiation.

Angioplasty catheters have the same outside diameter as normal arterial catheters when the balloon is deflated and can be passed into the arterial tree by the Seldinger technique. The catheter is passed over a guide wire and through the narrowed or occluded segment. The balloon is then inflated with dilute contrast medium, under radiological control for several periods of 15–30 s and, when the artery has been successfully dilated, the catheter is withdrawn. The procedure is carried out under local anaesthesia and is particularly attractive for treating patients in whom general anaesthesia would pose a risk. (Fig. 14.6).

Drainage Procedures

Renal Drainage

Percutaneous nephrostomy of an obstructed kidney is an alternative to surgical nephrostomy and is carried out under local anaesthesia. The technique was extensively reviewed in 1984 (Barbaric 1984). The renal pelvis is punctured from the loin, a guide wire is passed through the needle into the pelvis and a self-retaining catheter is passed over the guide wire. The procedure may be carried out with fluoroscopic control, but ultrasound is usually preferred.

Antegrade insertion of a double pigtail ureteric catheter is a more recent development and can replace retrograde insertion. The procedure is carried out under local anaesthesia and a guide wire is passed as for percutaneous nephrostomy. This is followed by a catheter which is manipulated within the renal pelvis so that the guide wire and catheter pass down the ureter, through the obstruction and into the bladder. The catheter is then removed and a double pigtail catheter of the appropriate length is passed over the guide wire and pushed as far as the bladder, when the guide wire is removed. The procedure can be difficult and the success rate is between 50% and 80% (Mitty et al. 1983).

Biliary Drainage

Obstruction of the biliary tract may be temporarily relieved by percutaneous insertion of a drainage catheter above the obstruction (external drainage) or by passing an endoprosthesis through the obstruction (internal drainage).

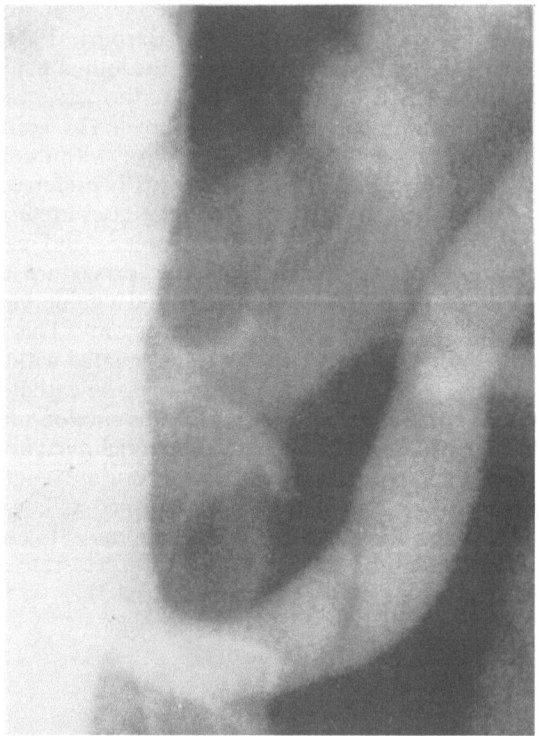

a

b

Fig. 14.6a,b. Before (**a**) and after (**b**) transluminal angioplasty of the left renal artery in a middle-aged man with severe hypertension and long-standing ischaemic heart disease. The blood pressure fell to normal after the procedure.

The techniques have been well described and illustrated (Dooley et al. 1981). Following a transhepatic cholangiogram, a modified Seldinger technique is used to pass a guide wire, dilator and catheter into the dilated biliary tract. Although preoperative external biliary drainage produces considerable biochemical improvement, it can result in cholangitis and there is no evidence that it prolongs survival (Dooley et al. 1986).

For internal drainage it is necessary to pass the guide wire and catheter through the obstruction, which often requires general anaesthesia, as the tract through the skin and liver has to be dilated to 12G before inserting the prosthesis. A prosthesis should remain patent for several months, even in the presence of malignant disease, and this will usually relieve the patient's symptoms for the last few months of life (Fig. 14.7). There have been some long-term successes using an endoprosthesis to relieve benign strictures.

Digital Subtraction Angiography

Digital subtraction angiography (DSA) allows the arterial tree to be demonstrated by intravenous injection of contrast medium and avoids the risk of arterial damage caused by arterial puncture and catheterisation. The investigation is readily carried out on outpatients and often avoids hospital admission, but this is of no relevance when managing patients in intensive care. However, the ability to visualise arteries with an intravenous injection is valuable in patients where access to the arterial tree is difficult owing to widespread arterial disease, and in patients with clotting defects where arterial catheterisation would carry a risk of severe haemorrhage.

The technique is widely used to demonstrate the carotid arteries in patients with cerebrovascular disease as it avoids the risks of catheterising the aortic arch and carotid arteries (Earnest et al. 1984). In severely ill patients the procedure is often used to outline aortic aneurysms and to show the origins of the iliac and other arteries (Fig. 14.8).

Intravenous DSA suffers from the disadvantage that it opacifies the aorta and its main branches at the same time and the technique does not replace selective arteriography. Another limitation is that investigations may require multiple injections of contrast medium (30–40 ml) which can be hazardous in patients with border-line renal failure as large doses of contrast medium can reduce renal function. The technique requires 30–40 ml of con-

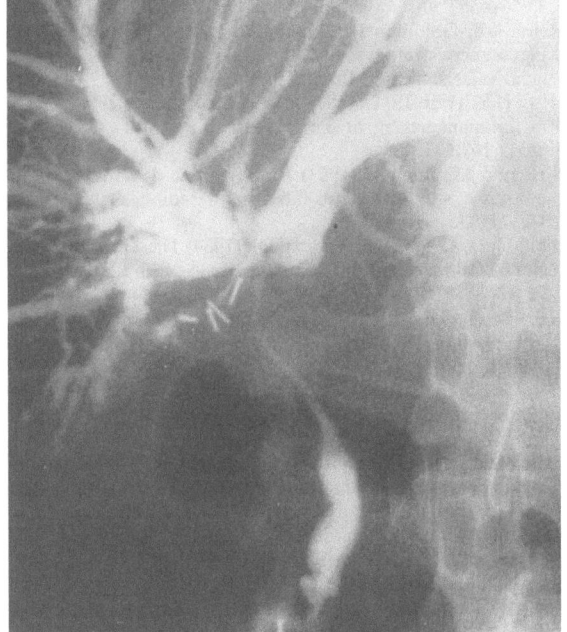

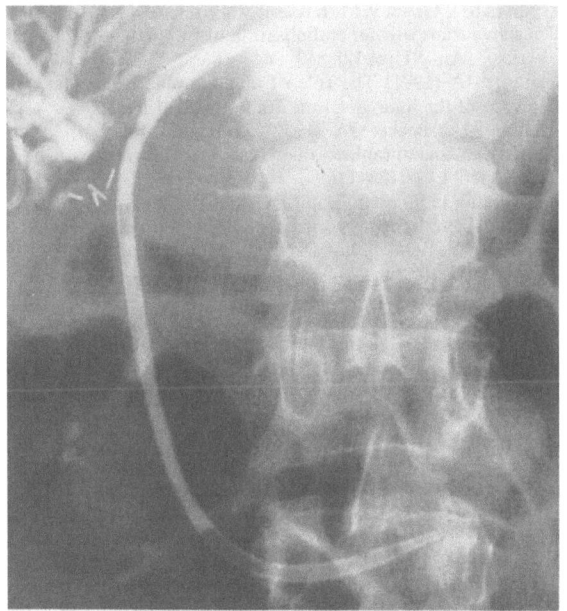

Fig. 14.7a,b. Before (**a**) and after (**b**) percutaneous insertion of an endoprosthesis from the left hepatic duct into the duodenum to relieve obstruction due to cholangiocarcinoma. The symptoms were relieved for several months, although the right hepatic duct remained obstructed.

trast medium to be injected over a period of 2–3 s and contrast extravasation is always a risk. To reduce this, a FG5 catheter is usually passed into the superior vena cava, inferior vena cava or right atrium from an anticubital vein. This can be time consuming and has resulted in cardiac arrhythmias,

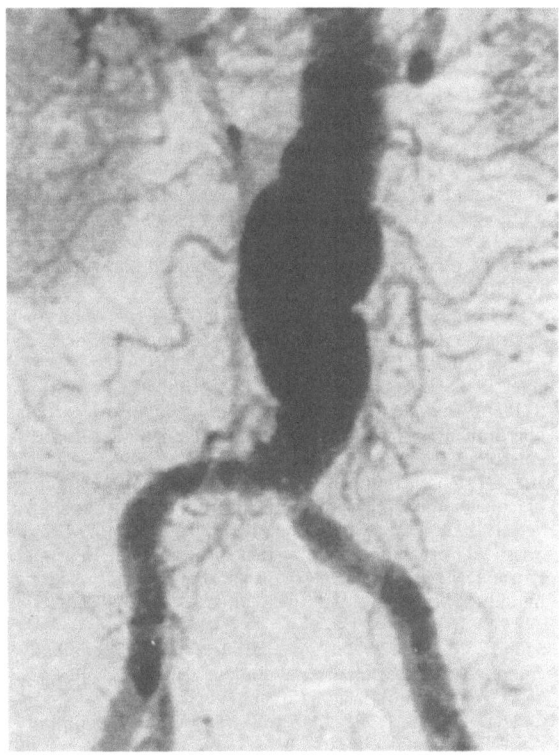

Fig. 14.8. Intravenous DSA demonstrating an aneurysm of the lower abdominal aorta.

thrombophlebitis, hypertension and pulmonary oedema (Pinto et al. 1984).

Intra-arterial DSA allows arteriograms to be carried out with dilute contrast medium (25%–30% normal) which is an advantage in patients who require complicated arteriograms, particularly if hypertensive or azotemic (Illescas et al. 1984). The resolution of the resultant image is slightly poorer than the resolution of an arteriogram recorded on conventional radiographic film, but this rarely affects the diagnostic value of the examination.

References

Allison DJ (1980) Gastro-intestinal bleeding: radiological diagnosis. Br J Hosp Med 23:358–365

Allison DJ, Fletcher DR, Gordon Smith EC (1981) Therapeutic arterial embolisation of the spleen: a new cause of free intraperitoneal gas. Clin Radiol 32:617–621

Athanasoulis CA, Baum S (1975) Mesenteric arterial infusion of vasopressin for haemorrhage from colonic diverticulum. Am J Surg 129:212–216

Barabric ZL (1984) Percutaneous nephrostomy for urinary tract obstruction. Am J Roentgenol 143:803–809

Bernhardt LC, Wegner GP, Mendenhall JT (1970) Intravenous catheter embolisation to pulmonary artery. Chest 57:329–332

Braf ZF, Koontz WW (1977) Gangrene of bladder: complication of hypogastric artery embolisation. Urology 9:670–671

Carmignani G, Belgrano E, Puppo P, Chicher A, Giuliani L (1980) Transcatheter embolisation of the hypogastric arteries in cases of bladder haemorrhage from advanced pelvic cancers: follow-up in 9 cases. J Urol 124:196–200

Chuang VP, Reuter SR, Walter J, Foley WD, Bookstein JJ (1975) Control of renal haemorrhage by selective arterial embolisation. Am J Roentgenol 125:300–306

Cumberland DC (1983) Percutaneous transluminal angioplasty: a review. Clin Radiol 34:25–38

Davies J, Alvares R, Allison JD (1981) An intracardiac foreign body: diagnosed non-invasively and removed non-surgically. Br J Radiol 54:987–989

Dooley JS, Dick R, Irving D, Sherlock S (1981) Relief of bileduct obstruction by the percutaneous transhepatic insertion of an endoprosthesis. Clin Radiol 32:163–172

Dooley JS, Dick R, George P, Kirk RM, Hobbs KEF, Sherlock S (1986) An evaluation of the results of percutaneous external bile drainage in patients with obstructive jaundice. Gastroenterology (In press 1986).

Dotter CT, Rosch J, Bilbao MK (1971) Transluminal extraction of catheter and guide wire fragments from the heart and great vessels: 29 collected cases. Am J Roentgenol 111:467–472

Earnest F, Forbes G, Sandok BA, Piepgras DG, Faust RJ, Ilstrup DM, Arndt LJ (1984) Complications of cerebral arteriography: prospective assessment of risk. Am J Roentgenol 142:247–253

Ekelund L, Mansson W, Olsson AM, Stigsson L (1979) Palliative embolisation of arterial renal tumour supply: results in 10 cases. Acta Radiol [Diagn] (Stockh) 20:323–336

Grüntzig AR (1981) Percutaneous transluminal angioplasty. Am J Roentgenol 136:216–217

Hare WSC, Holland CJ (1983) Paresis following internal iliac artery embolisation. Radiology 146:47–51

Harley JD, Shen FH, Carter SJ (1980) Transcatheter infarction of a polycystic kidney for control of recurrent haemorrhage. Am J Roentgenol 134:818–820

Helliwell M, Irving JD (1981) Haemorrhage from gastric artery aneurysms. Br Med J 282:460–461

Hietala S (1978) Urinary bladder necrosis following selective embolisation of the internal iliac artery. Acta Radiol [Diagn] (Stockh) 19:316–320

Illescas FF, Ford K, Braun SD, Dunnick NR (1984) Intra-arterial digital subtraction angiography in hypertensive azotemic patients. Am J Roentgenol 143:1065–1067

Irving JD, Northfield TC (1976) Emergency arteriography in acute gastro-intestinal bleeding. Br Med J i:929–931

Keller FS, Rosch J, Dotter CT (1983) Transhepatic obliteration of gastro-intestinal varices with absolute alcohol. Radiology 146:615–619

Kobayashi T, Kusano S, Matusbayashi T, Uchida T (1980) Selective embolisation of the vesical artery in the management of massive bladder haemorrhage. J Urol 121:30–36

Lang EK (1981) Transcatheter embolisation of pelvic vessels for control of intractable haemorrhage. Radiology 140:331–339

Lang EK, Deutch JS, Goodman JR, Barnett TF, Lanassa JA, Dupleiss GH (1979) Transcatheter embolisation of hypogastric branch arteries in the management of intractable bladder haemorrhage. J Urol 121:30–36

Macerlean DP, Owens AP, Bryan PJ (1980) Hypernephroma embolisation – is it worthwhile? Clin Radiol 31:297–300

Matalon TSA, Athanasoulis CA, Margolies MN, Waltman AC, Novelline RD, Greenfield AJ, Miller SE (1979) Haemorrhage with pelvic fractures: efficacy of transcatheter embolisation. Am J Roentgenol 133:859–864

McIvor J, Williams G, Southcott RCC (1982) Control of severe vesical haemorrhage by therapeutic embolisation. Clin Radiol 33:561–567

Mehta AB, Goldman JM, Hemingway AP, Allison DJ (1983) Percutaneous retrieval of catheter fragments from heart and great vessels: 5 cases. Br Med J 286:937

Mitty HA, Train JS, Dan SJ (1983) Antegrade ureteral stenting in the management of fistulas, strictures and calculi. Radiology 149:433–438

Nusbaum M, Baum S (1963) Radiographic demonstration of unknown sites of gastro-intestinal bleeding. Surg Forum 14:374–375

O'halpin D, Legge D, Macerlean DP (1984) Therapeutic arterial embolisation: report of 5 years experience. Clin Radiol 35:85–93

Pais SO, Glickman MG, Schwartz PE (1980) Embolisation of pelvic arteries for control of postpartum haemorrhage. Radiology 136:817

Pinto RS, Manuell M, Kricheff II (1984) Complications of digital intravenous angiography: experience in 2488 cervicocranial examinations. Am J Roentgenol 143:1295–1299

Rahn NH, Tishler JM, Han SY, Russinovich NAE (1982) Diagnostic and interventional angiography in acute gastro-intestinal haemorrhage. Radiology 143:361–366

Remy J, Arnauld A, Fardon H, Girard R, Voisin C (1977) Treatment of haemoptysis by embolisation of bronchial arteries. Radiology 122:33–38

Remy J, Smith M, Lamaitre L, Marache P, Fournier E (1980) Treatment of massive haemoptysis by occlusion of a Rasmussen aneurysm. Am J Roentgenol 135:605–606

Richman SD, Green WM, Krole R, Casarella WJ (1977) Superselective transcatheter embolisation of traumatic renal haemorrhage. Am J Urol 128:843–844

Sclafani SJA (1981) The role of angiographic haemostasis in salvage of the injured spleen. Radiology 141:645–650

Sclafani SJA, Becker JA (1982) Traumatic presacral haemorrhage: angiographic diagnosis and therapy. Am J Roentgenol 138:123–126

Smith-Laing G, Scott J, Long RG, Dick R, Sherlock S (1981) Role of Percutaneous transhepatic obliteration of varices in the management of haemorrhage from gastro-oesophageal varices. Gastroenterology 80:1031–1036

Spigos DG, Jonasson O, Mozes M, Capek V (1979) Partial splenic embolisation in the treatment of hypertension. Am J Roentgenol 132:777–782

Tegtmeyer CJ, Keelum CD, Ayers MD (1984) Percutaneous transluminal angioplasty of the renal artery. Radiology 153:77–84

Thompson JN, Hemingway AP, MacPherson GAD, Rees HC, Allison DJ, Spencer J (1984) Obscure gastro-intestinal haemorrhage of small bowel origin. Br Med J 288:1663–1665

Uflacker R (1983) Percutaneous transhepatic obliteration of gastro-oesophageal varices using absolute alcohol. Radiology 146:621–625

Vujic I, Pyle R, Hungerford GD, Griffin CN (1982) Angiography and therapeutic blockade in the control of haemoptysis; the importance of non-bronchial systemic arteries. Radiology 143:19–23

Wallace S, Schwarten DE, Smith DC, Gerson LP, Davis LJ (1978) Intrarenal arteriovenous fistulas: transcatheter steel coil occlusion. J Urol 120:282–286

White RI, Lundell C (1984) Prevention of complications during embolotherapy of the lung. Ann Radiol 27:310–315

Yoshioka H, Kuroda C, Hori S, Tokunaga K, Tanaka T et al. (1985) Splenic embolisation for hypersplenism using steel coils. Am J Roentgenol 144:1269–1274

Zeitler E, Richter EI, Roth FJ, Scloop W (1983) Results of percutaneous transluminal angioplasty. Radiology 146:57–60

Chapter 15

Radiolabelled Blood Cells in the Investigation of the Critically Ill

C. N. McCollum

The patient in the intensive therapy unit (ITU) is rarely able to give a history and is usually on a ventilator and therefore sufficiently suppressed by medication that clinical signs depending on the recognition of pain, tenderness or peritonitis cannot be elicited. It is for these reasons that the diagnosis of the many complications that may occur in such patients depends heavily on the various imaging techniques described in this book. There can be no doubt that immense progress has been made over the last decade in the quality of anatomical images that can be obtained using grey-scaled ultrasound, computed tomography (CT) scanning, digital subtraction angiography and magnetic resonance imaging. Abnormalities can usually be clearly seen and as they can be precisely located the clinician has greater confidence in directing aspiration or advising surgery in a severely ill and debilitated patient. Nevertheless, these anatomical images fail to distinguish the nature of various fluid collections where it would be important to know whether the lesion contained haematoma or pus. In these cases a functional investigation, which recognises the involvement of various blood cell types in the pathology, may prove critical in recognising occult sepsis or the source of emboli. Although radiolabelled leucocytes are by far the most useful of these techniques for ITU patients we will also briefly describe the value of radiolabelled platelets in various specific applications.

Blood cell kinetics were initially studied only by platelet or leucocyte survival using cells labelled with ^{51}Cr which was limited to the recognition of abnormal consumption of these cells. More recently labelling techniques have evolved so that the isotope indium-111 can be used as a stable label for both platelets and leucocytes (Thakur et al. 1976a,b). This isotope has many advantages which include a half-life of 2.81 days (permitting the study of in vivo changes over a period of one week) and high energy gamma emissions which produce good quality images on gamma camera. As a result of the latter characteristic blood-cell kinetics may be extended to localise precisely any area in the body where platelets or leucocytes are accumulating. Indium-111-labelled blood cells have gained wide applications in surgical research and their role in the field of clinical diagnosis has now become apparent. In this chapter we shall briefly consider the value of radiolabelled platelets in the detection of thrombosis and the sources of emboli before examining in more detail the role of radiolabelled leucocytes in assessing inflammatory processes and distinguishing abscess from other collections of fluid.

Radiolabelled Platelets

The use of ^{111}In as a platelet label was first described by Matthew Thakur in 1976 (Thakur et al. 1976a). This technique has now been substantially improved for the labelling of platelets from small volumes of venous blood by incubating the platelets with ^{111}In-oxine in a plasma-free suspension (Hawker et al. 1980). More recently, monoclonal antibodies have been used to achieve in vivo labelling of platelets but this technique must still be considered experimental and should not yet be generally used in clinical practice (Peters et al. 1986). The dose of isotope that may be safely administered is limited by splenic irradiation at 7.4 mGy^{-1}MBq^{-1} (27.4 rad^{-1}mCi^{-1}) which is a splenic dose very similar to that we have observed in our own studies on patients (Van Reenan et al. 1980). This permits the safe administration of approximately 200 μCi for routine diagnostic and research purposes although the clinician may obviously assess the need to administer higher doses in individual patients. Radiolabelled platelets may be used for the detection of either arterial or venous thrombi and as a result their main clinical application is in the detection of deep vein thrombosis and the sources of both arterial and venous emboli. Their reliability in the detection of thrombosis may be emphasised by their research applications where the rate of ^{111}In-platelet deposition on vascular grafts predicts the risk of graft failure (Goldman et al. 1983). Where blood containing radiolabelled platelets flows over the surface of a thrombus sufficient platelets are deposited for clear imaging on gamma camera. The quantification of this process that is possible in research applications has no value in the clinical problems that may be encountered in the ITU patient.

Locating the Source of Emboli

The vascular surgeon is often confronted by a patient with an ischaemic lesion but no evidence of significant occlusive arterial disease. In these cases there is either thrombosis or arteritis affecting the small distal vessels or an embolus has lodged in these vessels arising from the heart or a source within the proximal arterial tree. The assessment of potential sources of emboli in the large arteries has been particularly difficult, especially as arteriography may demonstrate severe anatomical disease throughout the arterial tree thereby giving no help in localising that part of the disease that is giving rise to thrombus formation and subsequent embolisation. Specific applications in the detection of sources of emboli include the diagnosis of aneurysm, carotid disease and deep vein thrombosis. Aneurysms may be imaged as the widened lumen causes turbulence with stagnant blood flow near the arterial wall. As a result thrombus is usually deposited in the lumen and autologous radiolabelled platelets become incorporated in this thrombus. The images obtained may be dramatic but in practice the diagnosis of aneurysm is very much more easily achieved by ultrasound or CT examination (Fig. 15.1).

In the ITU the value of radiolabelled platelets is limited and largely confined to localising the source of multiple pulmonary emboli, either simple or

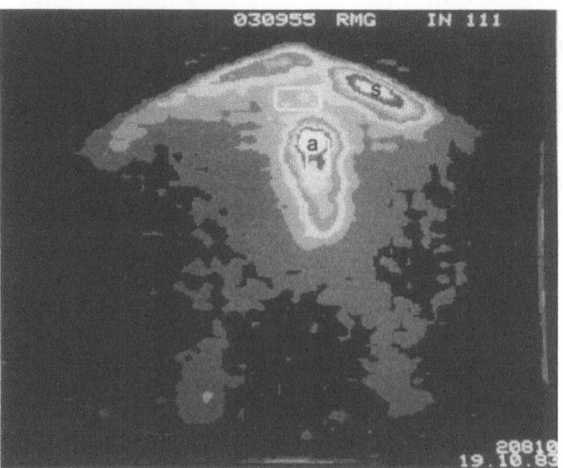

Fig. 15.1. On gamma imaging radiolabelled platelet deposition in an abdominal aortic aneurysm can easily be seen. The radioactivity in the aneurysm (a) approaches that in the spleen (s) and is considerably greater than that in the adjacent aorta just above the aneurysm.

mycotic. It is well recognised that clinical signs are inadequate in the diagnosis of deep vein thrombosis. This is particularly true following pulmonary emboli where there may be little or no sign in the legs. The plethora if diagnostic techniques available include Doppler flow studies, impedance plethysmography, thermography and various isotope methods; none of which are entirely satisfactory. Although ^{125}I-fibrinogen has been widely used as a research method for detecting deep vein thrombosis it has little value in clinical diagnosis as the isotope must be circulating before the thrombus forms, gives poor gamma images and is excreted in the bladder effectively obscuring the pelvic veins. ^{111}In-platelets have been used in sufficient numbers of patients to confirm their precision particularly in the diagnosis of extensive pelvic vein thrombosis (Grimly et al. 1981; Fenech et al. 1981). The sensitivity and specificity reported by Dr Fenech were 95% and 100% respectively (Fenech et al. 1981) but false-negative images may be obtained when patients have already been on heparin for up to three weeks before the injection of autologous ^{111}In-platelets (Grimly et al. 1981). This disadvantage is not a problem in the type of patient seen in ITU where multiple pulmonary emboli are arising from an unknown source. The use of this technique may best be illustrated by a brief case history.

Case History

A 67-year-old man progressively developed pulmonary failure and corpulmonale over a period of three months. Unfortunately, the possibility that this may have been due to multiple small pulmonary emboli was not considered until his pulmonary function had deteriorated sufficiently that ventilation was required. Although he was already anticoagulated, gamma images of the lung following the infusion of autologous ^{111}In-platelets demonstrated a small pulmonary embolus in the right upper lobe (Fig. 15.2a). The source of embolism was found to be a dramatic "hot spot" in the left femoral region (Fig. 15.2b). This was confirmed by venography (Fig. 15.2c) but the patient had deteriorated such that it was no longer thought reasonable to extract the causative thrombus and ligate the deep femoral vein. On post-mortem examination the presence of a thrombus arising from the deep femoral vein and protruding into the superficial femoral vein was confirmed (Fig. 15.2d).

We have also found radiolabelled platelets useful in the detection of the source of mycotic pulmonary emboli leading to multiple pulmonary abscesses of the sort seen in intravenous drug users (Fig. 15.3a). In these patients the pulmonary abscesses are best demonstrated with ^{111}In-leucocytes but there may be little or no pus in the region of the infected thrombophlebitis that leads to this embolism. It is not necessary to do a separate ^{111}In-platelet study as in preparing the leucocyte label it is easy to retain 30% platelets which will easily take up sufficient radioactivity to demonstrate the source of these mycotic emboli (Fig. 15.3b).

Research Applications of ^{111}In-Platelets

Both radiolabelled platelets and leucocytes are taken up in damaged organs. One of the best examples of this is in transplantation where one of the earliest features of the rejection process is damage to the endothelium of the microvasculature. This leads to early and rapid platelet accumulation over a large surface area such that the transplanted organ becomes dramatically radioactive within hours of onset of acute rejection. This technique has already been applied to renal and pancreatic transplant rejection and could potentially be of immense value in cardiac transplantation (Buckels et al. 1983; Jurewicz et al. 1985). In severe shock it is possible that one of the contributory causes to organ dysfunction and particularly to adult respiratory distress syndrome or shock lung may be microembolisation of circulating aggregated blood cells. A close relationship between the development of intravascular platelet aggregates and postoperative pulmonary dysfunction in

patients undergoing major surgery has been demonstrated (McCollum and Campbell 1979). The use of radiolabelled cells to measure platelet or leucocyte accumulation in the vital organs is beyond the scope of this chapter but the relationship between radiolabelled platelet accumulation in the vital organs and subsequent pulmonary and renal failure has recently been described (McCollum and Poskitt 1987).

Radiolabelled Leucocytes

Intraabdominal sepsis remains a feared complication of most abdominal surgery, particularly that involving the biliary tract, colon and pelvic viscera. The mortality is around 30% in such patients (Altemeier et al. 1973; Fry et al. 1980) but is considerably greater in patients on intensive care where the immune system and leucocyte function are usually depressed. Even in survivors the morbidity is extensive with hospital in-patient treatment usually prolonged for more than six weeks and the more difficult to diagnose visceral or retroperitoneal abscesses extending in patient care to a mean of over 10 weeks (Altemeier et al. 1973; Fry et al. 1980). The main cause for both this high mortality and prolonged ill-health is the delay in reaching a firm diagnosis and localising sepsis. This delay is never more obvious than in the ITU where the traditional clinical signs of swinging pyrexia, leucocytosis, malaise and night sweats may be absent or fail to give any indication as to the site of sepsis. Frequently the only indication of intraabdominal sepsis may be a failure to improve on the anticipated clinical course or the unexpected development of pulmonary or renal failure which is a clear indication for urgent investigation. These investigations will clearly include plain X-ray, ultrasound examination and CT. The place of these anatomical investigations is well covered in the appropriate chapters in this book. Nevertheless, it is necessary to review their advantages and disadvantages so that the indications for ^{111}In-leucocyte studies may be placed in perspective.

Ultrasound and CT

Both these techniques have been extensively evaluated in the diagnosis of abdominal abscess and have proved effective in demonstrating the anatomy of selected sections of the body. There is a wide range of reported diagnostic accuracies peaking at over 90% when reported by enthusiastic proponents

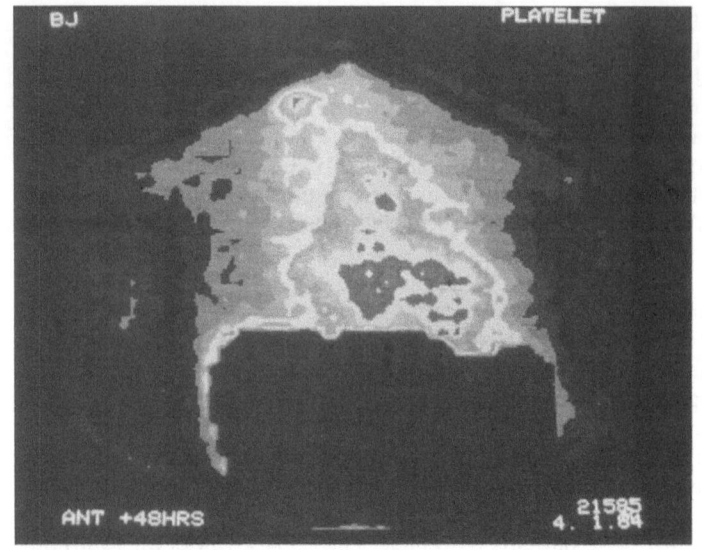

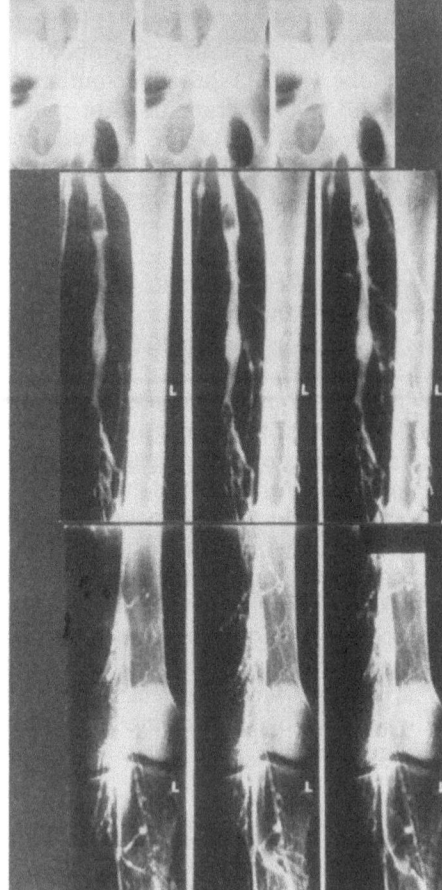

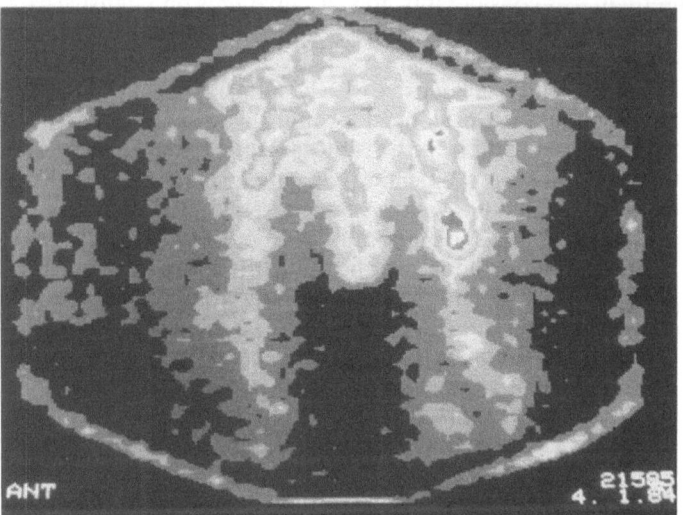

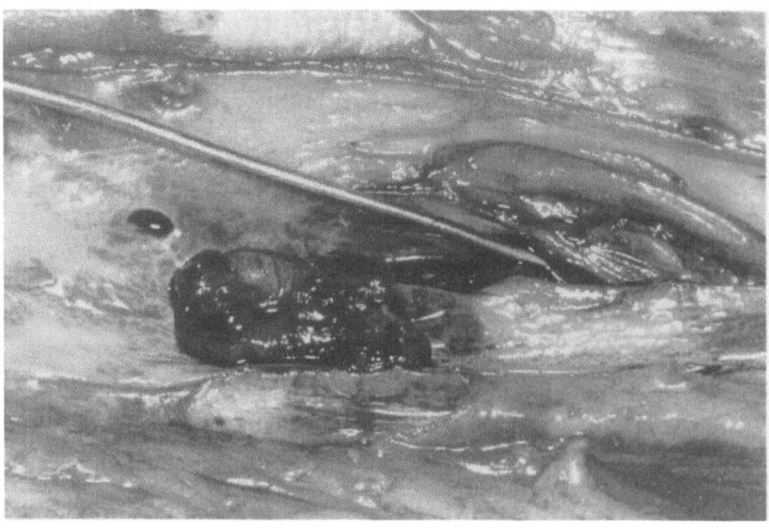

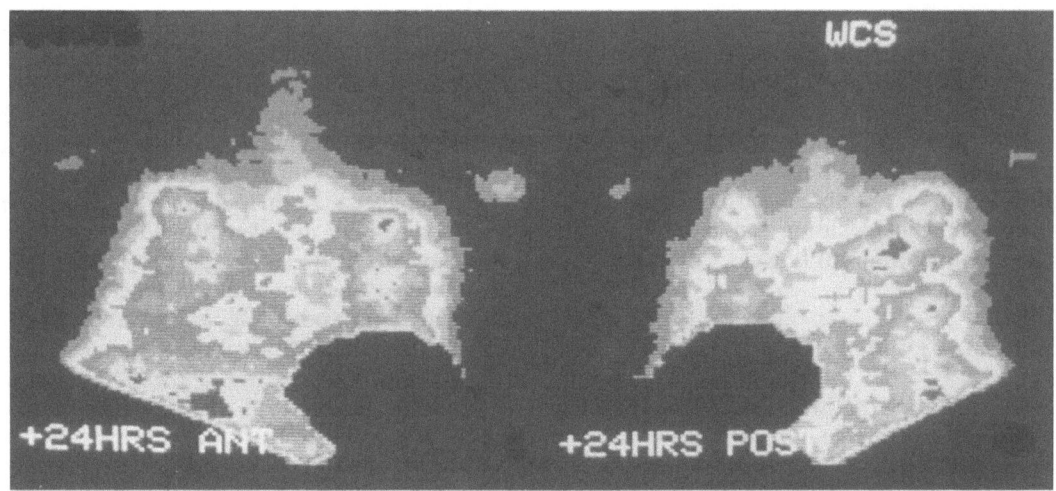

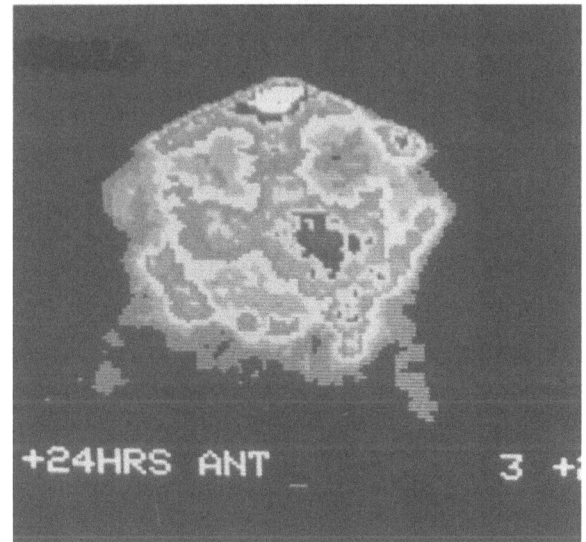

Fig. 15.3a,b. This 19-year-old drug addict had multiple mycotic pulmonary abscesses confirmed on this leucocyte study. **a** The source of these emboli was detected on the gamma image of the pelvic region **b** where marked uptake of radioactive platelets and leucocytes over the left iliac vessels clearly demonstrates the source of emboli. A history of difficult left femoral vein puncture two weeks previously was obtained.

(Koehler and Knochel 1980) but in our own experience and in comparative studies both the sensitivity and specificity is considerably lower in abdominal sepsis (Norton et al. 1978). The image definition is certainly clearer with CT, particularly when the retroperitoneal structures are involved where the transmission of ultrasound is impaired by gas in the gut. Both ultrasound and CT share one serious disadvantage: they cannot be relied upon to distinguish collections of serous fluid or haematoma from a collection of pus forming an abscess (Doust et al. 1977). Although they are more sensitive to the detection of small loculi of air within an abscess than is plain X-ray, an abscess in close proximity to the bowel presents immense difficulties as the gas, pus and abscess wall cannot be distinguished

Fig. 15.2.a On gamma image following injection of autologous ^{111}In-platelets a small pulmonary embolus can be seen in the right upper lobe of this 67-year-old man who was in progressive pulmonary failure. **b** In the same patient, the gamma image of the upper thigh region clearly shows marked platelet uptake localised to an area appropriate to the femoral vein 10cm below the inguinal ligament. **c** On venography in this patient thrombus can be seen within the popliteal and distal superficial femoral vein. There is a prominent filling defect distal to the junction of the common femoral vein and the long saphenous vein which represents the active thrombus on gamma imaging. **d** This man died in respiratory failure and on post mortem the thrombus can be seen arising from the profunda femoris vein and projecting into the superficial femoral vein. A probe has been placed down the profunda femoris vein.

from the normal contents and wall of small or large intestine. It is for these reasons that the functional approach of injecting radiolabelled leucocytes and monitoring first their sequestration in the inflammation around an abscess and then their accumulation within the pus has such immense value in distinguishing an abscess from other fluid collections and in localising sepsis in the abdominal cavity among loops of bowel.

Gallium-67 Citrate

The first isotope that was widely used for the detection of sepsis was gallium-67 citrate. The precise mechanism of accumulation in abscesses remains uncertain but it is thought that it may act as an in-vivo label for leucocytes although its attachment to various plasma proteins may also be important. Where the procedure was carefully undertaken with laxatives to purge the radioactivity from the bowel and gamma images taken between 24 and 72 h, accuracies of approaching 90% have been reported (Hopkins et al. 1975). However, over 15% of this isotope is excreted into the bowel and obscures the abdominal image. In much larger comparative series where more patients with intra-abdominal sepsis were included. [67]Ga achieved only slightly better than 80% sensitivity with an unacceptable rate of false-positive reports at 37% (Caffee et al. 1977). Gallium citrate may still have applications for sepsis outside the abdominal cavity but in practice its use has been superseded by the radiolabelling of leucocytes using [111]Indium.

[111]In-leucocytes

Over the last decade ^{111}In-oxine-labelled leucocytes have been increasingly used in the detection and quantification of inflammatory processes and in research relating to cell kinetics in these pathologies. As a powerful gamma-emitter this isotope is well suited for imaging by gamma camera and counting by standard probes and ratemeters. This "functional" approach to the diagnosis of sepsis has several advantages in that it gives clear information on any site within the body where leucocytes are accumulating.

Most of the mixed leucocyte labelling techniques are based on the method originally described by Thakur et al. in 1976b. Other techniques, such as the use of pure leucocytes or leucocytes labelled in the presence of plasma using ^{111}In-tropolonate give good results but do not appear to improve substantially the overall accuracy. For this reason we use a simple mixed leucocyte label that involves as little centrifugation as possible so that leucocyte damage is minimised. Venous blood (17 ml) is taken into 3 ml of acid citrate solution, mixed gently and allowed to sediment for 50 min at ambient temperature. The supernatant leucocyte- and platelet-rich plasma is then diluted with 20% modified tyrode buffer and centrifuged at 640 g for 10 min (Hawker et al. 1980). The platelet-rich plasma is removed and the residual leucocyte pellet resuspended in tyrode buffer and incubated with 150 μCi of ^{111}In-oxine (Mallinckrodt Diagnostica) for 2 min at room temperature. Plasma is then added to quench the reaction and the labelled mixed leucocytes obtained by repeat centrifugation are resuspended in 5 ml of tyrodes buffer for intravenous administration.

In our experience diagnostic accuracy depends on carefully timing the gamma scans. Rapid radiolabelled leucocyte uptake occurs at any site of inflammation within two or three hours (Fig. 15.4a). This early localisation of radioactivity does not indicate pus and it is only after further images have been taken at 24 h that the presence of pus may be confirmed. During this time, leucocytes mobilise from sites of inflammation but pass into the pus of an abscess where the radioactivity subsequently remains (Fig. 15.4b). This careful timing of gamma camera imaging is particularly important in patients with inflammatory bowel disease where the 4-h scans show radioactivity uptake at sites of active inflammation but the delayed images show both the excretion of radiolabelled cells into the bowel and intense accumulation in any abscesses that may be present (Fig. 15.5).

Even before the value of repeating scans at these time intervals had been appreciated the overall diagnostic accuracy of ^{111}In-leucocytes in patients with suspected abscess was reported to approach 90% (Ascher et al. 1980). I have been involved in two clinical series, the first at the Queen Elizabeth Hospital, Birmingham and the second at Charing Cross Hospital, London. The results of ^{111}In-leucocyte studies were compared with the final diagnosis after adequate follow up. In Birmingham, 100 consecutive patients were studied with the emphasis on suspected intra-abdominal sepsis: most of them were postoperative or had inflammatory bowel disease (Table 15.1). Abscess was confirmed by drainage of pus in 30 patients. In 28 of these, the abscess was reported on ^{111}In-leucocyte scans. The two false-negative reports were both in patients with pyonephroses where liver and spleen subtraction had not been performed and where the activity in these organs may have obscured renal uptake. In the remaining 70 patients the leucocyte

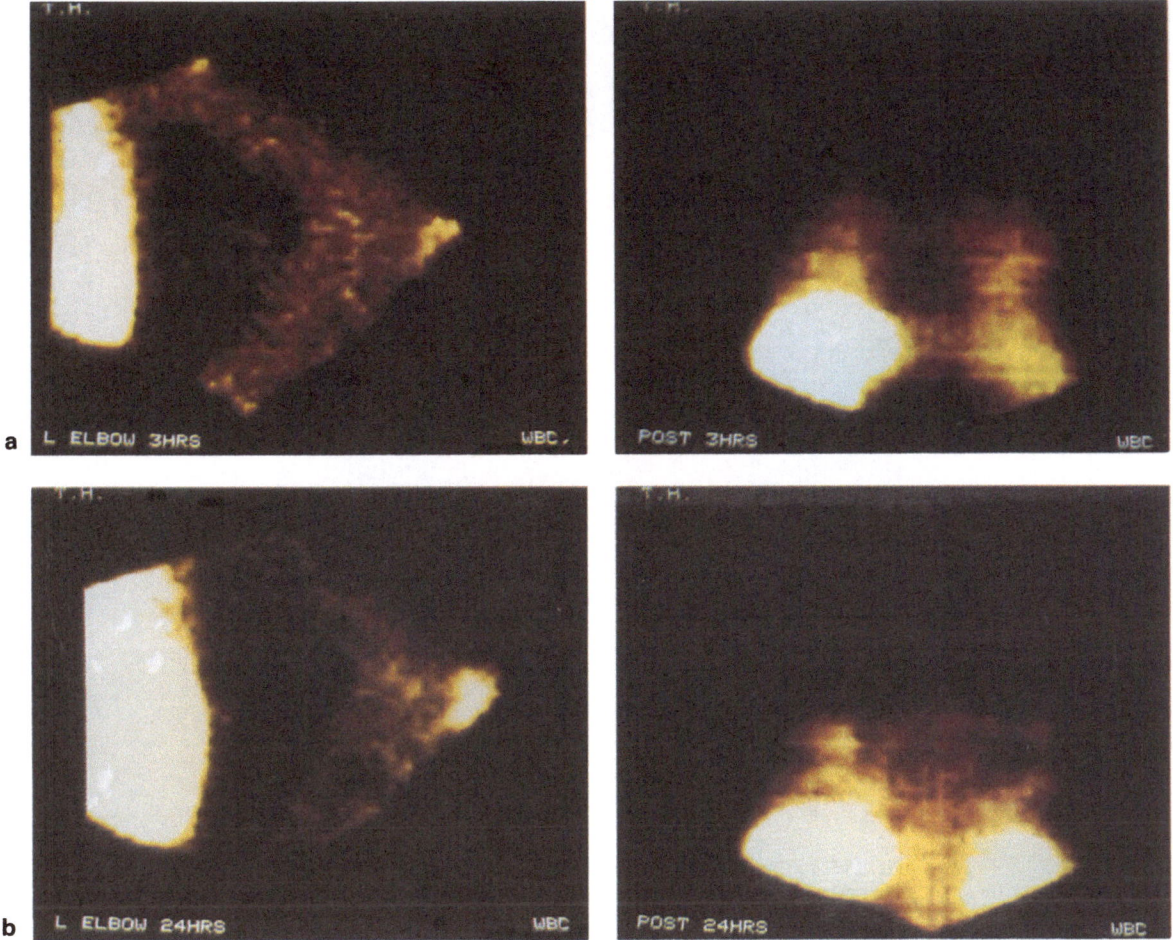

Fig. 15.4a,b. The timing of gamma images is critical to accurate interpretation of ^{111}In-mixed leucocyte studies. In this 18-year-old nurse an insect bite in Africa had led to an abscess at the left elbow, septicaemia, multiple pulmonary abscesses and peritonitis. Gamma images of the elbow at 3 h show uptake around the abscess and blood pool within the arm **a**. By 24 h the activity is concentrated in the pus of the abscess **b**. Posterior scans of the chest demonstrate the diffuse uptake of leucocytes in inflammation at 3 h **a** but by 24 h **b** the leucocytes have cleared from the inflammatory lung and concentrated only in the multiple abscesses which mainly affected the left lower lobe. Abdominal scans were clear and although she had peritonitis, laparotomy was avoided.

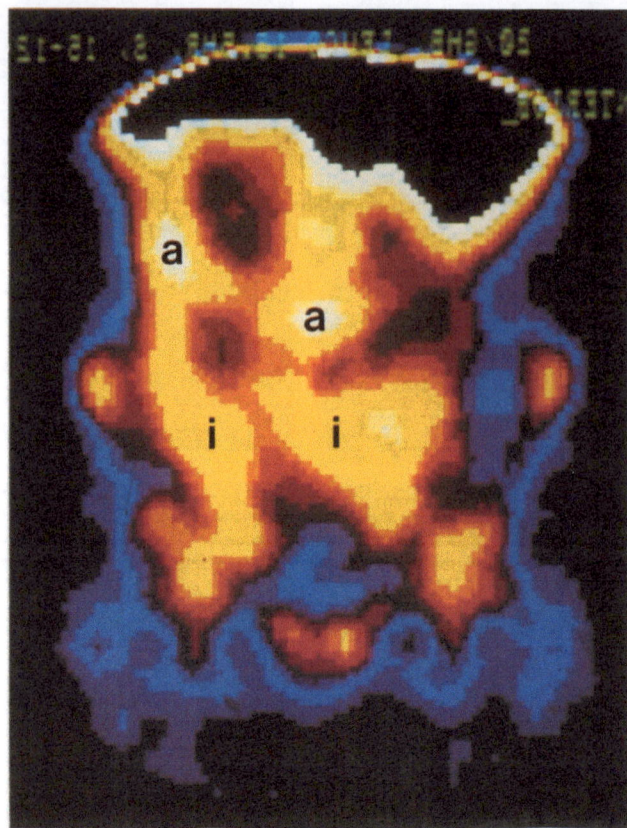

Fig. 15.5. In this patient with severe Crohn's disease the 4 h scans had demonstrated diffuse activity throughout the small bowel but by 24 h as shown in the above gamma scan the abscesses (*a*) can be distinguished from inflammation in surrounding bowel (*i*) as the radioactivity has increased to a level equivalent to that in the liver (rcp).

Table 15.1. One hundred patients investigated for abdominal sepsis (Birmingham series).

	Number	Total Number
Postoperative		34
Colonic surgery	12	
Appendicectomy	6	
Gastric and biliary	7	
Vascular	3	
Urological	3	
Miscellaneous	3	
Inflammatory bowel disease		36
Crohn's disease	33	
Ulcerative colitis	3	
Pyrexia of unknown origin		13
Miscellaneous abdominal and pelvic		17
Total		100

scans were reported as showing no abscess although inflammation was sufficiently intense to produce bowel uptake in 17 of the 36 patients with inflammatory bowel disease (Table 15.2). As has previously been reported in patients with inflammatory bowel disease, the diseased segment was usually imaged at 4 h but on subsequent scans at 24 h the activity had moved into the distal bowel (Segal et al. 1981). As there were no false-positive and only two false-negative reports the specificity was 100% and sensitivity 93% giving an overall diagnostic accuracy in abscess detection of 98% (Goldman et al. 1987).

Table 15.2. The result of leucocyte scans compared to clinical outcome in 100 patients (Birmingham series).

	Clinical outcome		
	Abscess	Inflammation	Normal
Leucocyte scan			
Abscess	28	—	—
Inflammation	—	17	—
Normal	2	26	27
Total	30	43	27

In a similar series of 100 consecutive patients at Charing Cross Hospital, the majority were again postoperative patients in whom intra-abdominal sepsis was suspected. In this series the importance of early and delayed gamma images had been fully appreciated and nearly every patient had images at 4 and 24 h. The results are shown in Table 15.3. Of the three false-negative reports one patient had a diffuse purulent peritonitis and the generalised abdominal uptake seen on the gamma image was not interpreted as pus. This emphasises that the pus must have localised into discrete abscesses before

Table 15.3. The result of leucocyte scans compared to clinical outcome in 100 patients (Charing Cross series).

	Clinical outcome	
	Abscess	Normal or Inflammation
Leucocyte scan		
Abscess	35	1
No abscess	3	61
Total	38	62

the technique can be relied upon. One further false-negative report was in a patient whose abscess had drained in the interval between the injection of radiolabelled leucocytes and the performance of the gamma scan. Of much more importance, we experienced our first false-positive report. This 34-year-old patient had a tender swelling in the left groin and on gamma imaging there was abnormal uptake of ^{111}In-leucocytes in this region (Fig. 15.6). However, no 4-h image had been taken and the less intense but equally abnormal uptake in the right groin was missed when the scan was reported. On exploration this patient was found to have leukaemic lymph nodes and we have on previous occasions found uptake of radioactivity in Hodgkin's disease although the intensity of this radioactivity is usually in the range compatible with inflammation rather than abscess. Usually an abscess is only reported where the radioactivity in the lesion approaches that of the liver and such a report may still be taken as a clear indication for either aspiration or surgical drainage.

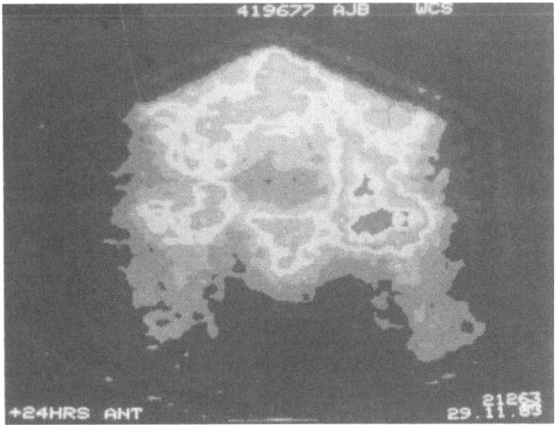

Fig. 15.6. This gamma image is important as it is the only false positive report that we have in over 200 patients. The activity in the left groin was reported as an abscess but was found to be an inflammatory response around leukaemic lymph nodes on exploration. The false-positive report might have been avoided if more importance had been attached to the clearly abnormal uptake also present in the right groin.

Further Observations on the ^{111}In-Leucocyte Technique

In seriously ill patients of the sort most frequently encountered on the ITU uptake of radioactivity in the abscess may be slow, presumably due to impaired immune or leucocyte function. Figure 15.7 depicts gamma images over 2 days in a 63-year-old lady referred from another hospital with suspected abdominal sepsis six weeks following chole-

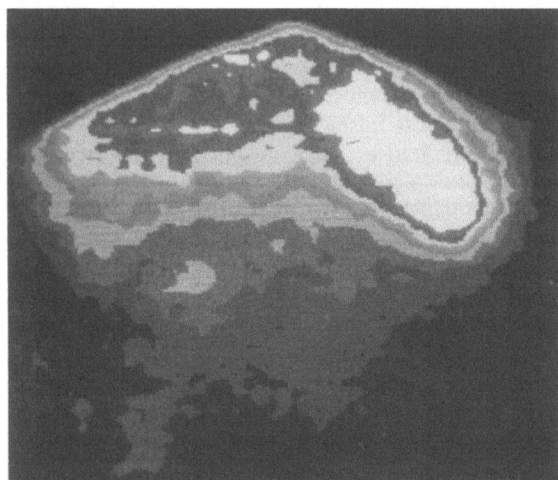

a

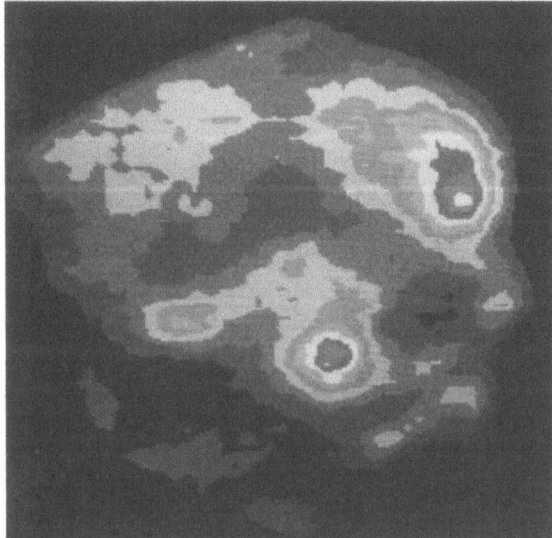

b

Fig. 15.7a,b. This 63-year-old lady deteriorated progressively following cholecystectomy. Despite multiple ultrasound and CT studies, the suspected abdominal sepsis could not be detected. Gamma images at 4 h (**a**) are unremarkable but by 24 h (**b**) an abscess can clearly be seen which was found on exploration to be between loops of small bowel. The danger inherent in delayed diagnosis is emphasised by this case as she died 48 h following exploration and surgical drainage.

cystectomy. She had deteriorated severely, required parenteral therapy and was hypoproteinaemic with gross loss of muscle bulk, ascites and generalised oedema. On the 4-h film there is little abnormal uptake of radioactivity (Fig. 15.7a) but by 24 h abnormal activity in the supraumbilical region was of sufficient intensity to confirm the presence of an abscess. This case serves as a good example of the dangers inherent in the delay in reaching a diagnosis as she did not survive operative drainage at her original hospital even though the abscess only contained 15–20 ml of pus. It is appropriate to comment that she had been intensively investigated during the six-week period before radiolabelled leucocyte studies having undergone ultrasound examination on several occasions and CT examination twice, illustrating the difficulty of detecting small abscesses in among the intestines.

Very delayed images may also be indicated where unusual movement of pus is identified. Gamma scans from a patient with a massive left retroperitoneal haematoma following rupture of an abdominal aortic aneurysm are shown in Fig. 15.8. This was repaired but five weeks later he developed symptoms of colitis and became pyrexial, toxic and unwell. The gamma image at 24 h demonstrates a massive left-sided abdominal abscess which we presumed to be infection in his haematoma (Fig. 15.8a). By 72 h a substantial proportion of this radioactivity had drained into the left colon (Fig. 15.8b). He was explored on the basis that his Dacron graft must also be involved and this was found to be the case. We believe that the mechanism of this sepsis was that the haematoma had ruptured into the colon creating the impression of colitis and causing secondary infection of the haematoma and then the graft. We do not agree with Saverymuttu et al.'s 1985 report, based on the appearance of radioactivity in the small or large bowel, that a substantial number of intra-abdominal abscesses have enteric drainage. Even when their own patients were explored a communication was not always found at surgery between the abscess and the bowel. We prefer to interpret their results as indicating that the inflammation in an abscess may be sufficient to cause adherent surrounding bowel to sequestrate radiolabelled leucocytes into its lumen. Certainly the presence of radiolabelled leucocytes in the lumen of the bowel in a patient with intra-abdominal abscess cannot be accepted as adequate evidence that drainage is occurring otherwise effective treatment will be delayed.

Finally, the development of tomographic gamma cameras allows more precise localisation of abnormal uptake of radioactivity. In Fig. 15.9a we show the AP view at 24 h of the lower abdomen in a

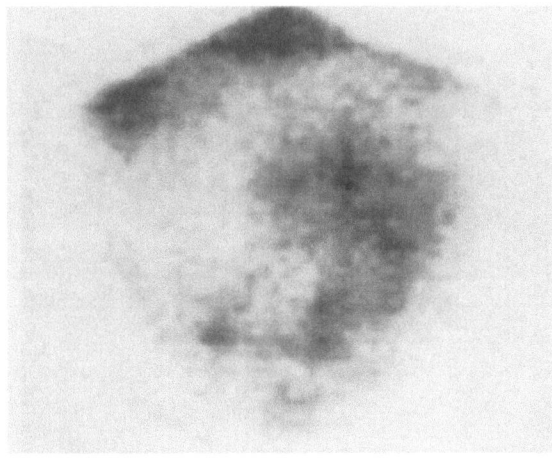

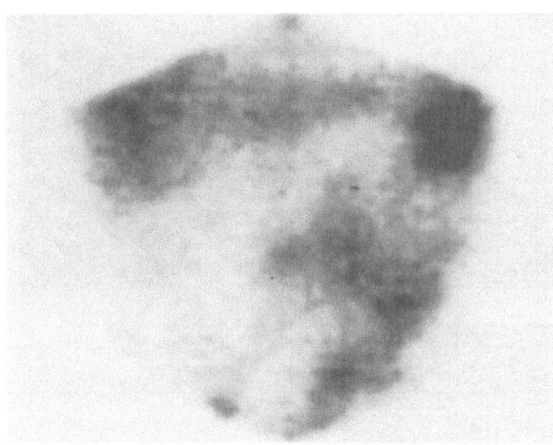

Fig 15.8a,b. This patient's gamma image at 24 h **a** clearly shows an abscess in the left retroperitoneal region which represented infection of a massive haematoma following rupture of an abdominal aortic aneurysm. By 72 h **b** a substantial part of this radioactivity has drained into the left bowel.

36-year-old lady with suspected intra-abdominal sepsis. The uptake in the left iliac fossa suggests a pyosalpinx. As she had previously had a laparoscopy performed by a gynaecologist we performed a further scan at 48 h and gamma camera tomography to be sure that this was not a retroperitoneal abscess (Fig. 15.9b, c). This confirmed the localisation of pus in the peritoneal cavity at the pelvic brim and on surgical exploration pyosalpinx was confirmed and drained.

The Importance of Simultaneous Ultrasound or CT Scanning

Despite their precision, radiolabelled leucocyte techniques should not replace the use of ultrasound and CT scanning. Both are noninvasive and give immediate, reliable information on the presence of abnormal fluid collections. It is essential to use one or other technique simultaneously with ^{111}In-leucocyte studies to detect fluid overlying the liver and spleen, especially as it is in these organs that high background radioactivity may obscure abscess uptake on ^{111}In leucocyte scans. Fortunately, it is in the regions overlying parenchymatous organs that the ultrasound technique is most reliable. Furthermore, both ultrasound and CT may be used to guide aspiration or catheter drainage for either diagnostic purposes or for definitive treatment (Johnson et al. 1981; Mandel et al. 1983). Where percutaneous drainage is planned, ^{111}In-leucocyte scanning provides insufficient definition to guide needle puncture but may usefully exclude other sites of intraabdominal sepsis reducing the need for full laparotomy. We view this as important as we have seen several patients succumb to the primary intraabdominal pathology following aspiration of a secondary or metastatic abscess either in the liver or elsewhere in the abdomen. This primary pathology would almost certainly have been recognised had a ^{111}In-leucocyte scan been performed and where this technique is not available we would still advise full laparotomy unless an intraabdominal cause of metastatic abscess can be excluded from the history or clinical features. CT examination also has the additional advantage that where a lesion is demonstrated it can be clearly seen by the surgeon which greatly increases his confidence in recommending exploration in severely debilitated patients.

Future Developments

Although the rapid development of imaging technology with increasing sophistication of ultrasound, CT and magnetic resonance imaging will continue to improve the definition in establishing anatomy it seems inevitable that we will continue to need techniques such as radiolabelled leucocytes to confirm the presence of pus. More importantly they will be required to exclude sepsis in other sites of the body that have not còme under clinical scrutiny. Despite this, cell labelling techniques are not widely used, being confined to a few centres with the necessary expertise and special facilities. The main limiting factor is the need for cell separation and in-vitro labelling. For this reason our research priority is to develop an isotopic substrate that may be used "off the shelf" and which achieves abscess radioactivity when simply injected intra-

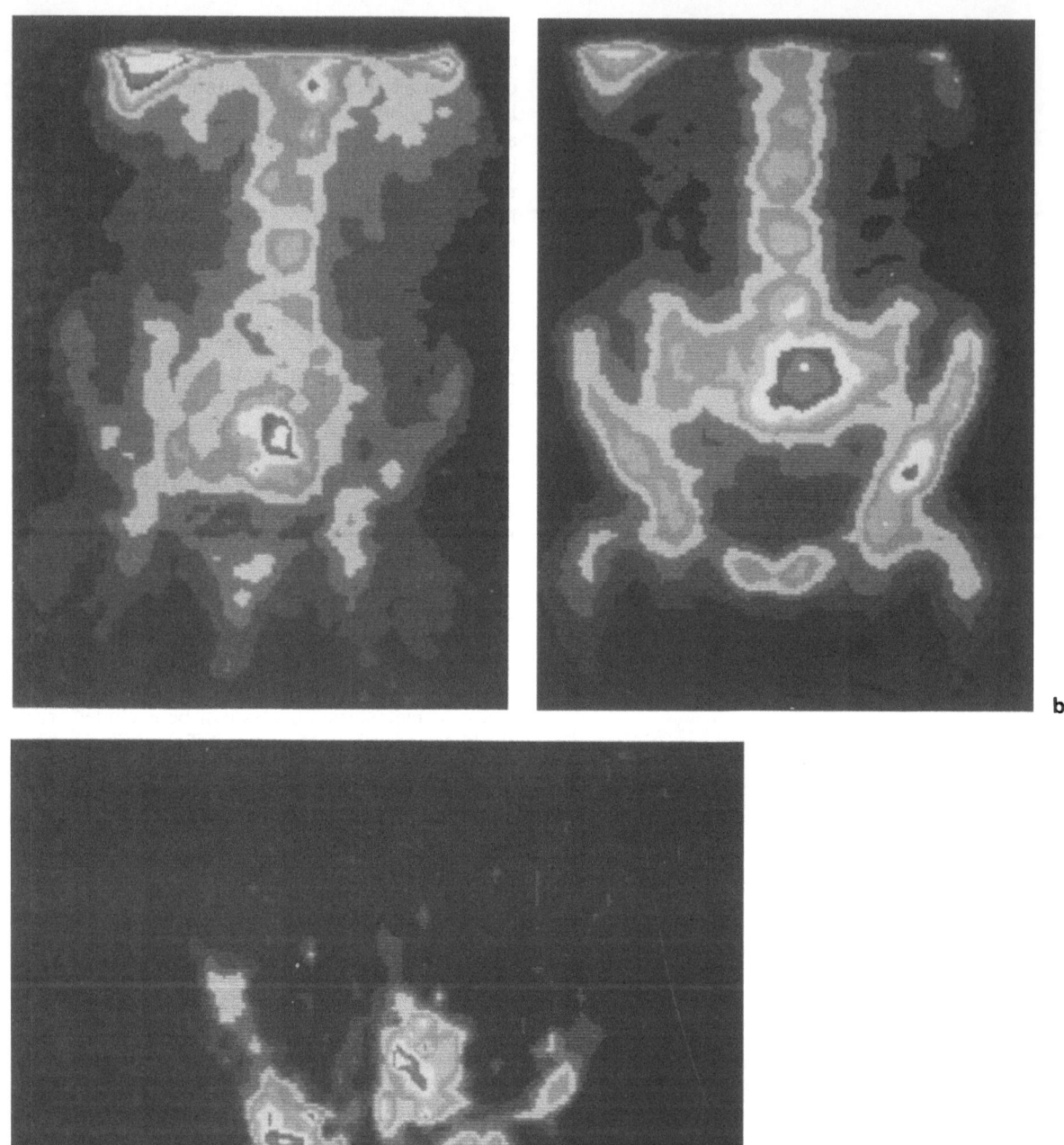

Fig. 15.9a–c. Occasionally, a very chronic low-grade abscess may produce an image that is difficult to interpret at 24 h **a** but which on further delayed imaging by 48 h **b** is clearly an abscess. As this patient has previously undergone laparoscopy by a gynaecologist a tomogram was performed **c** which confirmed the presence of pus within the peritoneal cavity at the pelvic brim. On laparotomy this was indeed a chronic pyosalpinx which was drained with complete recovery of the patient.

venously. One approach to achieving this may be the use of monoclonal antibodies labelled with indium. In the foreseeable future this will be expensive and it may be difficult to deliver sufficient radioactivity to the leucocytes with the technique. In our own studies we have concentrated on the potential of various plasma proteins such as lactoferrin in carrying radioactivity and achieving loose surface labelling of leucocytes in vivo. This technique has been successful in our animal models and we are starting clinical trials in patients. Should such an isotopic substrate be successfully developed then the precision of ^{111}In-leucocyte techniques may be made available for the early investigation of occult sepsis in any hospital possessing a gamma camera. Until then, referral to those centres with the necessary facilities for cell labelling must be rapid, if mortality is to be reduced.

References

Altemeier WA, Culbertson WR, Fullen WD, Shook CD (1973) Intra-abdominal abscesses. Am J Surg 125:70–79

Ascher NL, Forstrom L, Simmons RL (1980) Radiolabelled autologous leucocyte scanning in abscess detection. World J Surg 4:395–402

Buckels JAC, Chandler S, Hawker RJ, Barnes AD, McCollum CN (1983) The early diagnosis of acute renal transplant rejection using [111]Indium labelled platelets. Transplant Proc 15:1192–1194

Caffee HH, Watts G, Mena I (1977) Gallium 67 citrate scanning in the diagnosis of intra-abdominal abscess. Am J Surg 133:665–669

Doust BD, Quiroz F, Stewart JM (1977) Ultrasonic distinction of abscesses from other intra-abdominal fluid collections. Ultrasound 125:213–217

Fenech A, Hussey JK, Smith FW, Dendy PP, Bennett B, Douglas AS (1981) Diagnosis of deep vein thrombosis using autologous indium[−111] labelled platelets. Br Med J 282: 1020–1022

Fry DE, Garrison RN, Heitsch RC, Calhoun K, Polk HC (1980) Determinants of death in patients with intra-abdominal abscess. Surgery 88:517–523

Goldman M, Hall C, Dykes J, Hawker RJ, McCollum CN (1983) Does [111]Indium-platelet deposition predict patency in prosthetic arterial grafts? Br J Surg 70: 635–638

Goldman M, Ambrose NS, Drolc Z, Hawker RJ, McCollum CN (1987) ^{111}In-leucocytes in the diagnosis of abdominal abscess. Br J Surg 74:184–186

Grimly RP, Rafiqi E, Hawker RJ, Drolc Z (1981) Imaging of ^{111}In-labelled platelets – a new method for the diagnosis of deep vein thrombosis. Br J Surg 68:714–716

Hawker RJ, Hawker LM, Wilkinson AR (1980) Indium ([111]-In) labelled human platelets: optimal method. Clin Sci 58:243–248

Hopkins GB, Kan M, Mende CW (1975) Early 67Ga Scintigraphy for the localization of abdominal abscesses. J Nucl Med 16:990–992

Johnson WC, Gerzof SG, Robbins AH, Nabseth DC (1981) Treatment of abdominal abscesses. Ann Surg 194: 510–519

Jurewicz WA, Buckels JAC, Dykes JGA, McCollum CN, McMaster P (1985) [111]Indium platelets in monitoring pancreatic allografts in man. Br J Surg 72:228–231

Koehler PR, Knochel JQ (1980) Computed tomography in the evaluation of abdominal abscesses. AM J Surg 140:675–678

Mandel SR, Boyd D, Jaques PF, Mandell V, Staab EV (1983) Drainage of hepatic, intra-abdominal, and mediastinal abscesses guided by computerized axial tomography. Am J Surg 145:120–125

McCollum CN and Poskitt KR (1987) Intravascular microaggregates and pulmonary microembolisation in shock and surgery. In Bihari D and Kox W (eds) Shock and the Adult Respiratory Distress Syndrome. Springer-Verlag, New York, pp 43–64

McCollum CN, Campbell IT (1979) Value of measuring intravascular platelet aggregates in the prediction of postoperative pulmonary dysfunction. Br J Surg 66:703–707

Norton L, Eule J, Burdick D (1978) Accuracy of techniques to detect intraperitoneal abscess. Surgery 84:370–378

Peters AM, Lavender JP, Needham SG, Loutfi I, Snook D, Epenetos AA, Lumley P, Keery RJ, Hogg N (1986) Imaging thrombus with radiolabelled monoclonal antibody to platelets. Br Med J 293:1525–1527

Saverymuttu SH, Peters AM, Lavender JP (1985) Clinical importance of enteric communication with abdominal abscesses. Br Med J 290:23–26

Segal AW, Ensell J, Munro JM, Sarner M (1981) Indium[111] tagged leucocytes in the diagnosis of inflammatory bowel disease. Lancet ii: 230–232

Thakur ML, Welch MJ, Joist JH, Coleman RE (1976a) Indium[111] labelled platelets: studies on preparation and evaluation of in vitro and in vivo functions. Thromb Res 9:345–357

Thakur ML, Coleman RE, Mayhall G et al. (1976b) Preparation and evaluation of ^{111}In labelled leucocytes as an abscess imaging agent in dogs. Radiology 119: 731–732

Van Reenan OR, Lotter MG, Minnaar PC, Inst F, Heyns A, Path FF, Badenhorst PN, Pieters H. (1980) Radiation dose from human platelets labelled with indium[111]. Br J Rad 53:790–795

Chapter 16

Imaging and Investigating the Microcirculation in Intensive Care Patients

J. R. Weinberg and J. E. Tooke

The aim of intensive care medicine is to maintain a supply of adequately oxygenated, nutrient-containing blood to metabolically active tissue to reduce the occurrence of tissue damage or death. In spite of this being of primary importance we have no direct methods of measuring blood flow at the point where it matters, the nutritional capillaries. The great advances made in monitoring over the past decade mean that the oxygenation of the blood in the arteries can be accurately measured and the cardiac output and total peripheral resistance can be determined. However these measurements of the physiological state of the large vessels and the blood in them may have little relevance to events at capillary level. It may often be the case that treatments which improve the values associated with the central circulation are actually deleterious to the circulation at the capillary level. Increased blood pressure may reflect a rise in peripheral resistance with a reduction in nutritional flow, whilst an increased cardiac output may be the result of the opening of shunt vessels with a fall in afterload but a diversion of flow away from nutritional vessels.

There are no convenient ways of measuring directly nutritional capillary flow. Indirect methods, such as the measurement of skin temperature or transcutaneous oxygen diffusion which are both dependent upon a number of factors other than the state of the circulation, for example the environmental temperature and the state of tissue hydration, are inadequate (Tsuchida 1979, Eickhoff 1980). The measurement of transcutaneous oxygen diffusion involves local heating which may alter the capillary flow that is being measured. Therefore in this chapter we describe two relatively new methods of imaging the skin capillary circulation which are now starting to be used in the assessment of the microcirculation in disease. These are direct capillary microscopy and laser Doppler flowmetry.

Before we describe these techniques a note of caution is necessary. The skin is a specialised organ with a specialised capillary network. It would be wrong to extrapolate too widely from the capillary haemodynamics found in a few areas of the skin. However, the skin is accessible and changes in its microcirculation have profound effects upon the overall circulation. As the skin takes about 9% of the cardiac output at rest (Bard 1961) and skin blood flow can increase a hundred times (Burton 1962), changes in skin blood flow are of major haemodynamic importance. For example, it is suggested that an increase in shunt flow through the skin is responsible for the high output cardiac failure associated with sepsis (Parker and Parillo 1983). Although study of the skin microcirculation will enable us to understand only what is going on in a single microcirculatory bed, even that will contribute greatly to our understanding of the circulatory pathophysiology in critical illness.

The Anatomy of the Skin

Before describing the methods of assessing flow it is important to review the anatomy of the skin circulation. Over most of the body surface papillary capillary loops arise tangentially to the skin surface from a subpapillary arteriolar plexus. Each capillary drains back into the subpapillary venous plexus. In certain areas of the skin, particularly the acral areas, there are direct arteriovenous anastomoses which subserve the skin's thermoregulatory function. These shunts are arranged in parallel with the capillary bed and when heat loss is required can carry up to a hundred times the volume of the flow required for nutrition (Burton 1962; Roddie 1984). One of the problems with indirect measurements of skin blood flow is in differentiating nutritional from shunt flow.

If the skin is rendered relatively translucent by painting its surface with paraffin oil or clear varnish, the apices of the capillary loops can be seen by means of microscopy with indirect illumination and appear as black dots. In the toe and finger-nail fold the capillary loops lie parallel to the skin surface, an arrangement which means that the capillaries of the nail fold are available for noninvasive direct microvascular measurements.

Capillary Microscopy

Capillary microscopy can be either by means of still photography, which gives information on capillary density and morphology (Maricq 1986), or by means of a microscope-television system, which can be used to record dynamic images of the nail-fold circulation on to video tape for further analysis (Bollinger et al. 1974). Oil or clear varnish is applied to the nailfold which is illuminated by a strong oblique light. The light used is that from a mercury vapour lamp with an emission spectrum similar to the absorption spectrum of haemoglobin. In this way the contrast between the red cells and the background is maximised. The image is detected by a low intensity television camera and is stored on video tape. The image can be seen simultaneously on a television monitor (Fig. 16.1). The necessity for adequate contrast between the red cells and the background means that the technique is not suitable for sites where the skin is pigmented. As it is essential that the image is kept as still as possible, the arm is strapped on to a rest and a small metal bracket attached to the microscope is positioned so as to apply gentle pressure to the nail, thereby stabilising it (Ostergren and Fagrell 1986).

The image can be analysed off-line during playback of the video tape. The information available is the capillary blood cell velocity, the frequency of vasomotion and the capillary diameter (in practice the red cell column width, which is a close approximation). A value for capillary volume flow can be derived from the capillary blood cell velocity and red cell column width. The capillary diameter can be measured by using an image shear technique, or by using callipers to measure the image on the monitor. This measurement must be made at the point at which the velocity measurement is made if the intention is to derive flow, as the diameter of the capillary will vary along its length. There are various methods for measuring the capillary velocity. The most laborious is frame-by-frame analysis; however this has the advantage that even pictures of poor quality can be analysed. The flying spot technique consists of an electronically generated flying spot which can be superimposed upon the image of the capillary that is being analysed and the velocity of which can be matched with that of the red cells in the capillary in question (Bass et al. 1987). The method which gives the most information, but which is dependent upon good quality stable images, is that of video-photometric cross-correlation (Intaglietta et al. 1975). The passage of erythrocytes, leucocytes and plasma gaps through the capillary produces variations in the optical density of the image at a particular point along the capillary loop. The video-photometric analyser generates two windows which can be placed over the capillary that is being analysed. The changing pattern of optical density is the same in the upstream and downstream windows (as long as they are not too far apart) and the transit time between the windows is inversely proportional to the capillary blood flow. A cross-correlator can compute the delay between signals with maximal correlation and provide a continuous read-out of capillary velocity. The continuous read-out of capillary blood velocity means that information about the frequency of vasomotion can also be obtained. A mean capillary blood velocity can be derived by studying several capillaries in the nail fold and observing each one for at least 1 min in order to take the natural variation in capillary blood flow during vasomotion into account. It is important to standardise the investigation in either the arteriolar or venous limb of the capillary as the velocity may be 20% higher in the arteriolar limb.

Values for resting mean capillary blood velocity vary considerably both within and between individuals, the normal range being from almost zero to $3\,mm^{-1}s^{-1}$ (Ostergren and Fagrell 1986). There are spontaneous fluctuations in flow at a frequency of 5–8 cycles per minute (vasomotion) and therefore several estimations must be made over at least one minute from as many different capillaries as possible. As the wide variation of flow between individuals makes comparisons difficult, various provocation tests, such as the time to peak velocity following arterial occlusion (Tenlund et al. 1983),

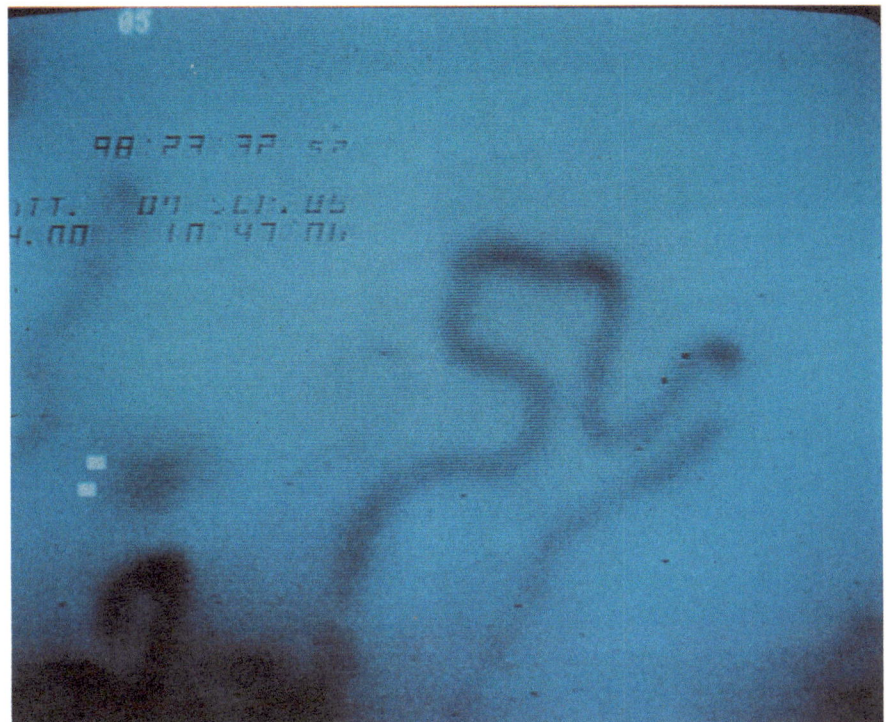

Fig. 16.1. Television capillaroscopy: Capillary loop showing plasma gap (space between columns of red cells). This gap will move with the same velocity as the red cells.

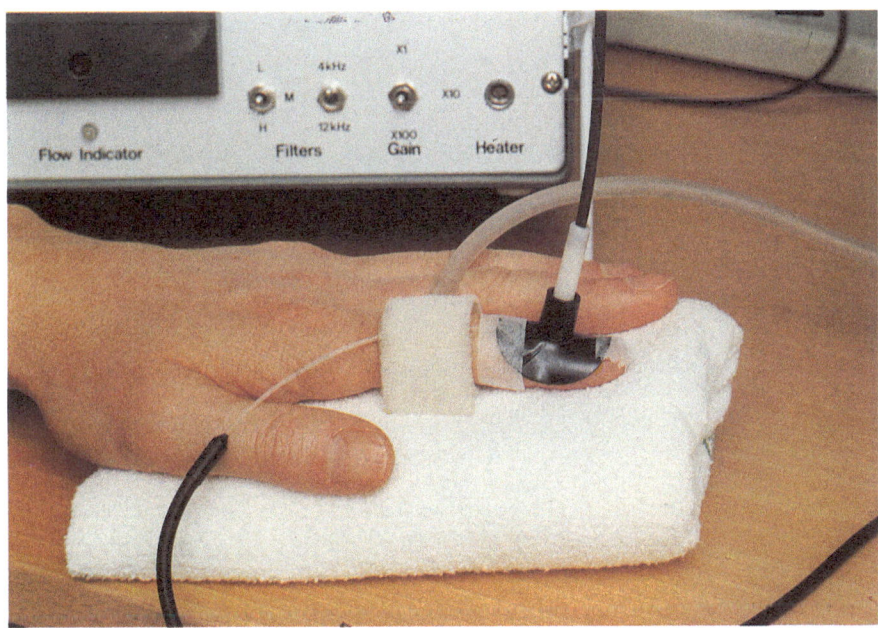

Fig. 16.2. Hand showing laser Doppler probe on index finger. Cuff for occlusion to determine time to maximum flow following occlusion.

have been employed. There is a weak correlation between resting capillary blood velocity and temperature, but the correlation is stronger when the time to reach peak velocity is compared with temperature. The within-individual variation means that the method is best used for comparing states (response to environment, drugs etc), when the control and test states are close together in time rather than separated by several hours.

Capillaroscopy in Clinical Practice

Hypertension (Williams and Tooke 1985). Capillary flow velocity in some patients with border-line hypertension has suggested an altered response to a variety of different agents with maldistribution of blood between shunt and nutritional flow.

Arterial occlusive disease (Ostergren and Fagrell 1985a). Capillary flow velocity in the toe-nail bed suggests that capillary hyperaemia at rest is a feature of atherosclerosis. However, the patients were unable to mount a hyperaemic response following arterial occlusion at the ankle and it has been suggested that this represents a disturbance of microvascular autoregulation.

Diabetes mellitus, Polycythaemia (Fagrell et al. 1984; Ostergren and Fagrell 1985b). Time to peak capillary blood velocity was prolonged in patients even though resting capillary blood velocity was similar to that of normal subjects.

Granulocytic leukaemia (Tooke and Milligan 1983). Resting capillary blood velocity was found to be reduced to very low levels; cytoreduction caused an increase in resting capillary blood velocity.

Raynaud's syndrome (Mahler et al. 1986). A cold-exposure test showed that cold-induced slowing of the erythrocyte velocity was significantly greater in patients with Raynaud's syndrome than in controls. Complete stand-still of the red cell column was seen.

Pharmacological agents. The technique is suited to the study of the acute effects of drugs on skin blood flow. Nifedipine taken sublingually has been shown to increase resting capillary blood velocity by 40% (Ostergren and Fagrell 1984). Insulin infusion in patients with type 1 diabetes has also been shown to increase resting nail-fold capillary blood velocity (Tooke et al. 1985).

Summary

A microscope television system can be used to visualise nail-fold capillaries and the image can be stored and analysed to provide data on capillary blood velocity, capillary blood flow and vasomotion. Although the system requires a skilled operator to acquire an adequate image the methodological difficulties are compensated for by the unambiguous nature of the data derived. This makes the method suitable for use in those situations in the intensive care unit where a better understanding of capillary flow would contribute to patient care.

Laser Doppler Flowmetry

Laser Doppler flowmetry is a simple noninvasive procedure to assess superficial blood flow at the surface of an organ, usually the skin. Coherent light back-scattered from the surface of the skin undergoes a spectral broadening. The laser light encounters moving red blood cells and undergoes a frequency shift which is related to the velocity of the moving particles (Riva et al. 1972; Tenlund 1982). Laser Doppler flow meters are commercially available. They contain a low-power Helium-Neon laser which emits monochromatic light at a frequency which is maximally reflected by the moving red cells. The light is conducted to the skin surface by a flexible fibre-optic light-guide. The light penetrates skin to a depth of about 1.5 mm and is back-scattered by both moving and stationary objects; however only the moving objects, largely red cells, produce a frequency shift. The red cells are moving at different speeds and in different directions and this results in a broad spectrum of Doppler-shifted frequencies. A proportion of this light of many different frequencies is returned to the instrument by efferent fibres in the fibre-optic bundle. Photodetectors within the instrument mix shifted and unshifted light to create beat frequencies which are proportional to the Doppler shifts. These beat frequencies produce a voltage output from the photodetectors. The final voltage output is theoretically proportional to the integrated velocities of all the moving red blood cells in the segment of skin that is being studied (Tenlund 1982).

The method has been validated in models of the microcirculation in which capillary blood flow and haematocrit can be varied and against direct methods of measuring capillary red cell flux (TV capillaroscopy). Broadly similar results have been obtained (Tenlund 1982; Fagrell et al. 1986) and such differences as have been observed have been interpreted as showing that laser Doppler also detects flow in deeper vessels such as arterio-venous anastomoses. Differences in the depth of penetration may also account for the differences in flow measured by other methods such as thermal clearance (Holti and Mitchell 1978). The penetration of the laser light is such that arterio-venous shunt flow influences the output of the flowmeter.

The major advantage of laser Doppler flow measurement is its ease of use (Fig. 16.2). However there are limitations. The probe needs to be fixed carefully to the surface where flow is being measured. Movement both of the probe relative to the skin and of the fibre-optic bundle creating internal reflection produce artefactual signals. The output of the instrument is in arbitrary units of volts and there is no calibration system to convert volts to flow. As has been discussed with capillaroscopy, the wide variation of normal flow makes absolute values unnecessary. Thus the arbitrariness of the units of volts is not an impediment to the use of the instrument as the clinician is largely interested in changes in flow consequent upon interventions.

Laser Doppler Flowmetry in Clinical Practice

Laser Doppler flowmetry has been used in a variety of different clinical applications: the assessment of the ischaemic limb (Ostergren and Fagrell 1987), the viability of skin grafts and arterial reconstruction (Roberts and Jones 1987; Svensson et al. 1985). In clinical research it has proved useful in investigating the vascular pathology of a number of diseases involving the microvasculature; Raynaud's syndrome (Jayson 1987), diabetes mellitus (Rayman et al. 1986), sickle cell disease (Rogers et al. 1984), and scleroderma (Serup and Kistensen 1984). Failure of the hyperaemic response to thermal injury is seen early in diabetes and may be useful as an early index of developing diabetic microangiopathy.

Summary

Laser Doppler flowmetry is a method of non-invasive measurement of skin blood flow which has proved to be useful in clinical physiology. The major disadvantage is that absolute values are not available with this method. However it is easy to use and shows changes in flow following interventions.

Future

Although useful information can be gained from both capillaroscopy and laser Doppler flow, a combination of the two modalities will provide a much better understanding of the pathophysiology of the skin. The available technology is now suitable for clinical studies and will probably improve in the near future. The assessment of treatment regimes designed to improve cardiac performance, the use of after-load reduction, inotropes, and intra-aortic balloon pumping, for example, has depended to date on measurements of central cardiovascular parameters, blood pressure cardiac output and pulmonary capillary wedge pressure. The techniques described give us the ability to study, in addition, one of the capillary beds. With the caveat that the skin microcirculation may not be representative of other capillary beds this information should be obtained in the course of the assessment of cardiovascular support as it is the capillary flow which is ultimately important. Alterations in capillary flow velocity and laser Doppler flow following the introduction of, or changes in, treatment may lead to better comparisons of different supportive regimes. In certain conditions pathological changes in the skin microcirculation may be responsible for cardiovascular collapse. In "septic shock" it is common to find a high cardiac output associated with the falling blood pressure. The total peripheral resistance is usually low and it has been suggested that this is due to shunting of blood through the skin following dilatation of arterio-venous shunts. Although there is a high cardiac output there may be diminished nutritional capillary flow if there is diversion of blood from the nutritional circuit to the low-resistance shunts. If this is true, laser Doppler flow should show high total skin flow as laser Doppler flow includes Doppler-shifted signals from the shunt vessels. As capillaroscopy reveals only the nutritional vessels a combination of these noninvasive methods may be a powerful way of analysing the changes within the skin microcirculation and assessing the treatment. If high shunt flow is the cause of cardiac failure, the rational treatment would not be to increase the cardiac output to raise the blood pressure but to reduce shunt flow to divert blood back into the nutritional capillaries. Simultaneous assessment using capillaroscopy and laser Doppler flow would thus be useful in the study of new treatments.

The flexibility of the laser Doppler flow probe and its amenability to sterilisation means that the technique may be used for measuring changes in blood flow in internal organs. Unfortunately the fibre-optic bundle is liable to be obscured by blood or exudate so that leaving probes behind at operation, to be withdrawn later like a drain, is probably impractical. However temporary percutaneous implantation of a special fine probe through a hollow needle under flouroscopic or ultrasound control may become useful, for example in the assessment of renal blood flow following transplantation. Prospects for the further improvement of capillaroscopy depend on the development of video-enhancement techniques so that more information can be extracted from poor-quality images and so that images that are now inadequate for automated analysis can be cleaned up sufficiently for analysis. The technology for on-line measurement of capillary blood flow is available but cumbersome.

We have described two methods of measuring skin blood flow that are currently moving from the research laboratory into clinical practice. We speculate about the value of these techniques in the practice of ITU medicine (Micheels et al. 1984) and believe that they will be of value in patient treatment and in the evaluation of new treatments.

References

Bard P. (1961). Medical Physiology, 11th edn Mosby, St Louis

Bollinger A, Batti P, Barrasal P, Traschler H, Siegenthaler W (1974) Red blood cell velocity in nailfold capillaries of man measured by a television microscope technique. Mirovasc Res 7: 61–72

Boss CH, Schneuly P, Mahler F (1987) Evaluation and clinical application of the flying spot method in clinical nailfold capillary TV-microscopy. Int J Microcirc 6: 15–23

Burton A (1962) Special features of the circulation of the skin. In: Advances in biology of skin, blood vessels and circulation. Montagna W. Ellis RA (eds) Pergamon, Oxford, vol 2 pp 117–122

Eickhoff JH, Jacobsen E (1980) Correlation of transcutaneous oxygen tension to blood flow in heated skin. Scand J Clin Lab Invest 40: 761–765

Fagrell B, Hermansson IL, Karlender SG, Ostergren J (1984) Vital capillary microscopy for assessment of skin viability and microangiopathy in patients with diabetes mellitus. Acta Med Scand 68: 25–28

Fagrell B, Intaglietta M, Tsai AG, Ostergren J (1986) Combination of laser Doppler flowmetry and capillary microscopy for evaluating the dynamics of skin microcirculation. In: Mahler F, Messmer K, Hammersen F (eds) Techniques in clinical capillary microscopy. Proc appl Microcirc 11: 11–27

Holti G, Mitchell KW (1978) Estimation of the nutrient skin blood flow using a segmental thermal clearance probe. Clin Exp Dermatol 3: 189–198

Intaglietta M, Silverman NR, Tompkins WR (1975) Capillary flow velocity measurements in vivo and in situ by television methods. Microvasc Res 10: 165–179

Jayson MIV (1987) Measurement of the microcirculation in Raynauds phenomenon. In: Tooke JE, Smaje LH (eds) Clinical Investigation of the microcirculation, Martinus Nijhoff, Boston pp 169–182

Mahler F, Saner H, Annaheim M, Linder HR (1986) Capillaroscopic examination of erythrocyte flow velocity in patients with Raynaud syndrome by means of a local cold exposure test. In: Mahler F, Messmer K, Hammersen F (eds) Techniques in Clinical Capillary Microscopy. Proc appl Microcirc 11: 47–59

Maricq HR (1986) Capillary Photography. In: Mahler F, Messmer K, Hammersen F (eds) Techniques in Clinical Capillary Microscopy. Proc appl Microcirc 11: 11–27

Micheels J, Alsbjorn B, Sorensen B (1984) Laser Doppler flowmetry: a non-invasive measurement of microcirculation in intensive care. Resuscitation 12: 31–39

Ostergren J, Fagrell B (1984) Videophotometric capillaroscopy for evaluating drug effects on skin microcirculation. A double blind study with Nifedipine. Clin Physiol 4: 169–176

Ostergren J, Fagrell B (1985a) Microvascular measurements in patients with arteriosclerosis. In: Tooke JE, Smaje LH Clinical investigation of the microcirculation. Martinus Nijhoff, Boston pp 157–167

Ostergren J, Fagrell B (1985b) Skin capillary blood velocity in patients with arterial obliterative disease and polycythaemia. A disturbed reactive hyperaemic response. Clin Physiol 5: 35–43

Ostergren J, Fagrell B (1986) Measurement of blood cell velocity in skin capillaries. In: Mahler F, Messmer K, Hammersen F. (eds) Techniques in Clinical Capillary Microscopy. Proc appl Microcirc; 11: 30–39

Ostergren J, Fagrell B (1987) Microvascular measurements in patients with arteriosclerosis. In: Tooke JE, Smaje LH (eds) Clinical investigation of the microcirculation. Martinus Nijhoff, Boston pp. 23–34

Parker MM, Parillo JE (1983) Septic Shock: Haemodynamics and Pathogenesis. JAMA 250: 3324–3327

Rayman G, Hassan AAK, Tooke JE (1986) Blood flow in the skin of the foot related to posture in diabetes mellitus. Br Med J 292: 87–90

Riva C, Ross B, Benedek GB (1972) Laser Doppler measurement of blood flow in capillary tubes and retinal arteries. Invest Ophthalmol Vis Sci 11: 936–944

Roberts JO, Jones BM (1987) Assessment and monitoring of microvascular free tissue transfers. In: Tooke JE, Smaje LH (eds) Clinical investigation of the microcirculation. Martinus Nijhoff, Boston, pp 199–224

Roddie IC (1984) Circulation in skin and adipose tissue. In: Shepherd JT, Abboud FM (eds) Handbook of Physiology, section 2: The Cardiovascular System; Vol 3, Part 1, Chapter 10. American Physiological Society, Baltimore

Rogers GB, Schechter AV, Noguch CT, Klein HG, Nienhuis AW, Bonner RF (1984) Periodic microcirculatory flow in patients with sickle cell disease. N Engl J Med 311: 1534–1538

Serup J, Kistensen JK (1984) Blood flow of morphoea plaques as measured by Laser Doppler flowmetry. Arch Dermatol Res 276: 322–325

Svensson L, Bergquist B, Takolander R, Svedman P. (1985) Laser Doppler flowmetry for blood flow monitoring in reconstructive vascular surgery. Presented at 5th Congress of European Section of International Conference of Plastic and Reconstructive Surgery. 16–20 June 1985. Stockholm

Tenlund T (1982) On laser Doppler flowmetry: methods and microvascular applications. Linköpping Studies in Science and technology Dissertations. No 83. University of Linköpping, Linköpping, Sweden

Tenlund T, Salerud EG, Nilsson GE, Oberg PA (1983) Spatial and temporal variations in human skin blood flow. Int J Microcirc Clin Exp; 2: 81–90

Tooke JE, Milligan DW (1983) Capillary flow velocity in leukaemia. Br Med J 286: 518–519

Tooke JE, Lins PE, Ostergren J, Adamson U, Fagrell B (1985)

Intravenous insulin and skin microcirculatory flow in type 1 diabetes. Int J Microcirc Clin Exp 4: 69–83

Tsuchida Y (1979) Rate of skin blood flow in various regions of the body. Plast Reconstr Surg 64: 505–508

Williams SA, Tooke JE (1985) Microvascular haemodynamics in hypertension. In Tooke JE, Smaje LH (eds) Clinical investigation of the microcirculation Martinus Nijhoff, Boston. pp 130–143

Subject Index